Melanoma: Current Status and Future Perspectives in Melanoma Management

Melanoma: Current Status and Future Perspectives in Melanoma Management

Edited by Riley Gibson

hayle
medical

New York

Hayle Medical,
750 Third Avenue, 9th Floor,
New York, NY 10017, USA

Visit us on the World Wide Web at:
www.haylemedical.com

ISBN: 978-1-63241-878-4

Cataloging-in-Publication Data

Melanoma : current status and future perspectives in melanoma management / edited by Riley Gibson.
  p. cm.
Includes bibliographical references and index.
ISBN 978-1-63241-878-4
1. Melanoma. 2. Melanoma--Treatment. 3. Cancer--Treatment.
4. Neuroendocrine tumors--Treatment. I. Gibson, Riley.
RC280.M37 M45 2020
616.994 77--dc23

Table of Contents

Preface

Every book is initially just a concept; it takes months of research and hard work to give it the final shape in which the readers receive it. In its early stages, this book also went through rigorous reviewing. The notable contributions made by experts from across the globe were first molded into patterned chapters and then arranged in a sensibly sequential manner to bring out the best results.

Melanoma is a form of cancer, which develops from melanocytes. It primarily occurs in the skin, but may occur rarely in the eye, mouth and intestines. Melanoma is caused mainly due to ultraviolet light exposure in individuals with low levels of skin pigment. It can also arise from a mole. Such a mole may exhibit changes in size and color, and develop irregular edges, skin breakdown or itchiness. Rare genetic defects like xeroderma pigmentosum, are associated with increased risk. The diagnosis of melanoma is through an analysis of skin lesions and biopsy. In cases where the melanoma has not spread, the prognosis is generally good, and most people survive. In people for whom the melanoma has spread, radiation therapy, immunotherapy, biologic therapy or chemotherapy can improve survival. Surgery is generally required to reduce the risk of recurrence. This book provides comprehensive insights into the current status and future perspectives in the management of melanoma. It is a collective contribution of a renowned group of international experts. This book elucidates new techniques of assessment, diagnosis and treatment of melanoma in a multidisciplinary manner.

It has been my immense pleasure to be a part of this project and to contribute my years of learning in such a meaningful form. I would like to take this opportunity to thank all the people who have been associated with the completion of this book at any step.

Editor

Autotaxin – An Enzymatic Augmenter of Malignant Progression Linked to Inflammation

David N. Brindley, Matthew G.K. Benesch and
Mandi M. Murph

1. Introduction

Malignant melanoma cells are incredibly hardy, stemming from their intrinsic defensive nature. These cells inherit unique characteristics, which allowed their non-malignant predecessors, melanocytes, to survive solar ultraviolet radiation and simultaneously provide protection to neighboring cells. Most other cell types would die after such harsh exposure. Unsurprisingly, melanoma cells, which survive ultraviolet radiation, are intrinsically resistant to most chemotherapy.

Although there are numerous molecular reasons for this reality, herein we focus on the causal role of autotaxin (ATX) in melanoma. ATX is a 125 kDa glycoprotein enzyme that was initially discovered in the serum-free medium of A2058 human melanoma cells by Stracke et al. in 1992 [1] (Figure 1). Today, we know much more about this glycoprotein enzyme and how it affects melanoma. Indeed, ATX is highly overexpressed among primary melanomas and metastatic melanomas, in comparison to melanoma *in situ* and in normal skin [2].

In fact, "autotaxin" derived its name based on its initial property as an "autocrine motility factor". The rationale is that A2058 melanoma cells secrete ATX into culture medium and then respond to it with self-stimulated random and directed motility. Even though the amount of ATX in conditioned medium is less than 0.005% of total protein, only miniscule amounts, detected in picomolar and nanomolar concentrations, are needed to promote motility. [1] This suggests a large role for a low-abundant secreted enzyme.

There are five alternatively-spliced isoforms of ATX that are catalytically active [3,4]. The original ATX protein described in 1992 is termed ATXα, whereas the most abundant isoform is ATXβ and is the same isoform responsible for plasma lysoPLD activity [5]. Full length ATX is synthesized as a pre-proenzyme and is secreted by the classical secretory pathway [6,7]. Secreted ATX binds to cell surface integrin or heparan sulfates through its somatomedin-B-like (SMB) domain. This surface binding is believed to localize LPA production adjacent to LPA receptors [8-12].

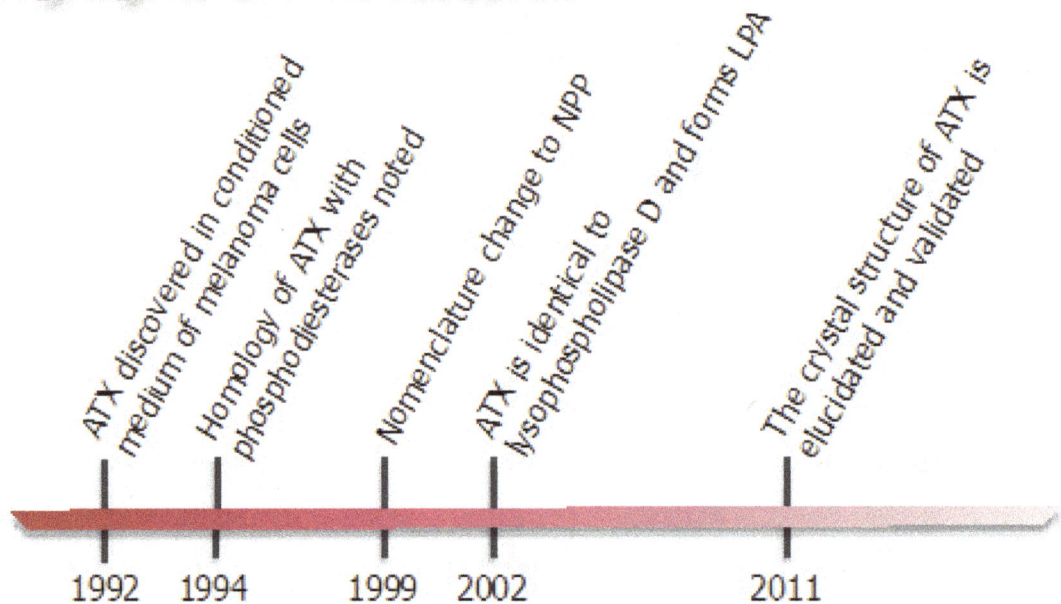

Figure 1. Major milestones in autotaxin (ATX) research. After the discovery of ATX in the conditioned medium of melanoma cells, it was not until a decade later that the enzyme was connected to lysophosphatidate. The elucidation of the crystal structure by two different groups caused a surge of novel inhibitors.

2. Multiple functions of ATX

In addition to the ability of ATX to stimulate motility, ATX also has ATPase, phosphodiesterase and ATP pyrophosphatase activities [13]. In other words, ATX releases nucleoside-5'-mono-phosphates from phosphodiester and pyrophosphate bonds [14], which is why it belongs to the family of ENPP (ectonucleotide pyrophosphatase/ phosphodiesterase) enzymes with ENPP1/PC-1, ENPP3/B10 [15], ENPP4 [14,16], ENPP6 [17], ENPP7 [18], and is also named ENPP2 (Table 1). Interestingly, all of the phosphodiesterase catalytic activity of ATX resides in one amino acid, threonine 210. Losing this phosphorylatable residue in the catalytic site results in a loss of phosphodiesterase activity and motility, but not ATP binding [19]. Theoretically, GTP, NAD, FAD, AMP and PPi are all susceptible to hydrolysis by ATX. However, the preferred substrate for ATX is lysophosphatidylcholine (LPC), which it converts to lysophosphatidate (LPA) (Figure 2). Since LPC concentrations in human plasma are greater than 200 μM, this should outcompete the hydrolysis of nucleotide phosphates and pyrophosphate, which are present in much lower concentrations.

Enzyme	Major Functions	Disease Association
ENPP1 / PC-1	Insulin signaling, glucose import, bone mineralization, immune response	Diabetes, obesity, stroke
ENPP2 / ATX	Vasculature formation, neural development, catalyzes lysophosphatidate production	Cancer, obesity, pulmonary fibrosis, arthritis, asthma, neuropathic pain, liver and colonic disorders
ENPP3 / B10	Basophil activation biomarker	Asthma, allergic reactions
ENPP4	Blood coagulant	Stroke
ENPP5	Putative neural glycoprotein	
ENPP6	Choline-specific hydrolysis of LPC, GPC and SPC	
ENPP7	Alkaline sphingomyelinase	

Table 1. Comparison between enzymes among the Ectonucleotide Pyrophosphatase/ Phosphodiesterase (ENPP) family

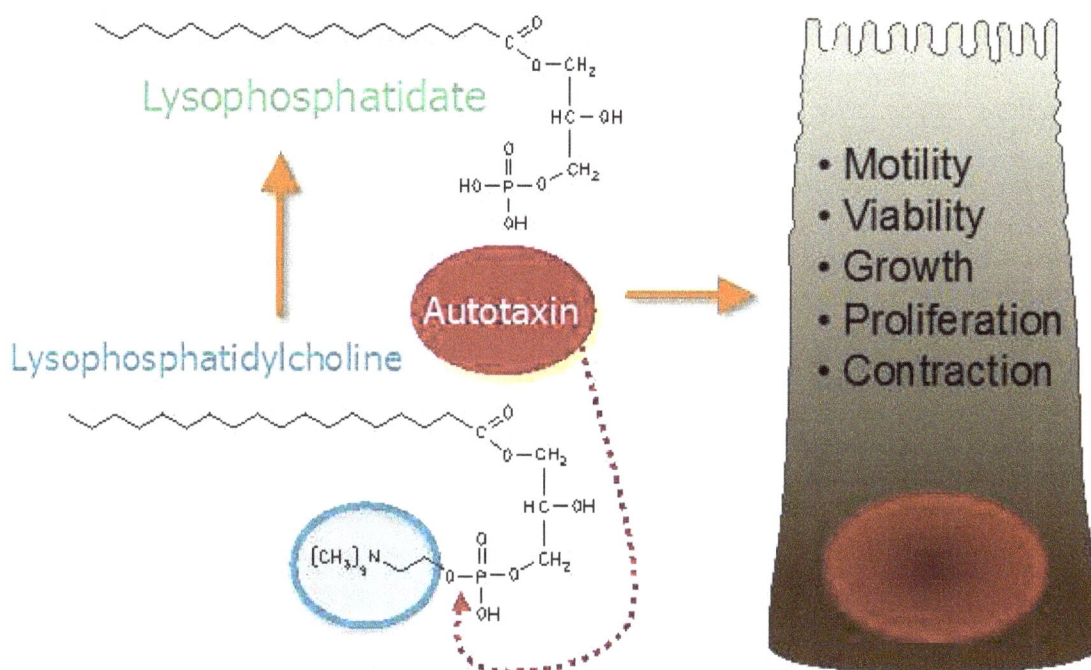

Figure 2. Autotaxin (ATX) catalyzes the biosynthesis of lysophosphatidiate (LPA). Since the lysophosphatidylcholine (LPC) concentrations in human circulation are >200 μM, ATX has abundantly available lipids to produce LPA. ATX hydrolyzes the choline head group from LPC to yield LPA. As a consequence of LPA signaling on cells, a multitude of various responses result, including motility, viability, growth, proliferation and contraction.

The ability of ATX to stimulate motility in melanoma cells can be modulated by chemical methods and genetic engineering. For example, ATX-meditated motility is inhibited by the PI3K inhibitors, wortmannin and LY294002, along with the catalytically inactive mutant of PI3K, PI3KK832R [20]. In addition, ras-transformed NIH3T3 cells become more motile and invasive in the presence of ATX. These cells also show enhanced colony formation in soft agar *in vitro* and produce significantly larger and metastatic tumors *in vivo* [21]. This suggests that while ATX alone may be insufficient to transform cells to a malignant phenotype, the presence of ATX significantly enhances malignant transformation among 'primed' cells.

3. Role as the main enzyme for the generation of extracellular LPA

The majority of LPA in the circulation is generated by ATX from the abundant LPC (>200 μM in human plasma) in the circulation. In fact, LPC is the major plasma phospholipid and it is bound to albumin [22]. Extracellular LPC is derived from two major routes of metabolism. The first is through the action of lecithin:cholesterol acyltransferase, which is present in plasma high-density lipoproteins. Lecithin:cholesterol acyltransferase, preferentially transfers unsaturated fatty acids from postion-2 of phosphatidylcholine to cholesterol, producing cholesterol ester and a mainly saturated LPC. However, a large proportion of circulating LPC is polyunsaturated [22] and this indicates another route for the production of extracellular LPC. Part of the polyunsaturated LPC is derived from secretion by hepatocytes, but it is possible that other cell types could produce polyunsaturated LPC. Since hepatocytes secrete a large quantity of arachidonoyl-LPC [22-26], it was originally postulated that this might represent a novel transport system for delivering choline and polyunsaturated fatty acids to the brain [22]. Although, this could still be true, we now know that LPC is an important substrate for ATX and that this is the major route for the production of extracellular LPA [27].

This predominant role of ATX in generating LPA is confirmed by circulating LPA concentrations that are 50% of normal levels among ATX heterozygous mice for a null-mutation for ATX [28,29]. Also, ATX inhibition produces a rapid decrease in plasma LPA of >95% [30-32]. The effects of ATX inhibition are more dramatic for the unsaturated species [33]. This is compatible with the substrate preference of ATX for unsaturated and polyunsaturated LPCs [34]. The crystal structures of ATX:LPA complexes show a hydrophobic pocket in the catalytic domain that is slightly U-shaped. This accommodates the kinked acyl chains of unsaturated fatty acids better than the linear conformations of saturated fatty acids [34].

Even though ATX is the major enzyme that generates LPA, other enzymes have a minor role in its biosynthesis. For example, saturated LPA species can also be derived through secretory phospholipase A_2, which hydrolyzes phosphatidate in microvesicles that are shed from cells during inflammation [35] and platelet aggregation [36]. In addition, LPA production by the Group VIA phospholipase A_2 (Ca^{2+}-independent) appears to be involved in the development of prostate cancers [37].

4. Crystal structure of ATX

The elucidation of the crystal structure of mouse and rat ATX revealed that the enzyme is composed of four domains [9,34]. The most important among these domains is the slightly U-shaped catalytic domain, which contains the enzyme's active site, a hydrophobic pocket and hydrophobic channel. Although ATX can hydrolyze both nucleotides and lysophospholipid substrates, when the unique hydrophobic pocket engages lysophospholipids, nucleotides are unable to bind to the active site. In addition, lipid acyl chains form further interactions with this pocket that nucleotides do not, which is also why ATX has a higher affinity for lysophospholipids [38]. The unique shape of the catalytic domain also accommodates the kinked acyl chains of unsaturated fatty acids better than the linear conformations of saturated fatty acids [34], which further explains substrate specificity for ATX.

ATX is the only member of the ENPP enzyme family that contains a hydrophobic pocket for lysophospholipids, thus giving it a unique capability over other ENPPs. Interestingly, one amino acid, asparagine 230, is required for ATX to recognize phosphate moieties and produce lysophosphatidate. Mutating asparagine to alanine inhibited all production. [34] Other single-point mutations deep within the hydrophobic pocket are capable of altering binding selectivity and reducing some of ATX's activity [9].

Perhaps the most exciting biological implication arising from the structural resolution of ATX is its proposed role as a directed transporter of LPA. In other words, ATX does not appear to arbitrarily release lysophospholipids from its hydrophobic pocket and channel them into solution. Rather, ATX is hypothesized to directly transfer LPA to its receptors along the plasma membrane. The flat surface of ATX on the side of the channel entrance facing the cell presumably facilitates this purpose [34]. This insinuates a role for ATX as an indirect initiator of cell signaling through its guided transport of an agonist to its receptor. It also further explains early observations of ATX as a motility-stimulating factor, even though it was actually due to LPA.

5. ATX Inhibitors

ATX, as an extracellular enzyme, is a very attractive drug candidate for reducing the abundance of extracellular LPA and subsequent signaling. Indeed, even a transient knockdown of ATX using siRNA is sufficient to significantly reduce melanoma cell viability [2]. Furthermore, the advantage of inhibiting ATX is the attenuation of signaling by all LPA receptors. This is considerably advantageous over the use of individual receptor antagonists because there are at least six and possibly eight confirmed LPA receptors with extensive redundancy. The design of ATX inhibitors has been reviewed previously [39-41] and so we will focus only those inhibitors that show utility *in vivo*.

Among the first ATX inhibitors was L-histidine, which was reported to have an ATX binding affinity (K_i) of about 1 mM *in vitro*, with 10 mM concentrations required to block ATX-stimulated migration in melanoma cells by 90% [42]. L-histidine inhibits ATX non-competitively by chelating cations such as Zn^{2+}, which are required for optimum catalytic rates [42]. Later work showed L-histidine administered intraperitoneally to rats limits thioacetamide-induced liver fibrosis [43]. Although L-histidine is required mM concentrations for activity *in vitro*, the authors cited its importance because it was the first "proof-of-principle" that inhibiting ATX was achievable.

Few studies have focused on inhibiting ATX transcription. However, one study showed that cholera toxin inhibits the proliferation of human hepatocellular carcinoma cells *in vitro* by suppressing the production of ATX through a TNF-α-dependent mechanism [44]. Cholera toxin increases the expression of anti-inflammatory cytokines (IL-4 and IL-10), which suppress ATX mRNA levels [45]. Knockdown of ATX expression with siRNA decreased the effects of cholera-toxin in suppressing the growth of Hep3B and Huh7 HCC cells [44]. Also, oral administration of the anti-inflammatory steroid, prednisolone, decreased serum ATX levels in a dose-dependent manner in patients treated for autoimmune skin diseases [46]. It is uncertain if suppressing ATX activity contributed to symptom relief since tapering the prednisolone dosage caused a rebound in serum ATX levels independently of disease severity. Significantly, the authors proposed that serum ATX levels could be used as a marker of compliance and/or efficacy of steroid therapy [46]. In addition, rifampicin, which is an inhibitor of DNA-dependent RNA polymerase, can be used to lower ATX mRNA transcription in the treatment of cholestatic pruritus. Cessation of rifampicin treatment led to both reoccurrence of pruritus and a rebound of ATX levels to pretreatment levels [47]. All of the treatment options for decreasing ATX expression appear to be effective in only specific diseases. By contrast, ATX inhibitors are designed to block LPA production and therefore this approach should have greater utility in multiple pathologies.

Major criteria for the efficacy of any therapeutic agent is a favorable therapeutic index and good bioavailability and potency. Reports on competitive ATX inhibitors began around 2006. These consisted of carba analogs of cyclic phosphatidate (cPA) with a K_i of approximately 100 nM (Table 2). These compounds inhibited metastasis of melanoma cells, which were injected in the tail vein in mouse models [48] and they inhibited chronic inflammation-induced C-fiber stimulation in rat neuropathic pain models [49]. However, cyclic phosphatidate analogs are also weak agonists of LPA receptors, which limits their utility [39].

Compound	Class	*In vivo therapeutic effects*
cPA	Lipid	• inhibits B16F10 melanoma metastasis in mouse tail vein model [48] • inhibits C-fiber stimulation by chronic inflammation in rat neuropathic pain models [49]
BrP-LPA	Lipid	• reduces MDA-MB-231 orthotopic breast tumor growth in mice [50] • inhibits A549 lung metastasis in engineered 3D mouse xenografts [51] • radiosensitizes GL-261 mouse glioma models [52] reduces collagen-induced arthritis in mice [53]
GWJ-A-23	Lipid	• reduces allergen-induced asthmatic phenotype in ATX-transgenic mice [54] • reduces fibrosis in bleomycin-treated mice [55]
PF-8380	Non-Lipid	• inhibits inflammatory hyperalgesia in rat air-pouch models [30] • radiosensitizes glioblastoma multiforme heteotropic mouse models [56]
ONO-8430506	Non-Lipid	• reduces tumor growth and metastasis in 4T1/Balb/c syngeneic and orthotopic mouse model and is synergistic with doxorubicin [33,57] • reduces urethral tension in rat benign prostatic hyperplasia models [58]

Table 2. ATX inhibitors used to effect a therapeutic response *in vivo*

A series of lipid-mimetic ATX inhibitors were developed in 2009 based on α-bromophosphonates (BrP-LPA). The *anti*-BrP-LPA isomer had IC_{50} of 22 nM in plasma, which was more potent than for *syn*-BrP-LPA [50] (Table 2). BrP-LPA is also a pan-antagonist of LPA_{1-3}, which is effective in decreasing to tumor growth in orthotopic xenograft models of breast cancer using MDA-MB-231 cells [50] and in metastasis of A549 lung cancer cells in nude mice [51]. We have also previously demonstrated that BrP-LPA is more effective than dacarbazine in reducing the viability of melanoma cells [59].

In addition to its efficacy against cancer cells, BrP-LPA had a radio-sensitizing effect on the tumor vasculature and delayed tumor growth by 7 days compared to radiation alone in a heterotopic murine glioma model using GL-261 cells [52]. This study was one of the first to demonstrate that ATX inhibitors can potential be used as an adjuvant therapy for cancer. A later report showed that BrP-LPA attenuated disease symptoms by diminishing synovial LPA signaling in a collagen-induced arthritis mouse model. Histological analysis of the joints showed a marked decrease in inflammation and synovial hyperplasia [53].

Several lipid-analogs of LPC, which have been used as ATX inhibitors, have relatively poor bioavailability, mainly because of the hydrophobic acyl tail [41]. This is illustrated by S32826, which is a benzyl phosphonic acid derivative (Figure 3). Despite having a very low nM IC_{50} *in vitro*, the long chain contributes to a very high lipophilicity and it cannot suppress circulating ATX activity for more than a few minutes [32]. Analogs of S32826, such as GWJ-A-23, were developed by shortening the hydrophobic chain and adding α-halo-or α-hydroxy-substituents to increase solubility. However, most of these compounds are less potent inhibitors of ATX compared to S32826 [60], but have been used in pulmonary studies of ATX [54,55]. Hence, much of the recent effort in discovering ATX inhibitors for use *in vivo* has concentrated on compounds that are more soluble and not based on lipid analogs.

There are numerous, small, non-lipid inhibitors of ATX that have been modified to increase potency [40,41]. These inhibitors tend to have better bioavailability because of decreased hydrophobicity and they are unlikely to be rapidly degraded by endogenous hydrolytic pathways [61]. One of these is PF-8380, which is a piperazinylbenzoxazolone derivative that was developed by Pfizer from compound library screening and optimization (Table 2). PF-8380 has an IC_{50} of 2.8 nM against recombinant human ATX and 101 nM for ATX in human whole blood. It was the first ATX inhibitor that was reported to decrease plasma LPA levels *in vivo* for an extended period [30]. In rat air-pouch models, 30 mg/kg PF-8380 inhibited inflammatory hyperalgesia with the same efficacy as 30 mg/kg naproxen, a routinely used nonsteroidal anti-inflammatory drug [30]. This dosage of PF-8380 produced a maximum decrease in LPA concentrations in plasma and also at the site of inflammation. Like BrP-LPA, PF-8380 had radio-sensitizing effects in a heterotopic mouse model of glioblastoma multiforme, delaying tumor growth by at least 20 days [52, 56]. In this study, inhibition of ATX by PF-8380 abrogated radiation-induced activation of Akt and subsequently decreased tumor vascularity and tumor growth [56]. Although we have *repeatedly* tested 30 mg/kg PF-8380 in animal models of melanoma, we have not observed a reduction of tumor growth (results not shown).

We have worked recently with another potent ATX inhibitor, which is a tetrahydrocarboline derivative (ONO-8430506) developed by Ono Pharmaceuticals Ltd. (Patent WO20120052227).

Oral dosing with 10 mg/kg ONO-8430506 suppressed plasma ATX activity as measured by choline release assay in the presence of 3 mM LPC by at least 90% at 6 h after administration in mice [33]. Plasma LPA levels were suppressed, especially the unsaturated species. C16:1-LPA and C20:5-LPA remained non-detectable at 6 and 24 h after ONO-8430506 administration. ONO-8430506 decreased the initial rate of tumor growth and subsequent lung metastasis by up to 60% in a syngeneic orthotopic model of breast cancer in BALB/c mice. This was accompanied by decreased concentrations of unsaturated LPA species in the breast tumors. These findings again confirm that ATX produces most of the extracellular LPA and that decreases in LPA concentrations in tissues mirror the decreases in plasma LPA levels following ATX inhibition [30, 33].

In other work, ONO-8430506 (30 mg/kg/day) decreased intra-urethral pressure and this was ascribed to urethral relaxation [58]. This work demonstrates the potential of ATX inhibition to decrease smooth muscle contraction by LPA. It also shows that ATX inhibition ameliorates urethral obstructive disease, such as benign prostatic hyperplasia.

6. Strategies to identify novel ATX inhibitors

So far, the most common technique for ATX inhibitor discovery and design is to screen libraries of compounds by using assays with ATX substrates such as Fluorescent Substrate-3 (FS-3). Inhibitors are then modified to increase potency. FS-3 is a fluorogenic substrate that is a doubly-labeled analogue of LPC. The fluorophore is quenched through intra-molecular energy transfer. Hydrolysis of FS-3 by ATX increases the fluorescent signal by removing the quencher [62]. The initial studies with this technique identified several inhibitors with an IC_{50} in the μM range [63, 64]. Later work with compounds designed from these studies developed nine pharmacophores for ATX inhibition and the results of these analyses were used to screen the National Cancer Institute's open chemical repository database to prioritize screening efforts [61]. This lead to the identification of several novel compounds with an IC_{50} in the high to low μM range [61, 65].

The identification of the crystal structure of ATX is also enabling structure-activity relationships to be established and more rational-design approaches towards optimizing inhibitor structures are now possible. The first study to report this approach was by Kawaguchi *et al.* who identified a thiazolone derivative from a 81,600-compound library, which inhibited ATX activity with an IC_{50} of 180 nM [66]. The authors proposed a series of side-chain modifications from the crystal structure of ATX complexed with this inhibitor. This led to the synthesis of a derivative compound, 3BoA, which has an IC_{50} of 13 nM [66]. More recent studies by Fells *et al.* combined large library screening results using the crystal structure of ATX with virtual screening tools to discover additional novel ATX inhibitors [67, 68]. This technique identified a common aromatic sulfonamide structural motif among potent inhibitors that targets the hydrophobic pocket of ATX. This accommodates the hydrocarbon tail of LPC/LPA [67, 68]. Similar techniques are expected to lead to the rapid development of ATX inhibitors for subsequent testing and development *in vivo*.

7. Physiological functions of ATX and LPA signaling

7.1. Vasculature system

Although studies *in vitro* detected no difference in the growth rate of *ras*-transformed NIH3T3 cells with or without ATX in culture, the growth rates in animals were significantly different, which suggested a role for ATX in blood vessel formation [21]. Indeed, Matrigel plugs of cells with ATX displayed extensive micro-aneurysms filled with red blood cells and more tumor cells, further corroborating this role. Furthermore, the ability of ATX to stimulate blood vessel formation in Matrigel plugs after 6 days was equivalent to VEGF, thus solidifying ATX as an angiogenesis-stimulating factor in the circulation [69].

Developmentally, the expression of ATX is indispensible. Beginning at 8.5 days, ATX expression is detectable in the early mouse embryo, within the floor plate of the neural tube [70]. Knocking out of ATX in mice causes embryonic lethality around 9.5 – 10.5 days with embryos exhibiting open, kinky neural tubes [28,71]. Although heartbeats are detected until 10.5 days *in utero*, contractions are weak, irregular and clearly abnormal. In addition, even the yolk sacs of ATX knockout embryos are irregular with a complete absence of blood vessels. [72] The role of ATX in vascular and neural development is also observed in zebrafish [72, 73]. ATX regulates the differentiation of oligodendrocytes in the hindbrain [74] and the correct left-right asymmetry for normal organ morphogenesis through Wnt-dependent pathways [75]. Taken together, these results definitively prove that the absence of ATX results in severe defects of the vasculature system and embryonic lethality. Organisms cannot develop without functional ATX expression.

Other groups have explored the parallel correlation by investigating the vasculature system when ATX is overexpressed in transgenic mice. Interestingly, ATX transgenic mice have an unusual susceptibility to bleeding and impaired platelet-dependent thrombus formation after injury [10]. Further studies have confirmed an important role for ATX in platelet activation through the production of LPA [76]. In addition, ATX binds to platelet β1-and β3-integrins, which localizes ATX to the cell surface of the appropriate microenvironment [11].

8. Adipose tissue regulation

An alternative, yet highly interesting function of ATX *in vivo* occurs in adipogenesis, obesity and the regulation of glucose homeostasis [77]. Foremost, ATX is expressed and secreted by adipose tissue. Its expression is also significantly upregulated during pre-adipocyte differentiation into adipocytes (adipogenesis) as well as in the adipose tissue of genetically obese diabetic mice [78]. In support of this finding, transgenic ATX mice accumulate more fat than littermates when they are fed a high-fat diet and thus, are more susceptible to diet-induced obesity [79]. Other work showed that ATX mRNA is upregulated in differentiating adipocytes but downregulated in hypertrophied adipocytes from obese mice [80]. Further, in humans, serum ATX levels and ATX mRNA expression in subcutaneous fat were negatively correlated with body mass index [80]. However this does not appear to be true if the subject is diabetic. Instead, these patients tend to have higher serum ATX levels [80]. In regards to the regulation of glucose metabolism, LPA produced by ATX is able to dose-dependently inhibit glucose-induced insulin secretion [77, 81]. Furthermore, knocking out the expression of ATX in adipose tissue results in a mouse with improved glucose tolerance [82].

9. Wound healing, tissue remodeling and inflammation

ATX and LPA facilitate critical processes necessary for skin re-epithelialization and wound healing. For example, among blister fluids, both ATX and LPA are produced and detected, originating *de novo* in the blister fluid and not from plasma. LPA is a potent activator of platelet aggregation and promotes keratinocyte migration, proliferation and differentiation. Thus, ATX and LPA facilitate critical processes necessary for skin re-epithelialization and wound healing [83]. ATX expression and LPA production are increased in rabbit aqueous humor following wounding by corneal freezing [84].

The range of physiological functions requiring ATX is quite diverse. For example, ATX and LPA signaling are involved in luteal tissue remodeling of regressing corpora lutea in rat ovaries. This occurs by recruiting phagocytes and proliferating fibroblasts, which are ultimately the factors involved in remodeling [85]. Other roles for ATX include hair follicle morphogenesis [86], bone mineralization [87] and myeloid differentiation in human bone marrow [88].

Another unique role of ATX occurs in response to oxidative stress in microglia, whereby ATX expression is increased. This protects microglia cells from damage by H_2O_2 and this effect is partially reversed by the mixed $LPA_{1/3}$ antagonist, Ki16425 [89]. Microglia cells overexpressing ATX show suppressed production of the pro-inflammatory cytokines, TNF-α and IL-6, and increases in the anti-inflammatory cytokine IL-10 upon treatment with lipopolysaccharide [90]. ATX is expressed in high endothelial venules in lymph nodes and other secondary lymphoid tissues [91]. This mediates lymphocyte extravasation, a process required for maintaining immune homeostasis [92, 93]. However, in chronically inflamed tissues, ATX mediates lymphocyte trafficking and increases cytokine production in response to repeated micro-injuries and incomplete tissue repair [94-96].

Interestingly, the catalytic activity of ATX has a dualistic role in wound healing. In this way, an ATX-like enzyme, SMaseD, is responsible for the pathology associated with venomous poisons through its dermonecrotic and hemolytic activities [97, 98]. In other words, the aberrant over-production of LPA by ATX cultivates an inappropriate immune response, similar to a wound that never heals, whereby overabundant inflammatory cytokines and chemokines are released. The damage is manifested in several ways, including the presence of severe dermonecrosis with blackened or missing skin appearing at the wounded site. The dermonecrosis can occur after envenomation by either *Loxosceles reclusa,* the brown recluse spider [97], or *Hemiscorpius lepturus,* a venomous scorpion [98]. Intriguingly, susceptibility to SMaseD is conferred by the LPA_1 receptor [99], suggesting a possible role for LPA receptor antagonists in this pathology.

As mentioned above, one of the main functions of ATX in adults is to repair damaged tissue. ATX is secreted in this situation partly in response to inflammation and the release of inflammatory cytokines. In normal wound healing, the production of LPA by ATX causes cells to migrate into the area of damage to effect wound repair and the formation of new blood vessels. In cases where the inflammation is not resolved, the process can result in tissue damage and fibrosis as in rheumatoid arthritis, atherosclerosis, organ fibrosis, diabetes and even obesity [100]. Cancer can be added to this list since it has been likened to "a wound that does not heal" [101]. The role of inflammatory cytokines in tumor progression [102-106] explains why inflammatory bowel disease and viral hepatitis can progress to cancer [107].

10. ATX in malignancy: Metastasis and angiogenesis

ATX is among the top 40 upregulated genes in metastatic cancer [108] and this is explained by the effects of LPA, which signals through at least six and putatively eight G-protein-coupled receptors. Through these receptors, LPA stimulates cell motility, cell survival/viability, cell proliferation, morphological changes, contraction, wound healing and invasion [109-118]. LPA achieves these effects by signaling through the relative activations of phosphatidylinositol 3-kinase (PI3K), $ERK_{1/2}$, mTOR, Ca^{2+}-transients, Rac, Rho and Ras [119].

The involvement of ATX and LPA in tumor progression affects multiple malignant processes and stages of tumor progression. For example, LPA increases the production of vascular endothelial growth factor, which stimulates angiogenesis [51, 120], a process required for tumor growth beyond 1 mm. However, in order for tumors to arise at all, tumor suppressors must be made ineffective. LPA levels can rise to 10 μM in the ascites fluid from advanced ovarian cancer patients [121]. Interestingly, LPA also decreases the abundance of the tumor suppressor, p53 [122], thus increasing cancer cell survival and proliferation, even in the presence of actinomycin D.

Pre-clinical models of disease and clinical pathology provide insight into the role of ATX and LPA receptors in cancer. For example, transgenic multiparous mice designed to overexpress ATX, LPA_1, LPA_2 or LPA_3 in mammary epithelium develop spontaneous metastatic mammary tumors as they age [123]. Women who express high levels of LPA_3 receptors in epithelial cells, or ATX in stromal cells, have larger breast tumors, nodal involvement, and higher stages of disease [124]. Since many early stage breast cancer patients are able to be cured using current treatment modalities, this suggests that the presence of ATX and/or LPA receptors has the ability to alter outcomes of malignancy.

The involvement of ATX and LPA in tumor progression can be understood in terms of a dysfunctional wound healing response. As mentioned above, one of the main functions of ATX in adults is to repair damaged tissue. ATX is secreted in this situation partly in response to inflammation and the release of inflammatory cytokines. In normal wound healing, the production of LPA by ATX causes cells to migrate into the area of damage to effect wound repair and the formation of new blood vessels. Cancer can be considered to be a case of unresolved inflammation and it has been likened to "a wound that does not heal" [101]. In fact, inflammation is now considered to be one of the "Hallmarks of Cancer" [125]. The secretion of ATX and increased LPA signaling should now be included as one of the inflammatory factors that drives tumor progression.

The role of ATX and LPA in this process is well illustrated in the case of work with mouse models of breast cancer. Most breast cancer cells do not themselves express ATX, but rather this is produced by fibroblasts within the breast tissue or by the surrounding adipose tissue [33] (Figure 3). The development of the breast tumor causes the release of inflammatory cytokines, which stimulate fibroblasts and adipose tissue to secrete ATX in a syngeneic orthotopic mouse model of breast cancer [33, 107]. This is part of a vicious cycle since LPA in turn stimulates the production of inflammatory cytokines [126-128]. This inflammatory cycle can be effectively blocked in a mouse by inhibiting ATX activity with ONO-8430506, which results in about a 60% decrease in tumor growth and lung metastasis.

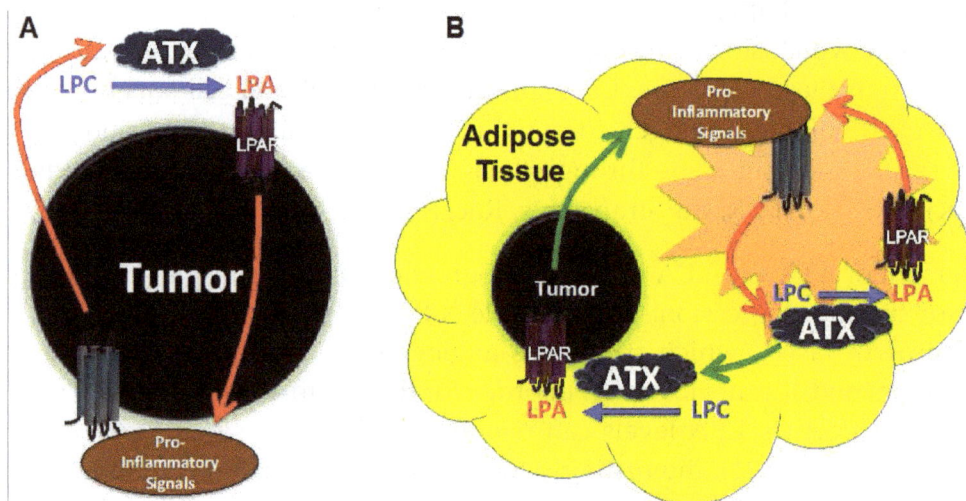

Figure 3. Proposed inflammatory-mediated models of ATX secretion. A) In cancer cells that overexpress ATX such as thyroid cancers, neuroblastomas and melanomas, autocrine-secreted ATX produces LPA, which signals through LPA receptors (LPARs) on the cancer cell surface. This signaling further increases the production of pro-inflammatory signals including growth factors, cytokines and chemokines. These molecules in turn can signal through specific receptors to increase ATX production. B) In breast cancer, a paracrine model of ATX secretion is possible since breast adipose tissue secretes high levels of ATX, whereas breast cancer cells normally produce negligible ATX. As the tumor grows, pro-inflammatory signals secreted by the tumor create an inflammatory environment within the surrounding adipose tissue (green arrows). This signaling increases ATX secretion and LPA production, which in turn can establish an autocrine feedback loop of increased pro-inflammatory signaling and ATX production (red arrows) within the adipose tissue. Increased ATX and LPA production can in turn contribute to tumor progression (green arrows). A combination of both autocrine and paracrine production of ATX is also possible when cancer cells produce significant quantities of ATX.

Although breast cancer cells do not do not express significant levels of ATX activity, this is not typical of other tumors where ATX activity is expressed in the cancer cells themselves. These cancers include thyroid [129], neuroblastomas [71, 130, 131] and melanomas [132-134]. However, in the case of melanomas, their normal predecessor cells, melanocytes, do not express ATX. Thus, the data suggests that ATX expression is acquired during the transition to malignancy in melanoma [2]. The secretion of inflammatory cytokines by cells in the tumor also produces a vicious cycle of ATX secretion and LPA production, which is a driving force in tumor progression [107]. In the case of breast tumors, we propose that the ATX come from surrounding adipose tissue, whereas in thyroid tumors, neuroblastomas and melanomas, ATX is secreted by the cancer cells (Figure 3).

11. ATX in chemo-resistance

Another important role of ATX expression and LPA signaling in malignancy occurs during the acquisition and manifestation of chemo-resistance. LPA facilitates chemo-resistance to the cytotoxic effects mediated by Taxol [119, 135, 136], doxorubicin [57], actinomycin D [122] and carboplatin [137]. These effects are mediated by LPA partly through activation of survival and viability pathways, such as ERK and PI3K. In addition, we previously demonstrated that LPA signaling does not encompass the entire molecular mechanism and there are other proteins, like the Regulators of G-protein Signaling proteins, which play a more dominant role [138]. Indeed, in the absence of appropriate Regulators of G-protein Signaling proteins, cells exposed to LPA have increased capacity to acquire chemo-resistance.

As chemo-resistance is a complex process, there are other molecular mechanisms involved. For example, among chemo-resistant cells, increased expression of multidrug resistance transporters enables toxins, like chemotherapeutic drugs, to be exported out of cancer cells. This is particularly problematic in the case of renal cell carcinomas, for which cytotoxic chemotherapy is largely ineffective, but also occurs widely in malignancy.

Recent work shows that the activation of PI3K by through LPA_1 receptors increases the stability of the transcription factor Nrf2, which increases the expression of antioxidant genes and multidrug resistant transporters [57]. The expression of antioxidant genes protects cancer cells against the oxidative damage caused by chemotherapeutic agents. Also, the expression of multidrug resistant transporters enables toxic oxidative products and chemotherapeutic drugs to be exported out of cancer cells. These effects explain why inhibiting ATX activity and blocking LPA signaling improves the efficacy of doxorubicin as a chemotherapeutic agent [57]. Thus blocking ATX activity can provide a novel adjuvant therapy for improving the efficacy of existing chemotherapeutic agents.

ATX inhibition could also have a beneficial effect as an adjuvant for improving the effects of radiotherapy as discussed above. This is possible since LPA, through activation of LPA_2 receptors, also protects against radiation-induced cell death. This action depends on the depletion Siva-1, which is a pro-apoptotic signaling protein [139].

The function of ATX in aggravating resistance to chemotherapy and radiotherapy can be understood in terms of the vicious cycle of inflammation caused by repeated bouts of therapy as described above [140] (Figure 3). Cancer therapy itself causes damage to the tumor and surrounding tissue, which responds by producing inflammatory cytokines resulting in increased ATX production [107]. This explains why blocking this cycle by inhibiting LPA formation can improve the sensitivity to chemotherapy by attenuating the effects of increased Nrf2 expression.

12. ATX in melanoma

Although accumulating studies suggest that inhibiting ATX activity could provide a novel adjuvant therapy for improving the efficacy of existing chemotherapeutic agents, we have previously demonstrated a role for ATX inhibitors as monotherapy against advanced cutaneous melanoma [2,48,59]. After injecting B16F10 metastatic melanoma cells into the tail veins of C57/Bl6 mice, we observed a significant reduction in the number of lung nodules, which represent metastatic melanoma tumors, after treatment with a phosphonothionate analogue of carba cyclic phosphatidic acid, thio-ccPA 18:1 [2]. This compound was synthesized for improved metabolic stability and activity, based on our previous results [48]. In addition to being an inhibitor of ATX, thio-ccPA 18:1 is a direct antagonist of LPA_1 and LPA_3 receptors [141].

As mentioned previously, melanomas are notoriously resistant to chemotherapy. In light of the role of ATX/LPA signaling in melanoma, perhaps it should not be surprising that melanoma cells, which produce high quantities of ATX, are resistant to chemotherapy, since excessive LPA signaling contributes to this phenotype. Only a few chemotherapy agents are approved options against melanoma, these include dacarbazine and temozolomide. Thus, we compared these single agents against both the anti-BrP-LPA and the mixed diastereomers BrP-LPA on the viability of MeWo melanoma cells. Indeed, both BrP-LPA compounds were more effective single-agents at 10 μM and 100 μM than either dacarbazine or temozolomide, at concentration ranging from 10-1000 μM [59]. This suggests that targeted approaches against ATX in melanoma have potential and further results will be reported in due time.

Besides cutaneous melanoma, in a study on uveal melanoma, ATX was the only gene among 32 candidate genes whose expression was sufficient to distinguish classes representing metastasis and prognosis. Paradoxically, "underexpression" of ATX correlated with poor prognosis and metastatic death among 27 samples [132]. Based on the discussion provided above it is tempting to propose that melanocytes evolved to survive solar ultraviolet radiation and simultaneously provide protection to neighboring cells by producing ATX and thus providing LPA. However, with repeated DNA damage and incomplete repair from excessive UV radiation, melanocytes are malignantly transformed into melanoma cells. At this point, the increased production of ATX and signaling by inflammatory cytokines, which are meant to facilitate repair, could be subverted into promoting cancer progression.

13. Summary and conclusions

Advanced metastatic melanoma is an incurable disease in dire need of additional therapeutic options. Although many newly targeted inhibitors have extended the life of patients with *BRAF* mutations, they do not achieve cure due to chemo-resistance, and they are not applicable to patients with Wild-type B-Raf. Thus, additional therapeutics are desperately needed to treat this growing population. Herein we have summarized the current state of ATX inhibitors and what we currently know about the role of ATX in melanoma and malignancy.

The original ATX inhibitors had little utility *in vivo* because of the very low bioavailability. However, as described above, potent ATX inhibitors are now being developed, which are effective *in vivo* for longer than 24 h. These inhibitors appear to be well tolerated by animals and the next stage is to take such inhibitors through Phase 1 clinical trials. These ATX inhibitors should be effective in improving the outcomes for which the ATX/LPA axis is involved. These include various forms of cancer whereby an ATX inhibitor could be used as a monotherapy or as an adjuvant to improve existing chemotherapies or radiation treatment. The ATX inhibitors should also be effective in improving the treatment of a variety of inflammatory conditions. These compounds deserve further examination.

Acknowledgements

This work was supported by research grants from the National Institutes of Health (1R15CA151006-01 American Recovery and Reinvestment Act and 1R15CA176653-01A1), a Research Scholar Grant 120634-RSG-11-269-01-CDD from the American Cancer Society and a Distinguished Scientist award from the Georgia Research Alliance to MMM. MGKB received a Vanier Canada Graduate Scholarship from the Government of Canada, a Killam Trust Award and an MD/PhD scholarship from Alberta Innovates-Health Solutions. DNB was supported by grants from the Canadian Breast Cancer Foundation, Women and Children's Health Research Institute of the University of Alberta and CIHR with the Alberta Cancer Foundation. DNB declares a conflict of interest in having received a consulting fee from Ono Pharmaceuticals.

Author details

David N. Brindley[1], Matthew G.K. Benesch[1] and Mandi M. Murph[2*]

*Address all correspondence to: mmurph@uga.edu

1 Signal Transduction Research Group, Department of Biochemistry, University of Alberta, Heritage Medical Research Center, Edmonton, Alberta, Canada

2 Department of Pharmaceutical and Biomedical Sciences, The University of Georgia, College of Pharmacy, Athens, Georgia, USA

References

[1] Stracke ML, Krutzsch HC, Unsworth EJ, Arestad A, Cioce V, Schiffmann E, Liotta LA (1992) Identification, purification, and partial sequence analysis of autotaxin, a novel motility-stimulating protein. J Biol Chem 267: 2524-2529.

[2]   Altman MK, Gopal V, Jia W, Yu S, Hall H, Mills GB, McGinnis AC, Bartlett MG, Jiang G, Madan D, Prestwich GD, Xu Y, Davies MA, Murph MM (2010) Targeting melanoma growth and viability reveals dualistic functionality of the phosphonothionate analogue of carba cyclic phosphatidic acid. Mol Cancer 9: 140.

[3]   Hashimoto T, Okudaira S, Igarashi K, Hama K, Yatomi Y, Aoki J (2012) Identification and biochemical characterization of a novel autotaxin isoform, ATXdelta, with a four-amino acid deletion. J Biochem 151: 89-97.

[4]   Boutin JA, Ferry G (2009) Autotaxin. Cell Mol Life Sci 66: 3009-3021.

[5]   Hausmann J, Perrakis A, Moolenaar WH (2013) Structure-function relationships of autotaxin, a secreted lysophospholipase D. Adv Biol Regul 53: 112-117.

[6]   Jansen S, Stefan C, Creemers JW, Waelkens E, Van Eynde A, Stalmans W, Bollen M (2005) Proteolytic maturation and activation of autotaxin (NPP2), a secreted metastasis-enhancing lysophospholipase D. J Cell Sci 118: 3081-3089.

[7]   Koike S, Keino-Masu K, Ohto T, Masu M (2006) The N-terminal hydrophobic sequence of autotaxin (ENPP2) functions as a signal peptide. Genes Cells 11: 133-142.

[8]   Houben AJ, van Wijk XM, van Meeteren LA, van Zeijl L, van de Westerlo EM, Hausmann J, Fish A, Perrakis A, van Kuppevelt TH, Moolenaar WH (2013) The polybasic insertion in autotaxin alpha confers specific binding to heparin and cell surface heparan sulfate proteoglycans. J Biol Chem 288: 510-519.

[9]   Hausmann J, Kamtekar S, Christodoulou E, Day JE, Wu T, Fulkerson Z, Albers HM, van Meeteren LA, Houben AJ, van Zeijl L, Jansen S, Andries M, Hall T, Pegg LE, Benson TE, Kasiem M, Harlos K, Kooi CW, Smyth SS, Ovaa H, Bollen M, Morris AJ, Moolenaar WH, Perrakis A (2011) Structural basis of substrate discrimination and integrin binding by autotaxin. Nat Struct Mol Biol 18: 198-204.

[10] Pamuklar Z, Federico L, Liu S, Umezu-Goto M, Dong A, Panchatcharam M, Fulkerson Z, Berdyshev E, Natarajan V, Fang X, van Meeteren LA, Moolenaar WH, Mills GB, Morris AJ, Smyth SS (2009) Autotaxin/lysopholipase D and lysophosphatidic acid regulate murine hemostasis and thrombosis. J Biol Chem 284: 7385-7394.

[11] Fulkerson Z, Wu T, Sunkara M, Kooi CV, Morris AJ, Smyth SS (2011) Binding of autotaxin to integrins localizes lysophosphatidic acid production to platelets and mammalian cells. J Biol Chem 286: 34654-34663.

[12] Wu T, Vander Kooi C, Shah P, Charnigo R, Huang C, Smyth SS, Morris AJ (2013) Integrin-mediated cell surface recruitment of autotaxin promotes persistent directional cell migration. FASEB J: 10.1096/fj.1013-229211.

[13] Clair T, Lee HY, Liotta LA, Stracke ML (1997) Autotaxin is an exoenzyme possessing 5'-nucleotide phosphodiesterase/ATP pyrophosphatase and ATPase activities. J Biol Chem 272: 996-1001.

[14] Albright RA, Chang WC, Robert D, Ornstein DL, Cao W, Liu L, Redick ME, Young JI, De La Cruz EM, Braddock DT (2012) NPP4 is a procoagulant enzyme on the surface of vascular endothelium. Blood 120: 4432-4440.

[15] Stefan C, Gijsbers R, Stalmans W, Bollen M (1999) Differential regulation of the expression of nucleotide pyrophosphatases/phosphodiesterases in rat liver. Biochim Biophys Acta 1450: 45-52.

[16] Albright RA, Ornstein DL, Cao W, Chang WC, Robert D, Tehan M, Hoyer D, Liu L, Stabach P, Yang G, De La Cruz EM, Braddock DT (2014) Molecular basis of purinergic signal metabolism by ectonucleotide pyrophosphatase/phosphodiesterases 4 and 1 and implications in stroke. J Biol Chem 289: 3294-3306.

[17] Sakagami H, Aoki J, Natori Y, Nishikawa K, Kakehi Y, Natori Y, Arai H (2005) Biochemical and molecular characterization of a novel choline-specific glycerophosphodiester phosphodiesterase belonging to the nucleotide pyrophosphatase/phosphodiesterase family. J Biol Chem 280: 23084-23093.

[18] Duan RD, Bergman T, Xu N, Wu J, Cheng Y, Duan J, Nelander S, Palmberg C, Nilsson A (2003) Identification of human intestinal alkaline sphingomyelinase as a novel ecto-enzyme related to the nucleotide phosphodiesterase family. J Biol Chem 278: 38528-38536.

[19] Lee HY, Clair T, Mulvaney PT, Woodhouse EC, Aznavoorian S, Liotta LA, Stracke ML (1996) Stimulation of tumor cell motility linked to phosphodiesterase catalytic site of autotaxin. J Biol Chem 271: 24408-24412.

[20] Lee HY, Bae GU, Jung ID, Lee JS, Kim YK, Noh SH, Stracke ML, Park CG, Lee HW, Han JW (2002) Autotaxin promotes motility via G protein-coupled phosphoinositide 3-kinase gamma in human melanoma cells. FEBS Lett 515: 137-140.

[21] Nam SW, Clair T, Campo CK, Lee HY, Liotta LA, Stracke ML (2000) Autotaxin (ATX), a potent tumor motogen, augments invasive and metastatic potential of ras-transformed cells. Oncogene 19: 241-247.

[22] Brindley DN (1993) Hepatic secretion of lysphosphatidylcholine: a novel transport system for polyunsaturated fatty acids and choline. J Nutr Biochem 4: 442-449.

[23] Mangiapane EH, Brindley DN (1986) Effects of dexamethasone and insulin on the synthesis of triacylglycerols and phosphatidylcholine and the secretion of very-low-density lipoproteins and lysophosphatidylcholine by monolayer cultures of rat hepatocytes. Biochem J 233: 151-160.

[24] Graham A, Bennett AJ, McLean AA, Zammit VA, Brindley DN (1988) Factors regulating the secretion of lysophosphatidylcholine by rat hepatocytes compared with the synthesis and secretion of phosphatidylcholine and triacylglycerol. Effects of albumin, cycloheximide, verapamil, EGTA and chlorpromazine. Biochem J 253: 687-692.

[25] Graham A, Zammit VA, Brindley DN (1988) Fatty acid specificity for the synthesis of triacylglycerol and phosphatidylcholine and for the secretion of very-low-density lip-

oproteins and lysophosphatidylcholine by cultures of rat hepatocytes. Biochem J 249: 727-733.

[26] Graham A, Zammit VA, Christie WW, Brindley DN (1991) Sexual dimorphism in the preferential secretion of unsaturated lysophosphatidylcholine by rat hepatocytes but no secretion by sheep hepatocytes. Biochim Biophys Acta 1081: 151-158.

[27] Saulnier-Blache JS (2004) [Lysophosphatidic acid: a "bioactive" phospholipid]. Med Sci (Paris) 20: 799-803.

[28] van Meeteren LA, Ruurs P, Stortelers C, Bouwman P, van Rooijen MA, Pradere JP, Pettit TR, Wakelam MJ, Saulnier-Blache JS, Mummery CL, Moolenaar WH, Jonkers J (2006) Autotaxin, a secreted lysophospholipase D, is essential for blood vessel formation during development. Mol Cell Biol 26: 5015-5022.

[29] Tanaka M, Okudaira S, Kishi Y, Ohkawa R, Iseki S, Ota M, Noji S, Yatomi Y, Aoki J, Arai H (2006) Autotaxin stabilizes blood vessels and is required for embryonic vasculature by producing lysophosphatidic acid. J Biol Chem 281: 25822-25830.

[30] Gierse J, Thorarensen A, Beltey K, Bradshaw-Pierce E, Cortes-Burgos L, Hall T, Johnston A, Murphy M, Nemirovskiy O, Ogawa S, Pegg L, Pelc M, Prinsen M, Schnute M, Wendling J, Wene S, Weinberg R, Wittwer A, Zweifel B, Masferrer J (2010) A novel autotaxin inhibitor reduces lysophosphatidic acid levels in plasma and the site of inflammation. J Pharmacol Exp Ther 334: 310-317.

[31] Albers HM, Dong A, van Meeteren LA, Egan DA, Sunkara M, van Tilburg EW, Schuurman K, van Tellingen O, Morris AJ, Smyth SS, Moolenaar WH, Ovaa H (2010) Boronic acid-based inhibitor of autotaxin reveals rapid turnover of LPA in the circulation. Proc Natl Acad Sci U S A 107: 7257-7262.

[32] Ferry G, Moulharat N, Pradere JP, Desos P, Try A, Genton A, Giganti A, Beucher-Gaudin M, Lonchampt M, Bertrand M, Saulnier-Blache JS, Tucker GC, Cordi A, Boutin JA (2008) S32826, a nanomolar inhibitor of autotaxin: discovery, synthesis and applications as a pharmacological tool. J Pharmacol Exp Ther 327: 809-819.

[33] Benesch MGK, Tang X, Maeda T, Ohhata A, Zhao YY, Kok BPC, Dewald J, Hitt M, Curtis JM, McMullen TPW, Brindley DN (2014) Inhibition of autotaxin delays breast tumor growth and lung metastasis in mice. FASEB J 28: 2655-2666.

[34] Nishimasu H, Okudaira S, Hama K, Mihara E, Dohmae N, Inoue A, Ishitani R, Takagi J, Aoki J, Nureki O (2011) Crystal structure of autotaxin and insight into GPCR activation by lipid mediators. Nat Struct Mol Biol 18: 205-212.

[35] Fourcade O, Simon MF, Viode C, Rugani N, Leballe F, Ragab A, Fournie B, Sarda L, Chap H (1995) Secretory phospholipase A2 generates the novel lipid mediator lysophosphatidic acid in membrane microvesicles shed from activated cells. Cell 80: 919-927.

[36] Sano T, Baker D, Virag T, Wada A, Yatomi Y, Kobayashi T, Igarashi Y, Tigyi G (2002) Multiple mechanisms linked to platelet activation result in lysophosphatidic acid and sphingosine 1-phosphate generation in blood. J Biol Chem 277: 21197-21206.

[37] Li H, Zhao Z, Wei G, Yan L, Wang D, Zhang H, Sandusky GE, Turk J, Xu Y (2010) Group VIA phospholipase A2 in both host and tumor cells is involved in ovarian cancer development. FASEB J.

[38] Tabchy A, Tigyi G, Mills GB (2011) Location, location, location: a crystal-clear view of autotaxin saturating LPA receptors. Nat Struct Mol Biol 18: 117-118.

[39] Federico L, Pamuklar Z, Smyth SS, Morris AJ (2008) Therapeutic potential of autotaxin/lysophospholipase d inhibitors. Curr Drug Targets 9: 698-708.

[40] Albers HM, Ovaa H (2012) Chemical evolution of autotaxin inhibitors. Chem Rev 112: 2593-2603.

[41] Barbayianni E, Magrioti V, Moutevelis-Minakakis P, Kokotos G (2013) Autotaxin inhibitors: a patent review. Expert Opin Ther Pat 23: 1123-1132.

[42] Clair T, Koh E, Ptaszynska M, Bandle RW, Liotta LA, Schiffmann E, Stracke ML (2005) L-histidine inhibits production of lysophosphatidic acid by the tumor-associated cytokine, autotaxin. Lipids Health Dis 4: 5.

[43] El-Batch M, Ibrahim W, Said S (2011) Effect of histidine on autotaxin activity in experimentally induced liver fibrosis. J Biochem Mol Toxicol 25: 143-150.

[44] Xia Q, Deng AM, Wu SS, Zheng M (2011) Cholera toxin inhibits human hepatocarcinoma cell proliferation in vitro via suppressing ATX/LPA axis. Acta Pharmacol Sin 32: 1055-1062.

[45] Kehlen A, Lauterbach R, Santos AN, Thiele K, Kabisch U, Weber E, Riemann D, Langner J (2001) IL-1 beta-and IL-4-induced down-regulation of autotaxin mRNA and PC-1 in fibroblast-like synoviocytes of patients with rheumatoid arthritis (RA). Clin Exp Immunol 123: 147-154.

[46] Sumida H, Nakamura K, Yanagida K, Ohkawa R, Asano Y, Kadono T, Tamaki K, Igarashi K, Aoki J, Sato S, Ishii S, Shimizu T, Yatomi Y (2013) Decrease in circulating autotaxin by oral administration of prednisolone. Clin Chim Acta 415: 74-80.

[47] Kremer AE, van Dijk R, Leckie P, Schaap FG, Kuiper EM, Mettang T, Reiners KS, Raap U, van Buuren HR, van Erpecum KJ, Davies NA, Rust C, Engert A, Jalan R, Oude Elferink RP, Beuers U (2012) Serum autotaxin is increased in pruritus of cholestasis, but not of other origin, and responds to therapeutic interventions. Hepatology 56: 1391-1400.

[48] Baker DL, Fujiwara Y, Pigg KR, Tsukahara R, Kobayashi S, Murofushi H, Uchiyama A, Murakami-Murofushi K, Koh E, Bandle RW, Byun HS, Bittman R, Fan D, Murph M, Mills GB, Tigyi G (2006) Carba analogs of cyclic phosphatidic acid are selective

inhibitors of autotaxin and cancer cell invasion and metastasis. J Biol Chem 281: 22786-22793.

[49]   Kakiuchi Y, Nagai J, Gotoh M, Hotta H, Murofushi H, Ogawa T, Ueda H, Murakami-Murofushi K (2011) Antinociceptive effect of cyclic phosphatidic acid and its derivative on animal models of acute and chronic pain. Mol Pain 7: 1744-8069.

[50]   Zhang H, Xu X, Gajewiak J, Tsukahara R, Fujiwara Y, Liu J, Fells JI, Perygin D, Parrill AL, Tigyi G, Prestwich GD (2009) Dual activity lysophosphatidic acid receptor pan-antagonist/autotaxin inhibitor reduces breast cancer cell migration in vitro and causes tumor regression in vivo. Cancer Res 69: 5441-5449.

[51]   Xu X, Prestwich GD (2010) Inhibition of tumor growth and angiogenesis by a lysophosphatidic acid antagonist in an engineered three-dimensional lung cancer xenograft model. Cancer 116: 1739-1750.

[52]   Schleicher SM, Thotala DK, Linkous AG, Hu R, Leahy KM, Yazlovitskaya EM, Hallahan DE (2011) Autotaxin and LPA receptors represent potential molecular targets for the radiosensitization of murine glioma through effects on tumor vasculature. PLoS One 6: e22182.

[53]   Nikitopoulou I, Kaffe E, Sevastou I, Sirioti I, Samiotaki M, Madan D, Prestwich GD, Aidinis V (2013) A metabolically-stabilized phosphonate analog of lysophosphatidic acid attenuates collagen-induced arthritis. PLoS One 8: e70941.

[54]   Park GY, Lee YG, Berdyshev E, Nyenhuis S, Du J, Fu P, Gorshkova IA, Li Y, Chung S, Karpurapu M, Deng J, Ranjan R, Xiao L, Jaffe HA, Corbridge SJ, Kelly EA, Jarjour NN, Chun J, Prestwich GD, Kaffe E, Ninou I, Aidinis V, Morris AJ, Smyth SS, Ackerman SJ, Natarajan V, Christman JW (2013) Autotaxin production of lysophosphatidic Acid mediates allergic asthmatic inflammation. Am J Respir Crit Care Med 188: 928-940.

[55]   Oikonomou N, Mouratis MA, Tzouvelekis A, Kaffe E, Valavanis C, Vilaras G, Karameris A, Prestwich GD, Bouros D, Aidinis V (2012) Pulmonary autotaxin expression contributes to the pathogenesis of pulmonary fibrosis. Am J Respir Cell Mol Biol 47: 566-574.

[56]   Bhave SR, Dadey DY, Karvas RM, Ferraro DJ, Kotipatruni RP, Jaboin JJ, Hallahan AN, Dewees TA, Linkous AG, Hallahan DE, Thotala D (2013) Autotaxin Inhibition with PF-8380 Enhances the Radiosensitivy of Human and Murine Glioblastoma Cell Lines. Front Oncol 3: 00236.

[57]   Venkatraman G, Benesch MGK, Tang X, Dewald J, McMullen TPW, Brindley DN (2014) Lysophosphatidate signalling stabilizes Nrf2 and increases the expression of genes involved in drug resistance and oxidative stress responses: Implications for cancer treatment. FASEB J: Under Review.

[58]   Saga H, Ohhata A, Hayashi A, Katoh M, Maeda T, Mizuno H, Takada Y, Komichi Y, Ota H, Matsumura N, Shibaya M, Sugiyama T, Nakade S, Kishikawa K (2014) A nov-

el highly potent autotaxin/ENPP2 inhibitor produces prolonged decreases in plasma lysophosphatidic acid formation in vivo and regulates urethral tension. PLoS One 9: e93230.

[59] Nguyen D, Nguyen O, Zhang H, Prestwich GD, Murph MM (2011) A Bromophosphonate Analogue of Lysophosphatidic Acid Surpasses Dacarbazine in Reducing Cell Proliferation and Viability of MeWo Melanoma Cells. In: Murph MM, editor. Research on Melanoma-A Glimpse into Current Directions and Future Trends: InTech.

[60] Jiang G, Madan D, Prestwich GD (2011) Aromatic phosphonates inhibit the lysophospholipase D activity of autotaxin. Bioorg Med Chem Lett 21: 5098-5101.

[61] North EJ, Howard AL, Wanjala IW, Pham TC, Baker DL, Parrill AL (2010) Pharmacophore development and application toward the identification of novel, small-molecule autotaxin inhibitors. J Med Chem 53: 3095-3105.

[62] Ferguson CG, Bigman CS, Richardson RD, van Meeteren LA, Moolenaar WH, Prestwich GD (2006) Fluorogenic phospholipid substrate to detect lysophospholipase D/ autotaxin activity. Org Lett 8: 2023-2026.

[63] Saunders LP, Ouellette A, Bandle R, Chang WC, Zhou H, Misra RN, De La Cruz EM, Braddock DT (2008) Identification of small-molecule inhibitors of autotaxin that inhibit melanoma cell migration and invasion. Mol Cancer Ther 7: 3352-3362.

[64] Parrill AL, Echols U, Nguyen T, Pham TC, Hoeglund A, Baker DL (2008) Virtual screening approaches for the identification of non-lipid autotaxin inhibitors. Bioorg Med Chem 16: 1784-1795.

[65] Mize CD, Abbott AM, Gacasan SB, Parrill AL, Baker DL (2011) Ligand-based autotaxin pharmacophore models reflect structure-based docking results. J Mol Graph Model 31: 76-86.

[66] Kawaguchi M, Okabe T, Okudaira S, Nishimasu H, Ishitani R, Kojima H, Nureki O, Aoki J, Nagano T (2013) Screening and X-ray crystal structure-based optimization of autotaxin (ENPP2) inhibitors, using a newly developed fluorescence probe. ACS Chem Biol 8: 1713-1721.

[67] Fells JI, Lee SC, Norman DD, Tsukahara R, Kirby RJ, Nelson S, Seibel W, Papoian R, Patil R, Miller DD, Parrill AL, Pham T-C, Baker DL, Bittman R, Tigyi G (2013) Targeting the Hydrophobic Pocket of Autotaxin with Virtual Screening of Inhibitors Identifies a Common Aromatic Sulfonamide Structural Motif. FEBS Journal 281: 1017-1028.

[68] Fells JI, Lee SC, Fujiwara Y, Norman DD, Lim KG, Tsukahara R, Liu J, Patil R, Miller DD, Kirby RJ, Nelson S, Seibel W, Papoian R, Parrill AL, Baker DL, Bittman R, Tigyi G (2013) Hits of a high-throughput screen identify the hydrophobic pocket of autotaxin/lysophospholipase D as an inhibitory surface. Mol Pharmacol 84: 415-424.

[69] Nam SW, Clair T, Kim YS, McMarlin A, Schiffmann E, Liotta LA, Stracke ML (2001) Autotaxin (NPP-2), a metastasis-enhancing motogen, is an angiogenic factor. Cancer Res 61: 6938-6944.

[70] Bachner D, Ahrens M, Betat N, Schroder D, Gross G (1999) Developmental expression analysis of murine autotaxin (ATX). Mech Dev 84: 121-125.

[71] Kishi Y, Okudaira S, Tanaka M, Hama K, Shida D, Kitayama J, Yamori T, Aoki J, Fujimaki T, Arai H (2006) Autotaxin is overexpressed in glioblastoma multiforme and contributes to cell motility of glioblastoma by converting lysophosphatidylcholine to lysophosphatidic acid. J Biol Chem 281: 17492-17500.

[72] Yukiura H, Hama K, Nakanaga K, Tanaka M, Asaoka Y, Okudaira S, Arima N, Inoue A, Hashimoto T, Arai H, Kawahara A, Nishina H, Aoki J (2011) Autotaxin regulates vascular development via multiple lysophosphatidic acid (LPA) receptors in zebrafish. J Biol Chem 286: 43972-43983.

[73] Moolenaar WH, Houben AJ, Lee SJ, van Meeteren LA (2013) Autotaxin in embryonic development. Biochim Biophys Acta 1831: 13-19.

[74] Yuelling LW, Waggener CT, Afshari FS, Lister JA, Fuss B (2012) Autotaxin/ENPP2 regulates oligodendrocyte differentiation in vivo in the developing zebrafish hindbrain. Glia 60: 1605-1618.

[75] Lai SL, Yao WL, Tsao KC, Houben AJ, Albers HM, Ovaa H, Moolenaar WH, Lee SJ (2012) Autotaxin/Lpar3 signaling regulates Kupffer's vesicle formation and left-right asymmetry in zebrafish. Development 139: 4439-4448.

[76] Rother E, Brandl R, Baker DL, Goyal P, Gebhard H, Tigyi G, Siess W (2003) Subtype-selective antagonists of lysophosphatidic Acid receptors inhibit platelet activation triggered by the lipid core of atherosclerotic plaques. Circulation 108: 741-747.

[77] Rancoule C, Attane C, Gres S, Fournel A, Dusaulcy R, Bertrand C, Vinel C, Treguer K, Prentki M, Valet P, Saulnier-Blache JS (2013) Lysophosphatidic acid impairs glucose homeostasis and inhibits insulin secretion in high-fat diet obese mice. Diabetologia 56: 1394-1402.

[78] Ferry G, Tellier E, Try A, Gres S, Naime I, Simon MF, Rodriguez M, Boucher J, Tack I, Gesta S, Chomarat P, Dieu M, Raes M, Galizzi JP, Valet P, Boutin JA, Saulnier-Blache JS (2003) Autotaxin is released from adipocytes, catalyzes lysophosphatidic acid synthesis, and activates preadipocyte proliferation. Up-regulated expression with adipocyte differentiation and obesity. J Biol Chem 278: 18162-18169.

[79] Federico L, Ren H, Mueller PA, Wu T, Liu S, Popovic J, Blalock EM, Sunkara M, Ovaa H, Albers HM, Mills GB, Morris AJ, Smyth SS (2012) Autotaxin and its product lysophosphatidic acid suppress brown adipose differentiation and promote diet-induced obesity in mice. Mol Endocrinol 26: 786-797.

[80] Nishimura S, Nagasaki M, Okudaira S, Aoki J, Ohmori T, Ohkawa R, Nakamura K, Igarashi K, Yamashita H, Eto K, Uno K, Hayashi N, Kadowaki T, Komuro I, Yatomi

Y, Nagai R (2014) ENPP2 contributes to adipose tissue expansion in diet-induced obesity. Diabetes: doi: 10.2337/db2313-1694.

[81] Rancoule C, Dusaulcy R, Treguer K, Gres S, Attane C, Saulnier-Blache JS (2014) Involvement of autotaxin/lysophosphatidic acid signaling in obesity and impaired glucose homeostasis. Biochimie 96: 140-143.

[82] Dusaulcy R, Rancoule C, Gres S, Wanecq E, Colom A, Guigne C, van Meeteren LA, Moolenaar WH, Valet P, Saulnier-Blache JS (2011) Adipose-specific disruption of autotaxin enhances nutritional fattening and reduces plasma lysophosphatidic acid. J Lipid Res 52: 1247-1255.

[83] Mazereeuw-Hautier J, Gres S, Fanguin M, Cariven C, Fauvel J, Perret B, Chap H, Salles JP, Saulnier-Blache JS (2005) Production of lysophosphatidic acid in blister fluid: involvement of a lysophospholipase D activity. J Invest Dermatol 125: 421-427.

[84] Tokumura A, Taira S, Kikuchi M, Tsutsumi T, Shimizu Y, Watsky MA (2012) Lysophospholipids and lysophospholipase D in rabbit aqueous humor following corneal injury. Prostaglandins Other Lipid Mediat 97: 83-89.

[85] Masuda K, Haruta S, Orino K, Kawaminami M, Kurusu S (2013) Autotaxin as a novel, tissue-remodeling-related factor in regressing corpora lutea of cycling rats. FEBS J 280: 6600-6612.

[86] Grisanti L, Rezza A, Clavel C, Sennett R, Rendl M (2013) Enpp2/Autotaxin in dermal papilla precursors is dispensable for hair follicle morphogenesis. J Invest Dermatol 133: 2332-2339.

[87] Mebarek S, Abousalham A, Magne D, Do le D, Bandorowicz-Pikula J, Pikula S, Buchet R (2013) Phospholipases of mineralization competent cells and matrix vesicles: roles in physiological and pathological mineralizations. Int J Mol Sci 14: 5036-5129.

[88] Evseenko D, Latour B, Richardson W, Corselli M, Sahaghian A, Cardinal S, Zhu Y, Chan R, Dunn B, Crooks GM (2013) Lysophosphatidic acid mediates myeloid differentiation within the human bone marrow microenvironment. PLoS One 8: e63718.

[89] Awada R, Rondeau P, Gres S, Saulnier-Blache JS, Lefebvre d'Hellencourt C, Bourdon E (2012) Autotaxin protects microglial cells against oxidative stress. Free Radic Biol Med 52: 516-526.

[90] Awada R, Saulnier-Blache JS, Gres S, Bourdon E, Rondeau P, Parimisetty A, Orihuela R, Harry GJ, d'Hellencourt CL (2014) Autotaxin Downregulates LPS-Induced Microglia Activation and Pro-Inflammatory Cytokines Production. Journal of Cellular Biochemistry: doi: 10.1002/jcb.24889.

[91] Umemoto E, Hayasaka H, Bai Z, Cai L, Yonekura S, Peng X, Takeda A, Tohya K, Miyasaka M (2011) Novel regulators of lymphocyte trafficking across high endothelial venules. Crit Rev Immunol 31: 147-169.

[92] Bai Z, Cai L, Umemoto E, Takeda A, Tohya K, Komai Y, Veeraveedu PT, Hata E, Su-
      giura Y, Kubo A, Suematsu M, Hayasaka H, Okudaira S, Aoki J, Tanaka T, Albers
      HM, Ovaa H, Miyasaka M (2013) Constitutive lymphocyte transmigration across the
      basal lamina of high endothelial venules is regulated by the autotaxin/lysophosphati-
      dic acid axis. J Immunol 190: 2036-2048.

[93] Zhang Y, Chen YC, Krummel MF, Rosen SD (2012) Autotaxin through lysophospha-
      tidic acid stimulates polarization, motility, and transendothelial migration of naive T
      cells. J Immunol 189: 3914-3924.

[94] Nakasaki T, Tanaka T, Okudaira S, Hirosawa M, Umemoto E, Otani K, Jin S, Bai Z,
      Hayasaka H, Fukui Y, Aozasa K, Fujita N, Tsuruo T, Ozono K, Aoki J, Miyasaka M
      (2008) Involvement of the lysophosphatidic acid-generating enzyme autotaxin in
      lymphocyte-endothelial cell interactions. Am J Pathol 173: 1566-1576.

[95] van Meeteren LA, Moolenaar WH (2007) Regulation and biological activities of the
      autotaxin-LPA axis. Prog Lipid Res 46: 145-160.

[96] Budd DC, Qian Y (2013) Development of lysophosphatidic acid pathway modulators
      as therapies for fibrosis. Future Med Chem 5: 1935-1952.

[97] Lee S, Lynch KR (2005) Brown recluse spider (Loxosceles reclusa) venom phospholi-
      pase D (PLD) generates lysophosphatidic acid (LPA). Biochem J 391: 317-323.

[98] Borchani L, Sassi A, Ben Gharsa H, Safra I, Shahbazzadeh D, Ben Lasfar Z, El Ayeb
      M (2013) The pathological effects of Heminecrolysin, a dermonecrotic toxin from
      Hemiscorpius lepturus scorpion venom are mediated through its lysophospholipase
      D activity. Toxicon 68: 30-39.

[99] van Meeteren LA, Frederiks F, Giepmans BN, Pedrosa MF, Billington SJ, Jost BH,
      Tambourgi DV, Moolenaar WH (2004) Spider and bacterial sphingomyelinases D tar-
      get cellular lysophosphatidic acid receptors by hydrolyzing lysophosphatidylcholine.
      J Biol Chem 279: 10833-10836.

[100] Krishnamoorthy S, Honn KV (2006) Inflammation and disease progression. Cancer
      Metastasis Rev 25: 481-491.

[101] Dvorak HF (1986) Tumors: wounds that do not heal. Similarities between tumor stro-
      ma generation and wound healing. N Engl J Med 315: 1650-1659.

[102] Allavena P, Garlanda C, Borrello MG, Sica A, Mantovani A (2008) Pathways connect-
      ing inflammation and cancer. Curr Opin Genet Dev 18: 3-10.

[103] Chopra M, Riedel SS, Biehl M, Krieger S, von Krosigk V, Bauerlein CA, Brede C, Jor-
      dan Garrote AL, Kraus S, Schafer V, Ritz M, Mattenheimer K, Degla A, Mottok A,
      Einsele H, Wajant H, Beilhack A (2013) Tumor necrosis factor receptor 2-dependent
      homeostasis of regulatory T cells as a player in TNF-induced experimental metasta-
      sis. Carcinogenesis 34: 1296-1303.

[104] Germano G, Allavena P, Mantovani A (2008) Cytokines as a key component of cancer-related inflammation. Cytokine 43: 374-379.

[105] Grivennikov SI (2013) Inflammation and colorectal cancer: colitis-associated neoplasia. Semin Immunopathol 35: 229-244.

[106] Wu JM, Xu Y, Skill NJ, Sheng H, Zhao Z, Yu M, Saxena R, Maluccio MA (2010) Autotaxin expression and its connection with the TNF-alpha-NF-kappaB axis in human hepatocellular carcinoma. Mol Cancer 9: 71.

[107] Benesch MGK, Ko YM, McMullen TPW, Brindley DN (2014) Autotaxin in the crosshairs: Taking aim at cancer and other inflammatory conditions. FEBS Letters 588: 2712-2727.

[108] Euer N, Schwirzke M, Evtimova V, Burtscher H, Jarsch M, Tarin D, Weidle UH (2002) Identification of genes associated with metastasis of mammary carcinoma in metastatic versus non-metastatic cell lines. Anticancer Res 22: 733-740.

[109] Bollen M, Gijsbers R, Ceulemans H, Stalmans W, Stefan C (2000) Nucleotide pyrophosphatases/phosphodiesterases on the move. Crit Rev Biochem Mol Biol 35: 393-432.

[110] Debies MT, Welch DR (2001) Genetic basis of human breast cancer metastasis. J Mammary Gland Biol Neoplasia 6: 441-451.

[111] Brindley DN (2004) Lipid phosphate phosphatases and related proteins: signaling functions in development, cell division, and cancer. J Cell Biochem 92: 900-912.

[112] Moolenaar WH, van Meeteren LA, Giepmans BN (2004) The ins and outs of lysophosphatidic acid signaling. Bioessays 26: 870-881.

[113] Gendaszewska-Darmach E (2008) Lysophosphatidic acids, cyclic phosphatidic acids and autotaxin as promising targets in therapies of cancer and other diseases. Acta Biochim Pol 55: 227-240.

[114] Liu S, Murph M, Panupinthu N, Mills GB (2009) ATX-LPA receptor axis in inflammation and cancer. Cell Cycle 8: 3695-3701.

[115] Panupinthu N, Lee HY, Mills GB (2010) Lysophosphatidic acid production and action: critical new players in breast cancer initiation and progression. Br J Cancer 102: 941-946.

[116] Houben AJ, Moolenaar WH (2011) Autotaxin and LPA receptor signaling in cancer. Cancer Metastasis Rev 30: 557-565.

[117] Gotoh M, Fujiwara Y, Yue J, Liu J, Lee S, Fells J, Uchiyama A, Murakami-Murofushi K, Kennel S, Wall J, Patil R, Gupte R, Balazs L, Miller DD, Tigyi GJ (2012) Controlling cancer through the autotaxin-lysophosphatidic acid receptor axis. Biochem Soc Trans 40: 31-36.

[118] Peyruchaud O, Leblanc R, David M (2013) Pleiotropic activity of lysophosphatidic acid in bone metastasis. Biochim Biophys Acta 1831: 99-104.

[119] Samadi N, Bekele R, Capatos D, Venkatraman G, Sariahmetoglu M, Brindley DN (2011) Regulation of lysophosphatidate signaling by autotaxin and lipid phosphate phosphatases with respect to tumor progression, angiogenesis, metastasis and chemo-resistance. Biochimie 93: 61-70.

[120] So J, Wang FQ, Navari J, Schreher J, Fishman DA (2005) LPA-induced epithelial ovarian cancer (EOC) in vitro invasion and migration are mediated by VEGF receptor-2 (VEGF-R2). Gynecol Oncol 97: 870-878.

[121] Baker DL, Morrison P, Miller B, Riely CA, Tolley B, Westermann AM, Bonfrer JM, Bais E, Moolenaar WH, Tigyi G (2002) Plasma lysophosphatidic acid concentration and ovarian cancer. JAMA 287: 3081-3082.

[122] Murph MM, Hurst-Kennedy J, Newton V, Brindley DN, Radhakrishna H (2007) Lysophosphatidic acid decreases the nuclear localization and cellular abundance of the p53 tumor suppressor in A549 lung carcinoma cells. Mol Cancer Res 5: 1201-1211.

[123] Liu S, Umezu-Goto M, Murph M, Lu Y, Liu W, Zhang F, Yu S, Stephens LC, Cui X, Murrow G, Coombes K, Muller W, Hung MC, Perou CM, Lee AV, Fang X, Mills GB (2009) Expression of autotaxin and lysophosphatidic acid receptors increases mammary tumorigenesis, invasion, and metastases. Cancer Cell 15: 539-550.

[124] Popnikolov NK, Dalwadi BH, Thomas JD, Johannes GJ, Imagawa WT (2012) Association of autotaxin and lysophosphatidic acid receptor 3 with aggressiveness of human breast carcinoma. Tumour Biol 33: 2237-2243.

[125] Hanahan D, Weinberg RA (2011) Hallmarks of cancer: the next generation. Cell 144: 646-674.

[126] Zhao C, Fernandes MJ, Prestwich GD, Turgeon M, Di Battista J, Clair T, Poubelle PE, Bourgoin SG (2008) Regulation of lysophosphatidic acid receptor expression and function in human synoviocytes: implications for rheumatoid arthritis? Mol Pharmacol 73: 587-600.

[127] Nikitopoulou I, Oikonomou N, Karouzakis E, Sevastou I, Nikolaidou-Katsaridou N, Zhao Z, Mersinias V, Armaka M, Xu Y, Masu M, Mills GB, Gay S, Kollias G, Aidinis V (2012) Autotaxin expression from synovial fibroblasts is essential for the pathogenesis of modeled arthritis. J Exp Med 209: 925-933.

[128] Hartman ZC, Poage GM, den Hollander P, Tsimelzon A, Hill J, Panupinthu N, Zhang Y, Mazumdar A, Hilsenbeck SG, Mills GB, Brown PH (2013) Growth of triple-negative breast cancer cells relies upon coordinate autocrine expression of the proinflammatory cytokines IL-6 and IL-8. Cancer Research 73: 3470-3480.

[129] Kehlen A, Englert N, Seifert A, Klonisch T, Dralle H, Langner J, Hoang-Vu C (2004) Expression, regulation and function of autotaxin in thyroid carcinomas. Int J Cancer 109: 833-838.

[130] Kawagoe H, Stracke ML, Nakamura H, Sano K (1997) Expression and transcriptional regulation of the PD-Ialpha/autotaxin gene in neuroblastoma. Cancer Res 57: 2516-2521.

[131] Farina AR, Cappabianca L, Ruggeri P, Di Ianni N, Ragone M, Merolle S, Sano K, Stracke ML, Horowitz JM, Gulino A, Mackay AR (2012) Constitutive autotaxin transcription by Nmyc-amplified and non-amplified neuroblastoma cells is regulated by a novel AP-1 and SP-mediated mechanism and abrogated by curcumin. FEBS Lett 586: 3681-3691.

[132] Singh AD, Sisley K, Xu Y, Li J, Faber P, Plummer SJ, Mudhar HS, Rennie IG, Kessler PM, Casey G, Williams BG (2007) Reduced expression of autotaxin predicts survival in uveal melanoma. Br J Ophthalmol 91: 1385-1392.

[133] Jankowski M (2011) Autotaxin: its role in biology of melanoma cells and as a pharmacological target. Enzyme Res 8: 194857.

[134] Braeuer RR, Zigler M, Kamiya T, Dobroff AS, Huang L, Choi W, McConkey DJ, Shoshan E, Mobley AK, Song R, Raz A, Bar-Eli M (2012) Galectin-3 contributes to melanoma growth and metastasis via regulation of NFAT1 and autotaxin. Cancer Res 72: 5757-5766.

[135] Samadi N, Gaetano C, Goping IS, Brindley DN (2009) Autotaxin protects MCF-7 breast cancer and MDA-MB-435 melanoma cells against Taxol-induced apoptosis. Oncogene 28: 1028-1039.

[136] Samadi N, Bekele RT, Goping IS, Schang LM, Brindley DN (2011) Lysophosphatidate induces chemo-resistance by releasing breast cancer cells from taxol-induced mitotic arrest. PLoS One 6: e20608.

[137] Vidot S, Witham J, Agarwal R, Greenhough S, Bamrah HS, Tigyi GJ, Kaye SB, Richardson A (2010) Autotaxin delays apoptosis induced by carboplatin in ovarian cancer cells. Cell Signal 22: 926-935.

[138] Hooks SB, Callihan P, Altman MK, Hurst JH, Ali MW, Murph MM (2010) Regulators of G-Protein signaling RGS10 and RGS17 regulate chemoresistance in ovarian cancer cells. Mol Cancer 9: 289.

[139] Brindley DN, Lin FT, Tigyi GJ (2013) Role of the autotaxin-lysophosphatidate axis in cancer resistance to chemotherapy and radiotherapy. Biochim Biophys Acta 1831: 74-85.

[140] Schneider G, Sellers ZP, Abdel-Latif A, Morris AJ, Ratajczak MZ (2014) Bioactive Lipids, LPC and LPA, are Novel Pro-metastatic Factors and Their Tissue Levels Increase

in   Response   to   Radio/Chemotherapy.   Mol   Cancer   Res: doi:
10.1158/1541-7786.MCR-1114-0188.

[141] Prestwich GD, Gajewiak J, Zhang H, Xu X, Yang G, Serban M (2008) Phosphatase-
       resistant analogues of lysophosphatidic acid: agonists promote healing, antagonists
       and autotaxin inhibitors treat cancer. Biochim Biophys Acta 1781: 588-594.

2

Emerging Drug Combination Approaches in Melanoma Therapy

Jin Wang, Duane D. Miller and Wei Li

1. Introduction

The FDA approvals of ipilimumab targeting the cytotoxic T lymphocyte-associated antigen 4 (CTLA-4), pembrolizumab targeting the programmed cell death protein 1 (PD-1), BRAF inhibitors vemurafenib and dabrafenib, and MEK inhibitor trametinib represent significant milestones in more effective treatment of advanced melanoma. However, it is clear that the use of these single-agent therapies have limitation clinically. For example, ipilimumab only showed 4.5% objective response rate when used alone in a Phase II clinical trial [1]. The efficacy of vemurafenib lasts only 6.7 months before the disease relapses especially in patients with metastatic melanoma [2]. Therefore, rational combination approaches are strongly preferred in order to improve the overall patient progression-free survival (PFS), overcome or delay the development of multi-drug resistance and reduce the incidents of side effects [3-6].

In this chapter, we will summarize the emerging combination therapy approaches from both clinical trial and preclinical research in the past five years.

2. Combination of kinase inhibitors for melanoma treatment

2.1. Combined inhibitions targeting components within the Mitogen-Activated Protein Kinase (MAPK) signaling pathway

2.1.1. Targeting BRAF: Mechanism of action, toxicity and drug resistance

BRAF is a serine/threonine growth signal transduction protein kinase from RAF family which plays important roles in the RAS/RAF/MEK/ERK pathway and directs cell division, proliferation and secretion [7]. BRAF inhibitors (BRAFi) are ATP-competitive ligands which inactivate the function of BRAF protein by either stabilizing the inactive form of kinase domain (sorafenib) or preferentially inhibit the active form of the kinase (vemurafenib, dabrafenib) [8, 9]. Various mutations of *BRAF* gene have been identified in cancers including melanoma, colorectal and ovarian cancer. Around 60% of human melanoma adopted the T1799A transversion in exon 15, which lead to BRAF^{V600E} mutation and the over-activated monomer phosphorylation for BRAF^{V600E} [9, 10]. The two FDA approved BRAFi (Vemurafenib and dabrafenib) selectively and potently block the activation of BRAF^{V600E} and thus inhibit the MAPK signaling pathway. These drugs show very high clinical efficacy in metastatic melanoma patients harboring the BRAF^{V600E} mutation [11-13]. Interestingly, in a clinical study which treated 43 patients with any V600 BRAF mutation including the rare V600R variant, five out of the six melanoma patients having V600R mutation had clinical response to the therapy of vemurafenib or dabrafenib (response rate 86%) [14].

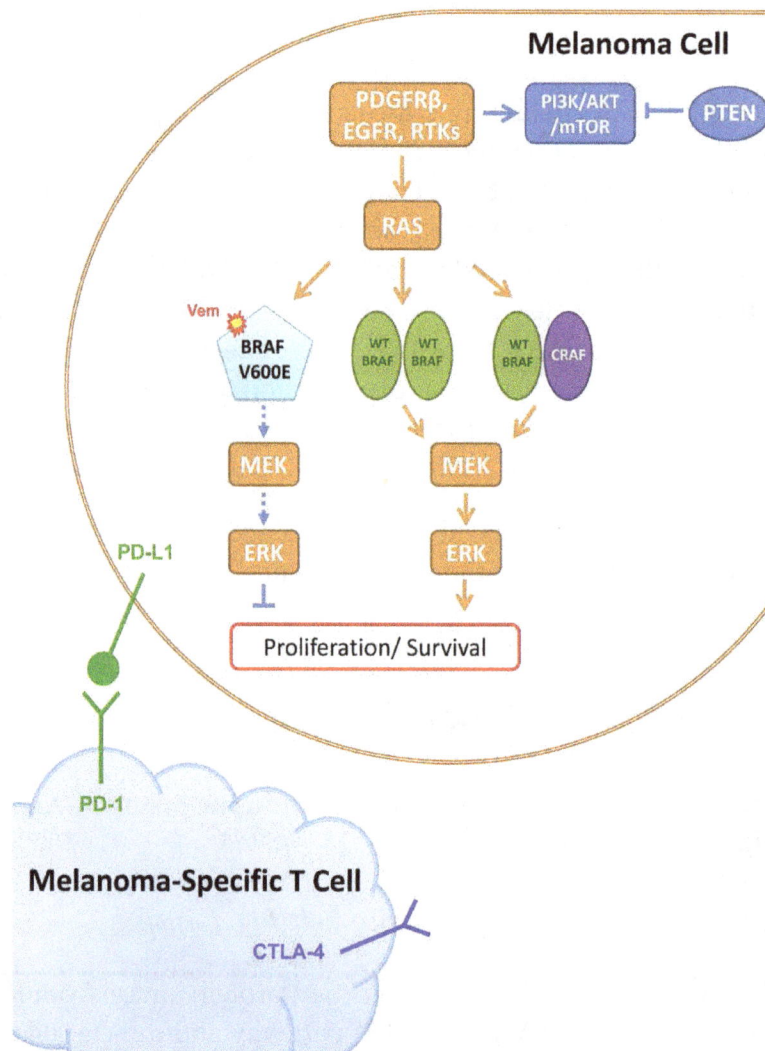

Figure 1. The mechanisms of BRAF inhibitor vemurafenib (Vem) action, toxicity and the interaction between melanoma cells with T lymphocytes.

However, wide type BRAF melanoma tumors do not respond to vemurafenib or dabrafenib inhibition, although they are sensitive to the MEK inhibitors [9]. Paradoxically, in cells with RAS mutation and wild-type BRAF, treatment with vemurafenib or dabrafenib will promote the formation of BRAF-CRAF heterodimer and lead to the activation of subsequent MEK/ERK signaling and cell proliferation as shown in Figure 1 [5]. This mechanism is used to explain the observation of typical clinical side effects associated with the use of vemurafenib: nearly 25% of patients developed skin lesions and even cutaneous squamous cell carcinoma (CSCC). In addition, *in vitro* study has revealed that vemurafenib inhibits multiple off-target kinases including c-Jun N-terminal kinase (JNK), suppresses JNK-dependent apoptosis, and generates CSCC toxicity [15].

2.1.2. Mechanisms of resistance to BRAF inhibition

In general, due to alternative pathway activations and inter-and intra-patients melanoma genetic heterogeneity, various mechanisms of resistance to BRAF inhibition have been identified [10, 16-19]. As we mentioned before, melanoma tumors bearing wide type BRAF are intrinsically resistant to vemurafenib and dabrafenib. Tumor micro-environment also contributes to the innate resistance to BRAF inhibition in melanoma. For example, stromal cells secrete hepatocyte growth factor (HGF), which activates the HGF-receptor MET, MAPK and PI3K-AKT pathways [20].

Eventually, nearly all BRAF mutated melanoma tumors develop acquired drug resistance upon treatment with BRAF inhibitors. The disease progression arises as early as two-month continuous treatment [18, 19]. The mechanisms of acquired resistance to BRAF inhibition can be generalized into two categories: BRAF^{V600E}-bypass mechanisms and MAPK-bypass mechanisms.

First, the BRAF^{V600E}-bypass mechanisms reactivate MAPK signaling and lead to ERK-dependent tumor cell survival and proliferation (Figure 2A). COT, which is coded by gene *MAP3K8*, is a MEK kinase. The overexpression of COT or amplification of *MAP3K8* directly activates MEK signaling without the participation of RAF protein [21]. The mutant of MEK1^{C121S} increases catalytic capability and circumvents BRAF to activate basal level of ERK phosphorylation [22]. Before the treatment of vemurafenib or dabrafenib, melanoma cells with BRAF^{V600E} mutation have over-activated monomer BRAF/MEK/ERK cascade which forms an ERK-dependent negative feedback loop. This negative feedback loop reduces the expression of the active RAS-GTP. In the presence of vemurafenib or dabrafenib, ERK phosphorylation level is rapidly reduced and the feed-back suppression on RAS activation is abolished (Figure 1). Therefore, eventually the ERK cascade level is restored through RAS over-activation. NRAS mutants including NRAS^{Q61K} and NRAS^{Q61R} can drive ERK activation through ARAF or CRAF homo-or hetero-dimers which are alternative MEK activators [23]. The combinations of BRAF inhibition plus MEK or ERK inhibition have showed efficacy of overcoming the resistance through these BRAF^{V600E}-bypass mechanisms [24-26], leading to the recent FDA approval of dabrafenib plus trametinib combination therapy for advanced melanoma.

Second, the MAPK-bypass mechanisms allow melanoma cells to escape from the cytotoxicity of BRAF or MEK inhibition through the activation of ERK-independent survival pathways

(Figure 2B). The PI3K-AKT signaling pathway can be activated through the overexpression of receptor tyrosine kinases (RTKs), for example, insulin-like growth factor 1 (IGF-1) receptor (IGF-1R) and platelet-derived growth factor receptor beta (PDGFRβ) [27]. The elevated levels of IGF-1R, PDGFRβ or HGF can also stimulate another receptor tyrosine kinase, MET, and increase the activity of PI3K. Phosphatase tensin (PTEN) is a negative regulator of PI3K. The PTEN loss-of-function mutation induces the resistance of BRAF inhibition and reduces the PFS of dabrafenib therapy in melanoma patients due to the PI3K activation [28]. Moreover, the upregulation of cyclin D1 can activate cyclin-dependent kinase 4 (CDK4) and 6 (CDK6) and make melanoma cells less dependent on MAPK signaling in cell cycle progressing [29].

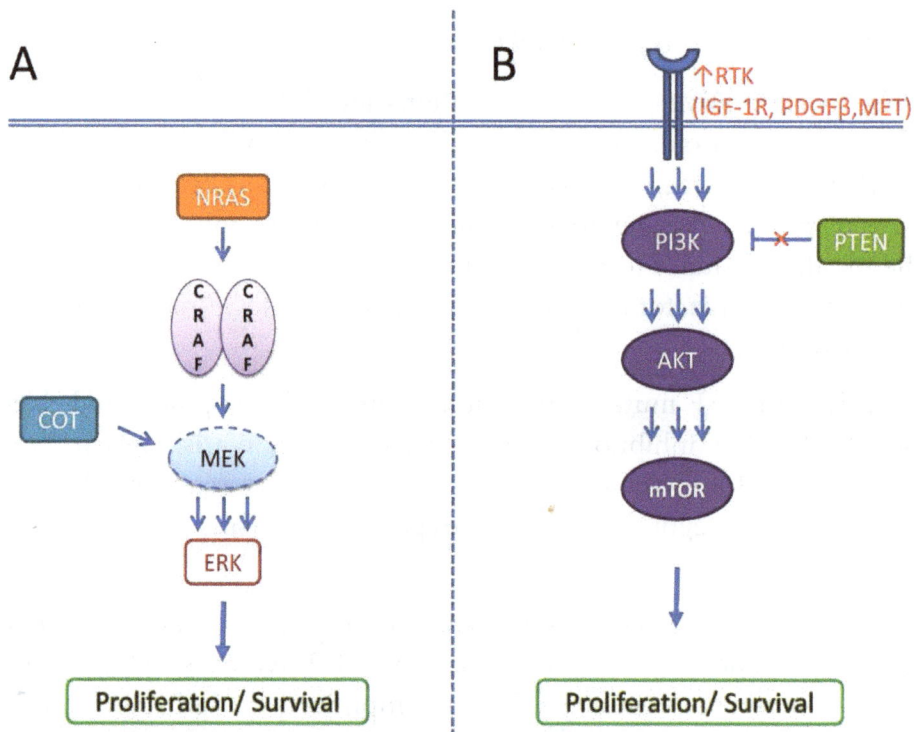

Figure 2. The mechanisms of acquired resistance to BRAF inhibition.

Additionally, Jaehyuk Choi *et al* has reported a BRAF^{L505H} mutation which changes an amino acid residue in BRAF-vemurafenib interface and causes the resistance to vemurafenib treatment *in vitro* [30]. Since vemurafenib is a substrate of the ATP-binding cassette sub-family G member 2 (ABCG2), the overexpression of ABCG2 in BRAF^{V600E} melanoma cell lines has caused the increasing of vemurafenib efflux *in vitro* [31]. The elucidation on the mechanism of acquired-resistance to BRAFi opens a door to rationally design and explore the proper combination strategies to overcome or delay the development of BRAFi resistance.

2.1.3. Targeting MEK: Mechanism of action, toxicity and resistance

Trametinib, which is approved by FDA in May 2013 as a monotherapy agent against advanced melanoma with BRAF^{V600E} and BRAF^{V600K} mutations, is a first-in-class, orally available, allosteric (non-ATP-competitive) MEK1/MEK2 inhibitor (MEKi) [32, 33]. It selectively inhibits

MEK, the down-stream kinase protein of RAF in the RAS-RAF-MEK-ERK pathway. As a result, melanoma cells with acquired resistance to BRAFi are commonly cross-resistant to MEKi such as trametinib or selumetinib, another selective allosteric MEKi [24, 34]. This mechanism explains the clinical trial results in which trametinib monotherapy fails to significantly benefit patients who have already developed acquired BRAFi resistance [35]. In contrast to the use of a BRAFi, no CSCC side effects are observed among the patients received trametinib treatment in clinical trials [13, 32]. However, similar to the use of vemurafenib, disease progression occurs within 6-7 months in patients receiving single-agent trametinib treatment [36]. Nevertheless, a retrospective analysis of 23 patients, who were first treated with MEKi and upon progression with a selective BRAFi, shows that the median time to progression (TTP) has been prolonged to 8.9 months from 4.8 months using a single-agent MEKi or 4.4 months for a single-agent BRAFi treatment, respectively [37]. However, a recent clinical trial indicated that if melanoma patients were treated with a BRAFi first then MEKi therapy, no confirmed response was observed [35]. This indicates that optimal treatment schedule and sequence is important for the melanoma therapy targeting the MAPK pathway.

2.1.4. Drug combination targeting MAPK pathway: From lab bench to clinical practice

Given that the mechanisms of tumor cells develop resistance to BRAFi partially by reactivating the ERK cascade and side effects such as CSCC are RAF-dependent, combining BRAFi with MEKi has attracted lots of research interest in order to further block the MAPK signaling pathway. In vitro and murine models first show the synergistic anti-proliferation and anti-tumor growth effects using the combined BRAFi and MEKi treatment [9, 27, 38, 39]. Further, this combination overcomes the acquired resistance to BRAFi [27, 38] in both cellular based assay and mouse xenograft models. In addition, the combined inhibition of BRAF-MEK suppresses the paradoxical BRAFi-induced MAPK signal elevation in melanoma cells and reduces the incidences of skin lesions in a rat model [9].

When it comes to the clinical trial data, the combined inhibition of BRAF-MEK has presented significant improvements of major patient benefits (PFS and overall survival). A phase I/II trial (ClinicalTrials.gov, NCT1072175) investigated the combination of oral dabrafenib (150 mg twice per day) plus oral trametinib (1 or 2 mg daily) (combination 150/1 and 150/2) versus monotherapy of dabrafenib (150 mg twice per day) over 108 metastatic melanoma patients bearing either V600E (92 patients) or V600K (16 patients) BRAF mutation [12, 36]. Median PFS in combination 150/2 group reached 9.4 months, compared to 5.8 months in the dabrafenib monotherapy group (hazard ratio 0.39, 95% confidence interval 0.25 to 0.62). The incidence of CSCC adverse events among combination 150/2 group is non-significantly lower than that among monotherapy group (7% versus 19%, P=0.09). But more frequent cases of pyrexia which is not common in trametinib single treatment have been reported in combination 150/2 group (71%, with recurrent rate 79%), as compared with dabrafenib monotherapy group (26%) [40]. These promising data lead to an accelerated FDA approval of the combination of dabrafenib (BRAFi) and trametinib (MEKi) for the treatment of unresectable or metastatic melanoma patients with BRAF V600E or V600K mutation, although further phase III studies with recruitment of more patients comparing the combination therapy with dabrafenib or vemurafenib single treatment (ClinicalTrials.gov, NCT01584648, NCT01597908) are still being assessed.

In addition, several ongoing phase I/II clinical trials now have shown that generally the combination of other BRAFi and MEKi is well tolerated in patients with or without receiving BRAFi treatment before (ClinicalTrials.gov, NCT01271803 vemurafenib (BRAFi)+cobimetinib (MEKi), NCT01543698 LGX818 (BRAFi)+MEK162 (MEKi)) [41-43] and overall response rate has increased comparing to the monotherapy groups, although the anti-tumor efficacy data haven't been released.

2.2. Combination targeted therapy using Phosphatidylinositol 3-Kinase (PI3K)/AKT/ mammalian Target of Rapamycin (mTOR) inhibitors

The activation of PI3K/AKT/mTOR pathway have been widely proved to be one of the major mechanisms of intrinsic or acquired resistance to both DNA-methylation agents (e.g. dacarbazine) and targeted BRAF inhibitor therapy (Figure 2). Some cell lines that are cross-resistant to both BRAFi and MEKi, are still sensitive to the inhibition of AKT/mTOR [34]. On the other hand, mechanistic study revealed evidences of a negative crosstalk between RAF/MEK/ERK and PI3K/AKT/mTOR pathways through RAS kinase. Therefore, when the downstream mTOR function is blocked, PI3K will be able to activate MAPK pathway via a switch of RAS [44, 45]. These investigations suggest a promising combination strategy of targeting MAPK pathway together with PI3K/AKT/mTOR cascade. Several preclinical studies widely proved that in MAPK inhibition sensitive melanoma cell lines, co-targeting PI3K/AKT/mTOR effectively induces cancer cell apoptosis with down-regulated anti-apoptotic BCL-2 family proteins [34, 46-48]. Such a co-targeting strategy can also postpone the emergence of acquired resistance to BRAFi dabrafenib mediated by PTEN mutation or disruption [49, 50]. Further, the dual inhibition of two pathways has successfully overcome NRAS mutation mediated resistance to MAPK blockade *in vitro* and induced xenograft tumor regression *in vivo* [34, 38, 51]. Finally, the combination of vemurafenib (BRAFi) or selumetinib (MEKi) with BEZ235 (dual PI3K and mTOR1/2 inhibitor) has been shown to overcome the PDGFRβ-driven resistance to MAPK pathway inhibition [52].

A series of Phase I studies have evaluated the clinical relevance of the combination therapy which co-targets PI3K/AKT/mTOR and RAF/MEK/ERK pathways in terms of the incidence on severe side effect and anti-tumor efficacy in 236 patients. These patients have advanced cancers including melanoma, colorectal, pancreatic and non-small cell lung cancers. Results from three combination groups (AKTi MK2206+MEKi selumetinib, NCT01021748; AKTi GSK2141795+MEKi trametinib, NCT01138085; mTOR inhibitor everolimus+MEKi trametinib, NCT 00955773) are compared to the single treatment groups [53]. Overall, the combination therapy did not provide significant increase of tumor control rate (64.6% for combination, 52.7% for monotherapy, $P=0.16$), although all five colorectal patients with co-activation of both pathways in combination group achieved tumor regression to varied extent between 2% and 64%. However, this combination strategy causes significant higher rates of drug-related grade III and above side effects (53.9% for combination, 18.1% for monotherapy, $P < 0.001$). Furthermore, two clinical trials which involve the combination therapy of BRAFi or MEKi with AKTi

DNE3 recently have been terminated due to the safety concerns of the toxic properties of DNE3 (ClinicalTrials.gov, NCT02087254 and NCT02095652). Nevertheless, in another ongoing phase I/II trial which measures the safety and efficacy of a well-tolerated pan-PI3K inhibitor BKM120 combined with vemurafenib therapy, preliminary data reveals that a vemurafenib-refractory melanoma patient with PTEN expression achieved a 35.9% reduction in target tumor (ClinicalTrials.gov, NCT01512251) [54]. In general, drug-related toxicity is one of the major issues for this cross-pathway targeted combination therapy and patients genetic profiling is very important to achieve the maximum objective response.

2.3. Combining targeted therapy with anti-angiogenic agents

Melanoma is a vascular tumor. The abnormal expression of the epidermal growth factor (EGF) family protein and the up-regulation of EGFR-mediated alternative survival pathway have critically shaped the response of melanoma to the current chemotherapy agents [55-58]. In a recent study by Sun *et al*, six out of sixteen melanoma cell lines display acquired EGFR expression after the development of resistance to BRAFi and MEKi [59]. Even before the FDA approval of BRAFi and MEKi, the combination of bevacizumab, a recombinant human monoclonal antibody VEGF inhibitor, with a specific chemotherapy agent (for example, fluorouracil [60] or fotemustine[61]), has become a first-line treatment for metastatic melanoma patients. Clinical trials that study the combination of anti-angiogenic agents with cytotoxic agents have achieved promising anti-tumor activity, although tolerability issues exist [62]. VEGF blockage has been shown to enhance the efficacy of a GM-CSF-secreting immunotherapy *in vitro* [63]. In addition, a VEGF receptor-2 inhibitor, semaxanib, prolonged both the complete and partial response time of an immunomodulatory drug, thalidomide, over 10 recurrent metastasis melanoma patients without showing significant drug-drug interaction toxicity in a phase II trial [64].

Along with the rapid development of targeted melanoma therapeutics, the combined inhibition of VEGFR plus PDGFR or mTOR has shown synergy anti-tumor effects on mouse models of B16 metastatic melanoma without increasing toxicity [65, 66]. A large-scale, unbiased drug screening study, which aims to discover effective genotype selective combinatorial therapeutics of vemurafenib-resistant BRAF and RAS mutant melanoma, identifies a triple BRAF+EGFR +AKT inhibition as highly effective approach [3]. In the year of 2010, combination of bevacizumab with an mTOR inhibitor, everolimus, was evaluated in a phase II trial for patients with metastatic melanoma [67]. The treatment was well tolerated in most patients. Seven out of fifty-seven patients (12%) receiving combination therapy have shown major responses, although the median PFS was only 4 months. This year (2014), in a phase II trial that combines bevacizumab and sorafenib, which is an inhibitor of both RAF kinase and VEGFR-2/PDGFRβ signaling, no objective tumor responses are seen in all the fourteen patients receiving treatment [68, 69]. Interestingly, the median TTP of patients with low VEGF (<300 pg/ml) was longer than that of patients with high VEGF (50 weeks versus 15 weeks, $P=0.02$). Therefore, the levels of VEGF in patients do influence the tumor progression profile (ClinicalTrials.gov, NCT00387751).

2.4. Combination therapy using targeted therapy with versatile chemotherapy agents

Since the abnormally activated (phosphorylation) of ERK and AKT constitutively exist in melanoma cells and promote the disease progression especially metastasis, blocking ERK or AKT pathway can sensitize the metastatic melanoma to the apoptosis induced by chemotherapeutic agents including cisplatin, temozolomide, DTIC and arsenite [70-72]. With the understanding of tumor biology about the programmed cell apoptosis and the rapid development of agents that can trigger the cell death process in melanoma, the combination of a MAPK inhibitor with a BCL-2 inhibitor (ABT-737 [73] or navitoclax [74]), or a MDM2 antagonist nutlin-3 [75], has synergistically induced apoptosis of melanoma *in vitro* and suppressed xenograft tumor growth *in vivo*. A comparative analysis on the samples collected from patients receiving vemurafenib or dabrafenib/trametinib combination treatment showed that BCL-2 expression level is closely related to the onset of MAPK inhibition resistance [74]. Clinical trials are being conducted to investigate the combination of BCL-2 inhibitor (BH3 mimetics) navitoclax and vemurafenib [74].

Due to the heterogenetic characteristics of melanoma disease, Vultur A *et al* [76] recently report that MEK or BRAF inhibition can potentially strengthen the invasion property of human melanoma cells by about 20%. As a result, co-inhibiting kinases that are actively involved in cell invasion process, such as RTK, STAT3 and Src, together with MEK inhibition has effectively abolished the invasive phenotype and further caused the tumor cell death in a 3D matrix model.

Metformin, a biguanide oral anti-diabetic drug, has been discovered with antitumor activity in various cancer types including melanoma. Although the exact mechanisms remain to be elucidated, accumulating data suggest that metformin can activate AMP-activated protein kinase (AMPK) and thus increase the activities of VEGF and ERK in BRAF^{V600E} mutated melanoma cells [77]. AMPK negatively regulates malignant cell proliferation and viability [78]. The combination of vemurafenib and metformin has shown synergistic anti-proliferative effects on six out of eleven tested BRAF^{V600E} melanoma cell lines [79]. Pilot clinical studies that evaluate the safety and efficacy of metformin combination therapies (plus dabrafenib or trametinib) are now recruiting patients (ClinicalTrials.gov, NCT0184000, NCT02143050).

Unlike the cutaneous melanoma, over-activation of MAPK pathway in uveal melanoma is associated GNAQ or GNA11 mutations instead of BRAF or RAS mutations [80]. Protein kinase C (PKC) inhibitors such as enzastaurin or AEB071 induce apoptosis in GNAQ-mutant but not in GNAQ wild type uveal melanoma cells [81]. The level of ERK phosphorylation also decreases in these cells when they are treated using PKC inhibitors [81]. Chen *et al.* has recently confirmed the synergy of the combination using a PKC inhibitor with a MEKi (PD0325901 or MEK162) in GNAQ/11 mutant uveal melanoma cells [82].

Understanding the mechanisms of resistance to MAPK inhibition in melanoma can lead to rational combination designs in order to overcome acquired drug resistance to BRAF inhibitors. For example, our lab recently identified a synergistic combination in which a novel tubulin inhibitor ABI-274 combined with vemurafenib could overcome the acquired vemurafenib-resistance [83]. This combination treatment effectively arrested the vemurafenib-resistant melanoma cells in both G_0/G_1 and G_2/M phases and induced strong apoptosis through the down-regulation of AKT phosphorylation. In addition, the combination of a MEKi (TAK-733) with an Hsp90 inhibitor (ganetespib) induces tumor regressions in vemurafenib-resistant xenograft models also through the depletion of AKT signaling [84]. With the finding that up-regulated cyclin D1 expression is critical for the survival of vemurafenib-resistant cells, a selective inhibitor of cyclin dependent kinase (CDK) 4/6, LY2835219, has been reported to overcome the reactivation of MAPK signaling in vemurafenib-resistant BRAF^{V600E} melanoma [85].

3. Combinations involving immunotherapy in melanoma treatment

3.1. Combined blockade of immuno-checkpoints

Given the unsatisfactory results of cytokine-based melanoma immunotherapy (recombinant interferon-α 2b and high dose interleukin-2) in the past decade, the development and approval of ipilimumab (anti-cytotoxic T lymphocyte-associated antigen 4 (CTLA-4) monoclonal antibody) in 2013 have marked a breakthrough of immune-checkpoints blockade therapy [86]. CTLA-4 (CD152) expresses on the surface of active T-lymphocytes and inhibits the initial T-cell proliferation and migration to the tumor tissue [87]. CTLA-4 antibodies preferentially target the suppressive regulatory T cells and prevent them from being hijacked by tumors [88]. In a double-blinded phase III study in 676 patients with pretreated and refractory metastatic melanoma, ipilimumab at the dose of 3 mg/kg achieved a median OS of 10 months [86]. In a meta-Kaplan-Meier-analysis of data collected from 1,861 melanoma patients in a clinical trial, a plateau of survival curve starts from around 3 years after ipilimumab treatment with follow-up extends as long as ten years, indicating a long-term survival benefits of ipilimumab therapy (ClinicalTrials.gov, NCT01844505). In addition, ipilimumab showed good tolerance and efficacy in several other clinical trials in which it was combined with a standard chemotherapy agent such as dacarbazine, fotemustine or temozolomide [89].

Another success of immune-check point blockade strategy is the development of anti-programmed death-1 (PD-1) antibodies, represented by pembrolizumab (MK-3475) and nivolumab [90, 91]. Pembrolizumab, as the first-in-class PD-1 inhibitor, has obtained FDA approval in September 2014 for patients with advanced or unresectable melanoma. The cDNA of PD-1 (CD279) is first cloned in programmed death T cells although PD-1 itself does not directly induce apoptosis. PD-1 is over-expressed on the surface of dysfunctional activated T-cells and contributes to the maintenance of T cell dysfunction (exhaust) phenotype and proliferation disability in the tumor site [92]. Two counter receptors of PD-1 have been identified: PD-L1 and PD-L2. PD-L1 is more frequently and exclusively expressed in various tumor cells; therefore, antibodies targeting PD-L1 (MPDL3280A and BMS-936559) also have anti-tumor activity in advanced cancer including melanoma [91, 93]. The PD-1-PD-L1 ligation retards the recognition and destroying of tumor cells by CD8+cytotoxic T-lymphocytes [87]. As a result, blocking PD-1 or PD-L1 will reverse the cancer cell immune escape. Because both CTLA-4 and PD-1 are key negative receptors that cooperatively modulate the adaptive immune response in tumor progression, their combination has been shown to be synergistic in B16 melanoma tumors without overt toxicity [94].

In a cohort phase I trial that studied the concurrent administration of ipilimumab and nivolumab to 53 patients with advanced, treatment-resistant melanoma, more than 80% tumor reduction was observed in 30% patients after 12 weeks treatment at the maximum tolerated dose. Twenty-one out of fifty-three patients had objective responses and over 80% of these patients had tumor regression. Grade 3/4 adverse events are diagnosed in 53% patients but the toxicities are manageable with immune-suppressants [95]. Consequential trials with more enrollment number of patients are necessary to further evaluate the safety and efficacy of this promising double immune-checkpoints blockage therapy comparing with each of its mono-therapy regiments.

Finally, combinatorial clinical trials using ipilimumab with other immunotherapy agents have shown some favorable therapeutic benefits. For example, combination of ipilimumab with peginterferon α-2b (pegylated interferon α-2b) in patients with unresectable melanoma both demonstrated significant increase of response rate and OS comparing with the monotherapy arm [96, 97] in recent phase I trials.

3.2. Combined therapy inhibiting both immuno-checkpoint and MAPK signaling pathway

Checkpoint blockade immunotherapy and MAPK targeted chemotherapy have distinct clinical profiles. For example, targeted therapy has relative higher initial response rate (~60% for BRAFi) with rapid onset of effect, but its efficacy restrictively rely on the continuous treatment and the therapeutic response is usually not durable due to the quick development of acquired drug resistance. In contrast, immunotherapy has much a lower response rate (4.5% for ipilimumab), delayed onset of effect and difficulty in predicting patient outcome, but it has shown potentially durable responses and long-term survival benefit even off treatment. In addition, since the MAPK pathway is not required in the process of anti-tumor immune response, blocking MAPK signaling should not interfere with the efficacy of checkpoint blockade immunotherapy. Therefore, it seems very rational that the combination of a MAPKi and an immunotherapy agent such as ipilimumab or pembrolizumab can maximize the therapeutic benefits in advance melanoma.

Interestingly, BRAF and MEK inhibition displayed an "endogenous vaccine-like" effects in melanoma cells [98]. Cytotoxic agents like BRAFi induce tumor cell death and promote the uptake and presentation of tumor antigens to the effector immune cells (T cells and B cells) through antigen-presenting cells [54]. MEK inhibition, BRAF[V600E] RNA silencing or BRAF inhibition by PLX4720 increases the CD4+ and CD8+ lymphocytes mediated T-cell infiltration and reduce the level of immune-suppressants including IL-6, IL-10 or VEGF [99-101] in mice. The expression of PD-L1 is found to be elevated in BRAFi-resistant melanoma cells and it is mediated through the off-target activity of BRAFi in JUN and STAT3 signaling [102]. However, Vella *et al* has published a paper in 2014 and stated that they have not found any impact of dabrafenib treatment on T lymphocytes. trametinib alone or in combination with dabrafenib has suppressed T lymphocyte proliferation, cytokine secretion and antigen-specific expansion in their isolated T lymphocyte and monocyte-derived dendritic cells. These findings should be carefully tested *in vivo* to evaluate the clinical relevance [103].

As for the clinical practice, dose-limiting hepatotoxicity issues have led to the premature termination of the first phase I study on combination of ipilimumab with vemurafenib (ClinicalTrials.gov, NCT01400451). This signified the complexity of adverse effect in combined therapy of immune-regulating agents and kinase inhibitors. Another phase I study of ipilimumab plus dabrafenib, or ipilimumab plus the combination of dabrafenib with trametinib is still active and a phase II study is exploring the safety and efficacy of sequential administration of vemurafenib followed by ipilimumab (ClinicalTrials.gov, NCT01767454, NCT01673854). The data of these most recent trials will be released in the near future.

4. Conclusions

Extensive efforts and remarkable progresses have been made to discover and investigate rational approaches in combination melanoma therapy since the recent approval of MAPKi and immune checkpoints blockade antibodies. A number of new targeted or immune drugs for metastatic melanoma are currently under commercial development or late stage clinical trials, some of which will likely be approved in the next few years. Quality of life for many melanoma patients has been dramatically increased. However, significant challenges still remain. While some clinical evidence has really raised the expectation of survivals for patients with advanced melanoma, the benefits of combination therapy are usually accompanied by limitations. Comprehensive genetic profile and tailored patient matching is essential for targeted therapy, while biomarkers are critical to predict the patient immunotherapy response. Drug-related toxicity for combination treatment usually is not a simple one-plus-one situation, and potential drug-drug interactions, especially the combination of a targeted agent with an immunotherapeutic agent must be carefully evaluated in order to achieve both fast and durable responses. Adverse effects should be closely monitored and potential alternative dosing regiments is worth further exploration. Optimized dose schedule may help to delay the resistance development and reduce the frequency of adverse effect. For example, intermittent doses of BRAFi was able to enhance the tolerance in combination with immunotherapy, decrease the paradoxical MAPK activation, which might be the main cause of severe toxicity in clinical trial [104]. Solid evidence of synergistic combination in preclinical research must be established before clinical trial conduction. In fact, with the relatively large number of available targeted agents and immunotherapeutic agents for metastatic melanoma, the huge number of possible drug combinations coupled with dosing sequences or schedules already presents a significant challenge in designing proper clinical trials. To test all the possible drug combinations along with different dosing sequences clinically will not only have low benefits to patients, but is also a huge financial burden to the society. Carefully designed, predictive preclinical studies will be essential to provide critical supports for rational prioritization of clinical trials using drug combinations. Finally, clear understandings of various combination mechanisms and patient genetic profiles are critically important for the development of new combination approaches, prediction of expected therapy response and potential side effects.

With the rapid advances in this field, it is likely that optimal combination treatments will great improve the management of advanced melanoma in cancer patients.

Abbreviations

AMPK: 5' adenosine monophosphate-activated protein kinase

BRAF: B-Raf protein

BRAFi: BRAF inhibitor

CDK: Cyclin dependent kinase

CR: Complete response

CTLA-4: Cytotoxic T lymphocyte-associated antigen 4

ERK: Extracellular signal-regulated kinase

HR: Hazard ratio

JNK: c-Jun N-terminal kinase

MAPK: Mitogen-activated protein kinase

MEKi: MEK inhibitor

MHC: Membrane histocompatibility complex

mTOR: Mammalian target of rapamycin

ORR: Overall response rate

OS: Overall survival

PD-1: Programmed cell death 1

PD-L1: Programmed cell death 1 ligand 1

PDGFR: Platete-derived growth factor receptor

PFS: Progression-free survival

PI3K: Phosphoinositide 3-kinase

PKC: Protein kinase C

PR: Partial response

RTKs: Receptor tyrosine kinases

TCR: T cell receptor

VEGF: Vascular endothelial growth factor

VEGFR: Vascular endothelial growth factor receptor

Acknowledgements

This work was supported by NIH grants R01CA148706. The content is solely the responsibility of the authors and does not necessarily represent the official views of the National Institutes of Health. Jin Wang acknowledges the support of the Alma and Hal Reagan Fellowship.

Author details

Jin Wang, Duane D. Miller* and Wei Li

*Address all correspondence to: dmiller@uthsc.edu or wli@uthsc.edu

Department of Pharmaceutical Sciences, College of Pharmacy. The University of Tennessee Health Science Center, Memphis, TN, USA

References

[1] Hersh, E.M.; O'Day, S.J.; Powderly, J.; Khan, K.D.; Pavlick, A.C.; Cranmer, L.D.; Samlowski, W.E.; Nichol, G.M.; Yellin, M.J.; Weber, J.S., A phase II multicenter study of ipilimumab with or without dacarbazine in chemotherapy-naive patients with advanced melanoma. *Investigational new drugs*, 2011, 29, (3), 489-498.

[2] Sosman, J.A.; Kim, K.B.; Schuchter, L.; Gonzalez, R.; Pavlick, A.C.; Weber, J.S.; McArthur, G.A.; Hutson, T.E.; Moschos, S.J.; Flaherty, K.T.; Hersey, P.; Kefford, R.; Lawrence, D.; Puzanov, I.; Lewis, K.D.; Amaravadi, R.K.; Chmielowski, B.; Lawrence, H.J.; Shyr, Y.; Ye, F.; Li, J.; Nolop, K.B.; Lee, R.J.; Joe, A.K.; Ribas, A., Survival in BRAF V600-mutant advanced melanoma treated with vemurafenib. *The New England journal of medicine*, 2012, 366, (8), 707-714.

[3] Al-Lazikani, B.; Workman, P., Unpicking the combination lock for mutant BRAF and RAS melanomas. *Cancer discovery*, 2013, 3, (1), 14-19.

[4] Hu-Lieskovan, S.; Robert, L.; Homet Moreno, B.; Ribas, A., Combining Targeted Therapy With Immunotherapy in BRAF-Mutant Melanoma: Promise and Challenges. *Journal of clinical oncology : official journal of the American Society of Clinical Oncology*, 2014, 32, (21), 2248-2254.

[5] Nijenhuis, C.M.; Haanen, J.B.; Schellens, J.H.; Beijnen, J.H., Is combination therapy the next step to overcome resistance and reduce toxicities in melanoma? *Cancer treatment reviews*, 2013, *39*, (4), 305-312.

[6] Voskoboynik, M.; Arkenau, H.T., Combination therapies for the treatment of advanced melanoma: a review of current evidence. *Biochemistry research international*, 2014, *2014*, 307059.

[7] Wan, P.T.; Garnett, M.J.; Roe, S.M.; Lee, S.; Niculescu-Duvaz, D.; Good, V.M.; Jones, C.M.; Marshall, C.J.; Springer, C.J.; Barford, D.; Marais, R.; Cancer Genome, P., Mechanism of activation of the RAF-ERK signaling pathway by oncogenic mutations of B-RAF. *Cell*, 2004, *116*, (6), 855-867.

[8] Tsai, J.; Lee, J.T.; Wang, W.; Zhang, J.; Cho, H.; Mamo, S.; Bremer, R.; Gillette, S.; Kong, J.; Haass, N.K.; Sproesser, K.; Li, L.; Smalley, K.S.; Fong, D.; Zhu, Y.L.; Marimuthu, A.; Nguyen, H.; Lam, B.; Liu, J.; Cheung, I.; Rice, J.; Suzuki, Y.; Luu, C.; Settachatgul, C.; Shellooe, R.; Cantwell, J.; Kim, S.H.; Schlessinger, J.; Zhang, K.Y.; West, B.L.; Powell, B.; Habets, G.; Zhang, C.; Ibrahim, P.N.; Hirth, P.; Artis, D.R.; Herlyn, M.; Bollag, G., Discovery of a selective inhibitor of oncogenic B-Raf kinase with potent antimelanoma activity. *Proceedings of the National Academy of Sciences of the United States of America*, 2008, *105*, (8), 3041-3046.

[9] King, A.J.; Arnone, M.R.; Bleam, M.R.; Moss, K.G.; Yang, J.; Fedorowicz, K.E.; Smitheman, K.N.; Erhardt, J.A.; Hughes-Earle, A.; Kane-Carson, L.S.; Sinnamon, R.H.; Qi, H.; Rheault, T.R.; Uehling, D.E.; Laquerre, S.G., Dabrafenib; preclinical characterization, increased efficacy when combined with trametinib, while BRAF/MEK tool combination reduced skin lesions. *PloS one*, 2013, *8*, (7), e67583.

[10] Solit, D.B.; Rosen, N., Towards a unified model of RAF inhibitor resistance. *Cancer discovery*, 2014, *4*, (1), 27-30.

[11] Hooijkaas, A.; Gadiot, J.; Morrow, M.; Stewart, R.; Schumacher, T.; Blank, C.U., Selective BRAF inhibition decreases tumor-resident lymphocyte frequencies in a mouse model of human melanoma. *Oncoimmunology*, 2012, *1*, (5), 609-617.

[12] Menzies, A.M.; Long, G.V., Dabrafenib and trametinib, alone and in combination for BRAF-mutant metastatic melanoma. *Clinical cancer research : an official journal of the American Association for Cancer Research*, 2014, *20*, (8), 2035-2043.

[13] Carlino, M.S.; Gowrishankar, K.; Saunders, C.A.; Pupo, G.M.; Snoyman, S.; Zhang, X.D.; Saw, R.; Becker, T.M.; Kefford, R.F.; Long, G.V.; Rizos, H., Antiproliferative effects of continued mitogen-activated protein kinase pathway inhibition following acquired resistance to BRAF and/or MEK inhibition in melanoma. *Molecular cancer therapeutics*, 2013, *12*, (7), 1332-1342.

[14] Klein, O.; Clements, A.; Menzies, A.M.; O'Toole, S.; Kefford, R.F.; Long, G.V., BRAF inhibitor activity in V600R metastatic melanoma. *European journal of cancer*, 2013, *49*, (5), 1073-1079.

[15] Vin, H.; Ojeda, S.S.; Ching, G.; Leung, M.L.; Chitsazzadeh, V.; Dwyer, D.W.; Adelmann, C.H.; Restrepo, M.; Richards, K.N.; Stewart, L.R.; Du, L.; Ferguson, S.B.; Chakravarti, D.; Ehrenreiter, K.; Baccarini, M.; Ruggieri, R.; Curry, J.L.; Kim, K.B.; Ciurea, A.M.; Duvic, M.; Prieto, V.G.; Ullrich, S.E.; Dalby, K.N.; Flores, E.R.; Tsai, K.Y., BRAF inhibitors suppress apoptosis through off-target inhibition of JNK signaling. *eLife*, 2013, *2*, e00969.

[16] Roesch, A., Tumor heterogeneity and plasticity as elusive drivers for resistance to MAPK pathway inhibition in melanoma. *Oncogene*, 2014.

[17] Yancovitz, M.; Litterman, A.; Yoon, J.; Ng, E.; Shapiro, R.L.; Berman, R.S.; Pavlick, A.C.; Darvishian, F.; Christos, P.; Mazumdar, M.; Osman, I.; Polsky, D., Intra-and inter-tumor heterogeneity of BRAF(V600E))mutations in primary and metastatic melanoma. *PloS one*, 2012, *7*, (1), e29336.

[18] Little, A.S.; Smith, P.D.; Cook, S.J., Mechanisms of acquired resistance to ERK1/2 pathway inhibitors. *Oncogene*, 2013, *32*, (10), 1207-1215.

[19] Tentori, L.; Lacal, P.M.; Graziani, G., Challenging resistance mechanisms to therapies for metastatic melanoma. *Trends in pharmacological sciences*, 2013, *34*, (12), 656-666.

[20] Straussman, R.; Morikawa, T.; Shee, K.; Barzily-Rokni, M.; Qian, Z.R.; Du, J.; Davis, A.; Mongare, M.M.; Gould, J.; Frederick, D.T.; Cooper, Z.A.; Chapman, P.B.; Solit, D.B.; Ribas, A.; Lo, R.S.; Flaherty, K.T.; Ogino, S.; Wargo, J.A.; Golub, T.R., Tumour micro-environment elicits innate resistance to RAF inhibitors through HGF secretion. *Nature*, 2012, *487*, (7408), 500-504.

[21] Johannessen, C.M.; Boehm, J.S.; Kim, S.Y.; Thomas, S.R.; Wardwell, L.; Johnson, L.A.; Emery, C.M.; Stransky, N.; Cogdill, A.P.; Barretina, J.; Caponigro, G.; Hieronymus, H.; Murray, R.R.; Salehi-Ashtiani, K.; Hill, D.E.; Vidal, M.; Zhao, J.J.; Yang, X.; Alkan, O.; Kim, S.; Harris, J.L.; Wilson, C.J.; Myer, V.E.; Finan, P.M.; Root, D.E.; Roberts, T.M.; Golub, T.; Flaherty, K.T.; Dummer, R.; Weber, B.L.; Sellers, W.R.; Schlegel, R.; Wargo, J.A.; Hahn, W.C.; Garraway, L.A., COT drives resistance to RAF inhibition through MAP kinase pathway reactivation. *Nature*, 2010, *468*, (7326), 968-972.

[22] Wagle, N.; Emery, C.; Berger, M.F.; Davis, M.J.; Sawyer, A.; Pochanard, P.; Kehoe, S.M.; Johannessen, C.M.; Macconaill, L.E.; Hahn, W.C.; Meyerson, M.; Garraway, L.A., Dissecting therapeutic resistance to RAF inhibition in melanoma by tumor genomic profiling. *Journal of clinical oncology : official journal of the American Society of Clinical Oncology*, 2011, *29*, (22), 3085-3096.

[23] Poulikakos, P.I.; Zhang, C.; Bollag, G.; Shokat, K.M.; Rosen, N., RAF inhibitors transactivate RAF dimers and ERK signalling in cells with wild-type BRAF. *Nature*, 2010, *464*, (7287), 427-430.

[24] Gowrishankar, K.; Snoyman, S.; Pupo, G.M.; Becker, T.M.; Kefford, R.F.; Rizos, H., Acquired resistance to BRAF inhibition can confer cross-resistance to combined

BRAF/MEK inhibition. *The Journal of investigative dermatology*, 2012, *132*, (7), 1850-1859.

[25] Carlino, M.S.; Todd, J.R.; Gowrishankar, K.; Mijatov, B.; Pupo, G.M.; Fung, C.; Snoyman, S.; Hersey, P.; Long, G.V.; Kefford, R.F.; Rizos, H., Differential activity of MEK and ERK inhibitors in BRAF inhibitor resistant melanoma. *Molecular oncology*, 2014, *8*, (3), 544-554.

[26] Sanchez-Laorden, B.; Viros, A.; Girotti, M.R.; Pedersen, M.; Saturno, G.; Zambon, A.; Niculescu-Duvaz, D.; Turajlic, S.; Hayes, A.; Gore, M.; Larkin, J.; Lorigan, P.; Cook, M.; Springer, C.; Marais, R., BRAF inhibitors induce metastasis in RAS mutant or inhibitor-resistant melanoma cells by reactivating MEK and ERK signaling. *Science signaling*, 2014, *7*, (318), ra30.

[27] Su, F.; Bradley, W.D.; Wang, Q.; Yang, H.; Xu, L.; Higgins, B.; Kolinsky, K.; Packman, K.; Kim, M.J.; Trunzer, K.; Lee, R.J.; Schostack, K.; Carter, J.; Albert, T.; Germer, S.; Rosinski, J.; Martin, M.; Simcox, M.E.; Lestini, B.; Heimbrook, D.; Bollag, G., Resistance to selective BRAF inhibition can be mediated by modest upstream pathway activation. *Cancer research*, 2012, *72*, (4), 969-978.

[28] Nathanson, K.L.; Martin, A.M.; Wubbenhorst, B.; Greshock, J.; Letrero, R.; D'Andrea, K.; O'Day, S.; Infante, J.R.; Falchook, G.S.; Arkenau, H.T.; Millward, M.; Brown, M.P.; Pavlick, A.; Davies, M.A.; Ma, B.; Gagnon, R.; Curtis, M.; Lebowitz, P.F.; Kefford, R.; Long, G.V., Tumor genetic analyses of patients with metastatic melanoma treated with the BRAF inhibitor dabrafenib (GSK2118436). *Clinical cancer research : an official journal of the American Association for Cancer Research*, 2013, *19*, (17), 4868-4878.

[29] Smalley, K.S.; Lioni, M.; Dalla Palma, M.; Xiao, M.; Desai, B.; Egyhazi, S.; Hansson, J.; Wu, H.; King, A.J.; Van Belle, P.; Elder, D.E.; Flaherty, K.T.; Herlyn, M.; Nathanson, K.L., Increased cyclin D1 expression can mediate BRAF inhibitor resistance in BRAF V600E-mutated melanomas. *Molecular cancer therapeutics*, 2008, *7*, (9), 2876-2883.

[30] Choi, J.; Landrette, S.F.; Wang, T.; Evans, P.; Bacchiocchi, A.; Bjornson, R.; Cheng, E.; Stiegler, A.L.; Gathiaka, S.; Acevedo, O.; Boggon, T.J.; Krauthammer, M.; Halaban, R.; Xu, T., Identification of PLX4032-resistance mechanisms and implications for novel RAF inhibitors. *Pigment cell & melanoma research*, 2014, *27*, (2), 253-262.

[31] Wu, C.P.; Sim, H.M.; Huang, Y.H.; Liu, Y.C.; Hsiao, S.H.; Cheng, H.W.; Li, Y.Q.; Ambudkar, S.V.; Hsu, S.C., Overexpression of ATP-binding cassette transporter ABCG2 as a potential mechanism of acquired resistance to vemurafenib in BRAF(V600E) mutant cancer cells. *Biochemical pharmacology*, 2013, *85*, (3), 325-334.

[32] Flaherty, K.T.; Robert, C.; Hersey, P.; Nathan, P.; Garbe, C.; Milhem, M.; Demidov, L.V.; Hassel, J.C.; Rutkowski, P.; Mohr, P.; Dummer, R.; Trefzer, U.; Larkin, J.M.; Utikal, J.; Dreno, B.; Nyakas, M.; Middleton, M.R.; Becker, J.C.; Casey, M.; Sherman, L.J.; Wu, F.S.; Ouellet, D.; Martin, A.M.; Patel, K.; Schadendorf, D.; Group, M.S., Im-

proved survival with MEK inhibition in BRAF-mutated melanoma. *The New England journal of medicine,* 2012, *367,* (2), 107-114.

[33] Wright, C.J.; McCormack, P.L., Trametinib: first global approval. *Drugs,* 2013, *73,* (11), 1245-1254.

[34] Atefi, M.; von Euw, E.; Attar, N.; Ng, C.; Chu, C.; Guo, D.; Nazarian, R.; Chmielowski, B.; Glaspy, J.A.; Comin-Anduix, B.; Mischel, P.S.; Lo, R.S.; Ribas, A., Reversing melanoma cross-resistance to BRAF and MEK inhibitors by co-targeting the AKT/mTOR pathway. *PloS one,* 2011, *6,* (12), e28973.

[35] Kim, K.B.; Kefford, R.; Pavlick, A.C.; Infante, J.R.; Ribas, A.; Sosman, J.A.; Fecher, L.A.; Millward, M.; McArthur, G.A.; Hwu, P.; Gonzalez, R.; Ott, P.A.; Long, G.V.; Gardner, O.S.; Ouellet, D.; Xu, Y.; DeMarini, D.J.; Le, N.T.; Patel, K.; Lewis, K.D., Phase II study of the MEK1/MEK2 inhibitor Trametinib in patients with metastatic BRAF-mutant cutaneous melanoma previously treated with or without a BRAF inhibitor. *Journal of clinical oncology : official journal of the American Society of Clinical Oncology,* 2013, *31,* (4), 482-489.

[36] Flaherty, K.T.; Infante, J.R.; Daud, A.; Gonzalez, R.; Kefford, R.F.; Sosman, J.; Hamid, O.; Schuchter, L.; Cebon, J.; Ibrahim, N.; Kudchadkar, R.; Burris, H.A., 3rd; Falchook, G.; Algazi, A.; Lewis, K.; Long, G.V.; Puzanov, I.; Lebowitz, P.; Singh, A.; Little, S.; Sun, P.; Allred, A.; Ouellet, D.; Kim, K.B.; Patel, K.; Weber, J., Combined BRAF and MEK inhibition in melanoma with BRAF V600 mutations. *The New England journal of medicine,* 2012, *367,* (18), 1694-1703.

[37] Goldinger, S.M.; Zimmer, L.; Schulz, C.; Ugurel, S.; Hoeller, C.; Kaehler, K.C.; Schadendorf, D.; Hassel, J.C.; Becker, J.; Hauschild, A.; Dummer, R.; Dermatology Cooperative Oncology, G., Upstream mitogen-activated protein kinase (MAPK) pathway inhibition: MEK inhibitor followed by a BRAF inhibitor in advanced melanoma patients. *European journal of cancer,* 2014, *50,* (2), 406-410.

[38] Greger, J.G.; Eastman, S.D.; Zhang, V.; Bleam, M.R.; Hughes, A.M.; Smitheman, K.N.; Dickerson, S.H.; Laquerre, S.G.; Liu, L.; Gilmer, T.M., Combinations of BRAF, MEK, and PI3K/mTOR inhibitors overcome acquired resistance to the BRAF inhibitor GSK2118436 dabrafenib, mediated by NRAS or MEK mutations. *Molecular cancer therapeutics,* 2012, *11,* (4), 909-920.

[39] Nakamura, A.; Arita, T.; Tsuchiya, S.; Donelan, J.; Chouitar, J.; Carideo, E.; Galvin, K.; Okaniwa, M.; Ishikawa, T.; Yoshida, S., Antitumor activity of the selective pan-RAF inhibitor TAK-632 in BRAF inhibitor-resistant melanoma. *Cancer research,* 2013, *73,* (23), 7043-7055.

[40] Lee, C.I.; Menzies, A.M.; Haydu, L.E.; Azer, M.; Clements, A.; Kefford, R.F.; Long, G.V., Features and management of pyrexia with combined dabrafenib and trametinib in metastatic melanoma. *Melanoma research,* 2014.

[41] Ribas, A.; Gonzalez, R.; Pavlick, A.; Hamid, O.; Gajewski, T.F.; Daud, A.; Flaherty, L.; Logan, T.; Chmielowski, B.; Lewis, K.; Kee, D.; Boasberg, P.; Yin, M.; Chan, I.; Musib,

L.; Choong, N.; Puzanov, I.; McArthur, G.A., Combination of vemurafenib and cobimetinib in patients with advanced BRAF(V600)-mutated melanoma: a phase 1b study. *The lancet oncology*, 2014, *15*, (9), 954-965.

[42] Kefford, R.; Miller, W.H.; Tan, D.S.W.; Sullivan, R.J.; Long, G.; Dienstmann, R.; Tai, W.M.D.; Flaherty, K.; Stutvoet, S.; Schumacher, K.M.; Wandel, S.; De Parseval, L.A.; Tabernero, J., Preliminary results from a phase Ib/II, open-label, dose-escalation study of the oral BRAF inhibitor LGX818 in combination with the oral MEK1/2 inhibitor MEK162 in BRAF V600-dependent advanced solid tumors. *Journal of Clinical Oncology*, 2013, 31, (15_supplement), abstract 9029.

[43] Dummer, R.; Robert, C.; Nyakas, M.; McArthur, G.A.; Kudchadkar, R.R.; Gomez-Roca, C.; Sullivan, R.J.; Flaherty, K.; Murer, C.; Michel, D.; Tang, Z.W.; De Parseval, L.A.; Delord, J.P., Initial results from a phase I, open-label, dose escalation study of the oral BRAF inhibitor LGX818 in patients with BRAF V600 mutant advanced or metastatic melanoma. *Journal of Clinical Oncology*, 2013, *31*, (15).

[44] Carracedo, A.; Pandolfi, P.P., The PTEN-PI3K pathway: of feedbacks and cross-talks. *Oncogene*, 2008, *27*, (41), 5527-5541.

[45] Villanueva, J.; Vultur, A.; Lee, J.T.; Somasundaram, R.; Fukunaga-Kalabis, M.; Cipolla, A.K.; Wubbenhorst, B.; Xu, X.; Gimotty, P.A.; Kee, D.; Santiago-Walker, A.E.; Letrero, R.; D'Andrea, K.; Pushparajan, A.; Hayden, J.E.; Brown, K.D.; Laquerre, S.; McArthur, G.A.; Sosman, J.A.; Nathanson, K.L.; Herlyn, M., Acquired resistance to BRAF inhibitors mediated by a RAF kinase switch in melanoma can be overcome by cotargeting MEK and IGF-1R/PI3K. *Cancer cell*, 2010, *18*, (6), 683-695.

[46] Lasithiotakis, K.G.; Sinnberg, T.W.; Schittek, B.; Flaherty, K.T.; Kulms, D.; Maczey, E.; Garbe, C.; Meier, F.E., Combined inhibition of MAPK and mTOR signaling inhibits growth, induces cell death, and abrogates invasive growth of melanoma cells. *The Journal of investigative dermatology*, 2008, *128*, (8), 2013-2023.

[47] Niessner, H.; Beck, D.; Sinnberg, T.; Lasithiotakis, K.; Maczey, E.; Gogel, J.; Venturelli, S.; Berger, A.; Mauthe, M.; Toulany, M.; Flaherty, K.; Schaller, M.; Schadendorf, D.; Proikas-Cezanne, T.; Schittek, B.; Garbe, C.; Kulms, D.; Meier, F., The farnesyl transferase inhibitor lonafarnib inhibits mTOR signaling and enforces sorafenib-induced apoptosis in melanoma cells. *The Journal of investigative dermatology*, 2011, *131*, (2), 468-479.

[48] Khalili, J.S.; Yu, X.; Wang, J.; Hayes, B.C.; Davies, M.A.; Lizee, G.; Esmaeli, B.; Woodman, S.E., Combination small molecule MEK and PI3K inhibition enhances uveal melanoma cell death in a mutant GNAQ-and GNA11-dependent manner. *Clinical cancer research : an official journal of the American Association for Cancer Research*, 2012, *18*, (16), 4345-4355.

[49] Lassen, A.; Atefi, M.; Robert, L.; Wong, D.J.; Cerniglia, M.; Comin-Anduix, B.; Ribas, A., Effects of AKT inhibitor therapy in response and resistance to BRAF inhibition in melanoma. *Molecular cancer*, 2014, *13*, 83.

[50] Byron, S.A.; Loch, D.C.; Wellens, C.L.; Wortmann, A.; Wu, J.; Wang, J.; Nomoto, K.; Pollock, P.M., Sensitivity to the MEK inhibitor E6201 in melanoma cells is associated with mutant BRAF and wildtype PTEN status. *Molecular cancer*, 2012, *11*, 75.

[51] Posch, C.; Moslehi, H.; Feeney, L.; Green, G.A.; Ebaee, A.; Feichtenschlager, V.; Chong, K.; Peng, L.; Dimon, M.T.; Phillips, T.; Daud, A.I.; McCalmont, T.H.; LeBoit, P.E.; Ortiz-Urda, S., Combined targeting of MEK and PI3K/mTOR effector pathways is necessary to effectively inhibit NRAS mutant melanoma in vitro and in vivo. *Proceedings of the National Academy of Sciences of the United States of America*, 2013, *110*, (10), 4015-4020.

[52] Shi, H.; Kong, X.; Ribas, A.; Lo, R.S., Combinatorial treatments that overcome PDGFRbeta-driven resistance of melanoma cells to V600EB-RAF inhibition. *Cancer research*, 2011, *71*, (15), 5067-5074.

[53] Shimizu, T.; Tolcher, A.W.; Papadopoulos, K.P.; Beeram, M.; Rasco, D.W.; Smith, L.S.; Gunn, S.; Smetzer, L.; Mays, T.A.; Kaiser, B.; Wick, M.J.; Alvarez, C.; Cavazos, A.; Mangold, G.L.; Patnaik, A., The clinical effect of the dual-targeting strategy involving PI3K/AKT/mTOR and RAS/MEK/ERK pathways in patients with advanced cancer. *Clinical cancer research : an official journal of the American Association for Cancer Research*, 2012, *18*, (8), 2316-2325.

[54] Frederick, D.T.; Piris, A.; Cogdill, A.P.; Cooper, Z.A.; Lezcano, C.; Ferrone, C.R.; Mitra, D.; Boni, A.; Newton, L.P.; Liu, C.W.; Peng, W.Y.; Sullivan, R.J.; Lawrence, D.P.; Hodi, F.S.; Overwijk, W.W.; Lizee, G.; Murphy, G.F.; Hwu, P.; Flaherty, K.T.; Fisher, D.E.; Wargo, J.A., BRAF Inhibition Is Associated with Enhanced Melanoma Antigen Expression and a More Favorable Tumor Microenvironment in Patients with Metastatic Melanoma. *Clinical Cancer Research*, 2013, *19*, (5), 1225-1231.

[55] Lev, D.C.; Ruiz, M.; Mills, L.; McGary, E.C.; Price, J.E.; Bar-Eli, M., Dacarbazine causes transcriptional up-regulation of interleukin 8 and vascular endothelial growth factor in melanoma cells: a possible escape mechanism from chemotherapy. *Molecular cancer therapeutics*, 2003, *2*, (8), 753-763.

[56] Ghosh, S.; Maity, P., Augmented antitumor effects of combination therapy with VEGF antibody and cisplatin on murine B16F10 melanoma cells. *International immunopharmacology*, 2007, *7*, (13), 1598-1608.

[57] Sini, P.; Samarzija, I.; Baffert, F.; Littlewood-Evans, A.; Schnell, C.; Theuer, A.; Christian, S.; Boos, A.; Hess-Stumpp, H.; Foekens, J.A.; Setyono-Han, B.; Wood, J.; Hynes, N.E., Inhibition of multiple vascular endothelial growth factor receptors (VEGFR) blocks lymph node metastases but inhibition of VEGFR-2 is sufficient to sensitize tu-

mor cells to platinum-based chemotherapeutics. *Cancer research,* 2008, *68*, (5), 1581-1592.

[58] Terheyden, P.; Hofmann, M.A.; Weininger, M.; Brocker, E.B.; Becker, J.C., Anti-vascular endothelial growth factor antibody bevacizumab in conjunction with chemotherapy in metastasising melanoma. *Journal of cancer research and clinical oncology,* 2007, *133*, (11), 897-901.

[59] Sun, C.; Wang, L.; Huang, S.; Heynen, G.J.; Prahallad, A.; Robert, C.; Haanen, J.; Blank, C.; Wesseling, J.; Willems, S.M.; Zecchin, D.; Hobor, S.; Bajpe, P.K.; Lieftink, C.; Mateus, C.; Vagner, S.; Grernrum, W.; Hofland, I.; Schlicker, A.; Wessels, L.F.; Beijersbergen, R.L.; Bardelli, A.; Di Nicolantonio, F.; Eggermont, A.M.; Bernards, R., Reversible and adaptive resistance to BRAF(V600E) inhibition in melanoma. *Nature,* 2014, *508*, (7494), 118-122.

[60] Motl, S., Bevacizumab in combination chemotherapy for colorectal and other cancers. *American journal of health-system pharmacy : AJHP : official journal of the American Society of Health-System Pharmacists,* 2005, *62*, (10), 1021-1032.

[61] Del Vecchio, M.; Mortarini, R.; Canova, S.; Di Guardo, L.; Pimpinelli, N.; Sertoli, M.R.; Bedognetti, D.; Queirolo, P.; Morosini, P.; Perrone, T.; Bajetta, E.; Anichini, A., Bevacizumab plus fotemustine as first-line treatment in metastatic melanoma patients: clinical activity and modulation of angiogenesis and lymphangiogenesis factors. *Clinical cancer research : an official journal of the American Association for Cancer Research,* 2010, *16*, (23), 5862-5872.

[62] Kottschade, L.A.; Suman, V.J.; Perez, D.G.; McWilliams, R.R.; Kaur, J.S.; Amatruda, T.T., 3rd; Geoffroy, F.J.; Gross, H.M.; Cohen, P.A.; Jaslowski, A.J.; Kosel, M.L.; Markovic, S.N., A randomized phase 2 study of temozolomide and bevacizumab or nab-paclitaxel, carboplatin, and bevacizumab in patients with unresectable stage IV melanoma : a North Central Cancer Treatment Group study, N0775. *Cancer,* 2013, *119*, (3), 586-592.

[63] Li, B.; Lalani, A.S.; Harding, T.C.; Luan, B.; Koprivnikar, K.; Huan Tu, G.; Prell, R.; VanRoey, M.J.; Simmons, A.D.; Jooss, K., Vascular endothelial growth factor blockade reduces intratumoral regulatory T cells and enhances the efficacy of a GM-CSF-secreting cancer immunotherapy. *Clinical cancer research : an official journal of the American Association for Cancer Research,* 2006, *12*, (22), 6808-6816.

[64] Mita, M.M.; Rowinsky, E.K.; Forero, L.; Eckhart, S.G.; Izbicka, E.; Weiss, G.R.; Beeram, M.; Mita, A.C.; de Bono, J.S.; Tolcher, A.W.; Hammond, L.A.; Simmons, P.; Berg, K.; Takimoto, C.; Patnaik, A., A phase II, pharmacokinetic, and biologic study of semaxanib and thalidomide in patients with metastatic melanoma. *Cancer chemotherapy and pharmacology,* 2007, *59*, (2), 165-174.

[65] Hasumi, Y.; Klosowska-Wardega, A.; Furuhashi, M.; Ostman, A.; Heldin, C.H.; Hellberg, C., Identification of a subset of pericytes that respond to combination therapy

targeting PDGF and VEGF signaling. *International journal of cancer. Journal international du cancer*, 2007, *121*, (12), 2606-2614.

[66] O'Reilly, T.; Lane, H.A.; Wood, J.M.; Schnell, C.; Littlewood-Evans, A.; Brueggen, J.; McSheehy, P.M., Everolimus and PTK/ZK show synergistic growth inhibition in the orthotopic BL16/BL6 murine melanoma model. *Cancer chemotherapy and pharmacology*, 2011, *67*, (1), 193-200.

[67] Hainsworth, J.D.; Infante, J.R.; Spigel, D.R.; Peyton, J.D.; Thompson, D.S.; Lane, C.M.; Clark, B.L.; Rubin, M.S.; Trent, D.F.; Burris, H.A., 3rd, Bevacizumab and everolimus in the treatment of patients with metastatic melanoma: a phase 2 trial of the Sarah Cannon Oncology Research Consortium. *Cancer*, 2010, *116*, (17), 4122-4129.

[68] Mahalingam, D.; Malik, L.; Beeram, M.; Rodon, J.; Sankhala, K.; Mita, A.; Benjamin, D.; Ketchum, N.; Michalek, J.; Tolcher, A.; Wright, J.; Sarantopoulos, J., Phase II study evaluating the efficacy, safety, and pharmacodynamic correlative study of dual anti-angiogenic inhibition using bevacizumab in combination with sorafenib in patients with advanced malignant melanoma. *Cancer chemotherapy and pharmacology*, 2014, *74*, (1), 77-84.

[69] Mittal, K.; Koon, H.; Elson, P.; Triozzi, P.; Dowlati, A.; Chen, H.; Borden, E.C.; Rini, B.I., Dual VEGF/VEGFR inhibition in advanced solid malignancies: Clinical effects and pharmacodynamic biomarkers. *Cancer biology & therapy*, 2014, *15*, (8), 975-981.

[70] Mirmohammadsadegh, A.; Mota, R.; Gustrau, A.; Hassan, M.; Nambiar, S.; Marini, A.; Bojar, H.; Tannapfel, A.; Hengge, U.R., ERK1/2 is highly phosphorylated in melanoma metastases and protects melanoma cells from cisplatin-mediated apoptosis. *The Journal of investigative dermatology*, 2007, *127*, (9), 2207-2215.

[71] Ivanov, V.N.; Hei, T.K., Combined treatment with EGFR inhibitors and arsenite up-regulated apoptosis in human EGFR-positive melanomas: a role of suppression of the PI3K-AKT pathway. *Oncogene*, 2005, *24*, (4), 616-626.

[72] Sinnberg, T.; Lasithiotakis, K.; Niessner, H.; Schittek, B.; Flaherty, K.T.; Kulms, D.; Maczey, E.; Campos, M.; Gogel, J.; Garbe, C.; Meier, F., Inhibition of PI3K-AKT-mTOR signaling sensitizes melanoma cells to cisplatin and temozolomide. *The Journal of investigative dermatology*, 2009, *129*, (6), 1500-1515.

[73] Keuling, A.M.; Andrew, S.E.; Tron, V.A., Inhibition of p38 MAPK enhances ABT-737-induced cell death in melanoma cell lines: novel regulation of PUMA. *Pigment cell & melanoma research*, 2010, *23*, (3), 430-440.

[74] Frederick, D.T.; Salas Fragomeni, R.A.; Schalck, A.; Ferreiro-Neira, I.; Hoff, T.; Cooper, Z.A.; Haq, R.; Panka, D.J.; Kwong, L.N.; Davies, M.A.; Cusack, J.C.; Flaherty, K.T.; Fisher, D.E.; Mier, J.W.; Wargo, J.A.; Sullivan, R.J., Clinical profiling of BCL-2 family members in the setting of BRAF inhibition offers a rationale for targeting de novo resistance using BH3 mimetics. *PloS one*, 2014, *9*, (7), e101286.

[75] Ji, Z.; Kumar, R.; Taylor, M.; Rajadurai, A.; Marzuka-Alcala, A.; Chen, Y.E.; Njauw, C.N.; Flaherty, K.; Jonsson, G.; Tsao, H., Vemurafenib synergizes with nutlin-3 to deplete survivin and suppresses melanoma viability and tumor growth. *Clinical cancer research : an official journal of the American Association for Cancer Research*, 2013, *19*, (16), 4383-4391.

[76] Vultur, A.; Villanueva, J.; Krepler, C.; Rajan, G.; Chen, Q.; Xiao, M.; Li, L.; Gimotty, P.A.; Wilson, M.; Hayden, J.; Keeney, F.; Nathanson, K.L.; Herlyn, M., MEK inhibition affects STAT3 signaling and invasion in human melanoma cell lines. *Oncogene*, 2014, *33*, (14), 1850-1861.

[77] Martin, M.J.; Hayward, R.; Viros, A.; Marais, R., Metformin accelerates the growth of BRAF V600E-driven melanoma by upregulating VEGF-A. *Cancer discovery*, 2012, *2*, (4), 344-355.

[78] Woodard, J.; Platanias, L.C., AMP-activated kinase (AMPK)-generated signals in malignant melanoma cell growth and survival. *Biochemical and biophysical research communications*, 2010, *398*, (1), 135-139.

[79] Niehr, F.; von Euw, E.; Attar, N.; Guo, D.; Matsunaga, D.; Sazegar, H.; Ng, C.; Glaspy, J.A.; Recio, J.A.; Lo, R.S.; Mischel, P.S.; Comin-Anduix, B.; Ribas, A., Combination therapy with vemurafenib (PLX4032/RG7204) and metformin in melanoma cell lines with distinct driver mutations. *Journal of translational medicine*, 2011, *9*, 76.

[80] Sagoo, M.S.; Harbour, J.W.; Stebbing, J.; Bowcock, A.M., Combined PKC and MEK inhibition for treating metastatic uveal melanoma. *Oncogene*, 2014.

[81] Wu, X.; Zhu, M.; Fletcher, J.A.; Giobbie-Hurder, A.; Hodi, F.S., The protein kinase C inhibitor enzastaurin exhibits antitumor activity against uveal melanoma. *PloS one*, 2012, *7*, (1), e29622.

[82] Chen, X.; Wu, Q.; Tan, L.; Porter, D.; Jager, M.J.; Emery, C.; Bastian, B.C., Combined PKC and MEK inhibition in uveal melanoma with GNAQ and GNA11 mutations. *Oncogene*, 2013.

[83] Wang, J.; Chen, J.; Miller, D.D.; Li, W., Synergistic combination of novel tubulin inhibitor ABI-274 and vemurafenib overcome vemurafenib acquired resistance in BRAFV600E melanoma. *Molecular cancer therapeutics*, 2014, *13*, (1), 16-26.

[84] Acquaviva, J.; Smith, D.L.; Jimenez, J.P.; Zhang, C.; Sequeira, M.; He, S.; Sang, J.; Bates, R.C.; Proia, D.A., Overcoming acquired BRAF inhibitor resistance in melanoma via targeted inhibition of Hsp90 with ganetespib. *Molecular cancer therapeutics*, 2014, *13*, (2), 353-363.

[85] Yadav, V.; Burke, T.F.; Huber, L.; Van Horn, R.D.; Zhang, Y.; Buchanan, S.G.; Chan, E.M.; Starling, J.J.; Beckmann, R.P.; Peng, S.B., The CDK4/6 Inhibitor LY2835219 Overcomes Vemurafenib Resistance Resulting from MAPK Reactivation and Cyclin D1 Upregulation. *Molecular cancer therapeutics*, 2014.

[86] Hodi, F.S.; O'Day, S.J.; McDermott, D.F.; Weber, R.W.; Sosman, J.A.; Haanen, J.B.; Gonzalez, R.; Robert, C.; Schadendorf, D.; Hassel, J.C.; Akerley, W.; van den Eert-wegh, A.J.; Lutzky, J.; Lorigan, P.; Vaubel, J.M.; Linette, G.P.; Hogg, D.; Ottensmeier, C.H.; Lebbe, C.; Peschel, C.; Quirt, I.; Clark, J.I.; Wolchok, J.D.; Weber, J.S.; Tian, J.; Yellin, M.J.; Nichol, G.M.; Hoos, A.; Urba, W.J., Improved survival with ipilimumab in patients with metastatic melanoma. *The New England journal of medicine,* 2010, *363,* (8), 711-723.

[87] Srivastava, N.; McDermott, D., Update on benefit of immunotherapy and targeted therapy in melanoma: the changing landscape. *Cancer management and research,* 2014, *6,* 279-289.

[88] Riley, J.L., Combination checkpoint blockade--taking melanoma immunotherapy to the next level. *The New England journal of medicine,* 2013, *369,* (2), 187-189.

[89] Maio, M.; Di Giacomo, A.M.; Robert, C.; Eggermont, A.M., Update on the role of ipi-limumab in melanoma and first data on new combination therapies. *Current opinion in oncology,* 2013, *25,* (2), 166-172.

[90] Topalian, S.L.; Hodi, F.S.; Brahmer, J.R.; Gettinger, S.N.; Smith, D.C.; McDermott, D.F.; Powderly, J.D.; Carvajal, R.D.; Sosman, J.A.; Atkins, M.B.; Leming, P.D.; Spigel, D.R.; Antonia, S.J.; Horn, L.; Drake, C.G.; Pardoll, D.M.; Chen, L.; Sharfman, W.H.; Anders, R.A.; Taube, J.M.; McMiller, T.L.; Xu, H.; Korman, A.J.; Jure-Kunkel, M.; Agrawal, S.; McDonald, D.; Kollia, G.D.; Gupta, A.; Wigginton, J.M.; Sznol, M., Safe-ty, activity, and immune correlates of anti-PD-1 antibody in cancer. *The New England journal of medicine,* 2012, *366,* (26), 2443-2454.

[91] Shah, D.J.; Dronca, R.S., Latest advances in chemotherapeutic, targeted, and immune approaches in the treatment of metastatic melanoma. *Mayo Clinic proceedings,* 2014, *89,* (4), 504-519.

[92] Perez-Gracia, J.L.; Labiano, S.; Rodriguez-Ruiz, M.E.; Sanmamed, M.F.; Melero, I., Orchestrating immune check-point blockade for cancer immunotherapy in combina-tions. *Current opinion in immunology,* 2014, *27,* 89-97.

[93] Brahmer, J.R.; Tykodi, S.S.; Chow, L.Q.; Hwu, W.J.; Topalian, S.L.; Hwu, P.; Drake, C.G.; Camacho, L.H.; Kauh, J.; Odunsi, K.; Pitot, H.C.; Hamid, O.; Bhatia, S.; Martins, R.; Eaton, K.; Chen, S.; Salay, T.M.; Alaparthy, S.; Grosso, J.F.; Korman, A.J.; Parker, S.M.; Agrawal, S.; Goldberg, S.M.; Pardoll, D.M.; Gupta, A.; Wigginton, J.M., Safety and activity of anti-PD-L1 antibody in patients with advanced cancer. *The New Eng-land journal of medicine,* 2012, *366,* (26), 2455-2465.

[94] Curran, M.A.; Montalvo, W.; Yagita, H.; Allison, J.P., PD-1 and CTLA-4 combination blockade expands infiltrating T cells and reduces regulatory T and myeloid cells within B16 melanoma tumors. *Proceedings of the National Academy of Sciences of the United States of America,* 2010, *107,* (9), 4275-4280.

[95] Wolchok, J.D.; Kluger, H.; Callahan, M.K.; Postow, M.A.; Rizvi, N.A.; Lesokhin, A.M.; Segal, N.H.; Ariyan, C.E.; Gordon, R.A.; Reed, K.; Burke, M.M.; Caldwell, A.;

Kronenberg, S.A.; Agunwamba, B.U.; Zhang, X.; Lowy, I.; Inzunza, H.D.; Feely, W.; Horak, C.E.; Hong, Q.; Korman, A.J.; Wigginton, J.M.; Gupta, A.; Sznol, M., Nivolumab plus ipilimumab in advanced melanoma. *The New England journal of medicine,* 2013, *369,* (2), 122-133.

[96] Kudchadkar, R.R.; Gibney, G.T.; Weber, J.; Chen, A.; Smith, K.; Merek, S., A phase IB study of ipilimumab with peginterferon alfa-2b in patients with unresectable melanoma. *Journal of Clinical Oncology,* 2013, *31,* (15).

[97] Hodi, F.S.; Lee, S.J.; McDermott, D.F.; Rao, U.N.M.; Butterfield, L.H.; Tarhini, A.A.; Leming, P.D.; Puzanov, I.; Kirkwood, J.M.; Grp, E.C.O., Multicenter, randomized phase II trial of GM-CSF (GM) plus ipilimumab (Ipi) versus ipi alone in metastatic melanoma: E1608. *Journal of Clinical Oncology,* 2013, *31,* (15).

[98] Kwong, M.L.; Neyns, B.; Yang, J.C., Adoptive T-cell transfer therapy and oncogene-targeted therapy for melanoma: the search for synergy. *Clinical cancer research : an official journal of the American Association for Cancer Research,* 2013, *19,* (19), 5292-5299.

[99] Wilmott, J.S.; Long, G.V.; Howle, J.R.; Haydu, L.E.; Sharma, R.N.; Thompson, J.F.; Kefford, R.F.; Hersey, P.; Scolyer, R.A., Selective BRAF Inhibitors Induce Marked T-cell Infiltration into Human Metastatic Melanoma. *Clinical Cancer Research,* 2012, *18,* (5), 1386-1394.

[100] Donia, M.; Fagone, P.; Nicoletti, F.; Andersen, R.S.; Hogdall, E.; Straten, P.T.; Andersen, M.H.; Svane, I.M., BRAF inhibition improves tumor recognition by the immune system: Potential implications for combinatorial therapies against melanoma involving adoptive T-cell transfer. *Oncoimmunology,* 2012, *1,* (9), 1476-1483.

[101] Liu, C.; Peng, W.; Xu, C.; Lou, Y.; Zhang, M.; Wargo, J.A.; Chen, J.Q.; Li, H.S.; Watowich, S.S.; Yang, Y.; Tompers Frederick, D.; Cooper, Z.A.; Mbofung, R.M.; Whittington, M.; Flaherty, K.T.; Woodman, S.E.; Davies, M.A.; Radvanyi, L.G.; Overwijk, W.W.; Lizee, G.; Hwu, P., BRAF inhibition increases tumor infiltration by T cells and enhances the antitumor activity of adoptive immunotherapy in mice. *Clinical cancer research : an official journal of the American Association for Cancer Research,* 2013, *19,* (2), 393-403.

[102] Jiang, X.; Zhou, J.; Giobbie-Hurder, A.; Wargo, J.; Hodi, F.S., The activation of MAPK in melanoma cells resistant to BRAF inhibition promotes PD-L1 expression that is reversible by MEK and PI3K inhibition. *Clinical cancer research : an official journal of the American Association for Cancer Research,* 2013, *19,* (3), 598-609.

[103] Vella, L.J.; Pasam, A.; Dimopoulos, N.; Andrews, M.; Knights, A.; Puaux, A.L.; Louahed, J.; Chen, W.; Woods, K.; Cebon, J.S., MEK inhibition, alone or in combination with BRAF inhibition, affects multiple functions of isolated normal human lymphocytes and dendritic cells. *Cancer immunology research,* 2014, *2,* (4), 351-360.

[104] Ribas, A.; Hodi, F.S.; Callahan, M.; Konto, C.; Wolchok, J., Hepatotoxicity with combination of vemurafenib and ipilimumab. The New England journal of medicine, 2013, 368, (14), 1365-1366.

3

RAGE and its Ligands in Melanoma

Estelle Leclerc

1. Introduction

Melanoma is a complex disease with both genetic and epigenetic components [1-3]. Once melanoma has formed distant metastases, melanoma patients have generally poor prognoses; less than 10% of these patients will survive 10 years [4]. For many years, treatment with the cytotoxic drug dacarbazine was the standard treatment for patients with metastatic melanoma, but the response rates were low and varied from 5-20% [4]. Intense research efforts on understanding the molecular mechanisms of melanoma progression led to the discovery and the approval by the FDA of two new drugs in 2011, vemurafenib and ipilimumab, which raised great hopes among melanoma patients [5-12]. Although treatment with vemurafenib has resulted in high overall responses rates [11], resistance against the drug appeared in treated melanoma patients within a year of treatment, leading to tumor regrowth [13-16]. On the other hand, treatment with ipilimumab does not result in resistance but can produce life threatening autoimmune adverse effects [17]. In addition, ipilimumab works best in patients whose tumors present abundant tumor infiltrated immune cells [18]. It is therefore essential to identify new therapeutic targets in melanoma.

One potential therapeutic target is the receptor for advanced glycation end products (RAGE). A possible role of RAGE in melanoma is emerging and has been the topic of a growing number of studies in the past decade [19-25]. These studies will be reviewed here and we will also discuss the RAGE ligands that play important roles in melanoma progression.

2. The Receptor for Advanced Glycation End Products (RAGE)

2.1. RAGE function

RAGE is an immunoglobulin-like cell-surface receptor that is involved in a large number of pathologies, including Alzheimer's disease, cancer, infectious diseases and complications of diabetes [31-38]. The ligands of RAGE are numerous (Table 1) and belong to distinct families of molecules. However, they also share structural features such as the propensity to form oligomers [39]. It is believed that RAGE recognizes similar structural elements or patterns within its numerous ligands and therefore RAGE is described as a pattern recognition receptor [40, 41].

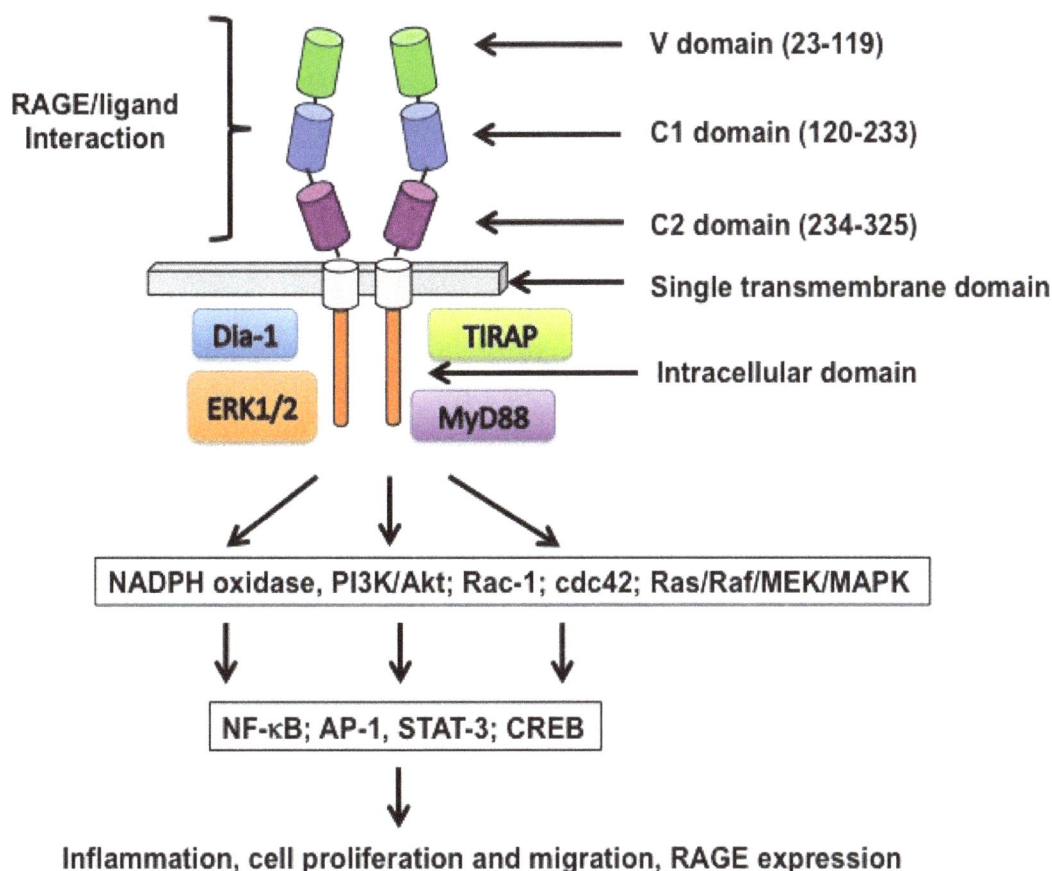

Figure 1. Schematic representation of RAGE. The extracellular part of RAGE is composed of three distinct immunoglobulin-like domains (V, C1 and C2). The V and C1 domains form a structural and functional unit [26]. Most ligands interact with the V-C1 domain. Four adaptor molecules have been suggested to bind to the intracellular domain of RAGE: ERK1/2 [27], diaphanous-1 (Dia-1) [28], TIRAP and MyD88 [29]. Following activation of RAGE by its ligands, multiple signaling pathways (MAPK, PI3K/Akt) or molecules (NADPH oxidase, Rac-1, cdc42) are activated and lead to the transcription of genes related to inflammation, cell proliferation and migration, and to the expression of RAGE itself, resulting in a positive feedback loop [30].

The physiological role of RAGE is not yet fully understood. Studies have shown that RAGE plays a role in the innate but not adaptive immunity and has been shown to play an important function in peripheral nerve repair [42-44]. A characteristic of RAGE is that it is expressed at low basal level in most tissues except in lungs where it has been suggested to exert a protective effect [45-48]. RAGE has also been shown to modulate the auditory system in mice [49].

Several spliced isoforms of RAGE have been described. Besides full-length RAGE, presented in Figure 1, RAGE exists as a soluble form (sRAGE) lacking the intracellular and transmembrane domains. The soluble form can result either from a splicing event or from the action of a metalloprotease such as ADAM 10 [50-58]. Other major identified spliced isoforms lack the N-terminal domain or present a deletion in the intracellular domain, resulting in abnormal ligand interaction and cell signaling activities, respectively [51, 56, 59]. sRAGE has been used in many animal experiments to validate the role of RAGE in various diseases such as Alzheimer's disease, atherosclerosis or encephalomyelitis [60-62]. Two different models explaining the mechanism of action of sRAGE have been proposed. The "classic" mechanism suggests that sRAGE acts as a decoy receptor and interacts with circulating RAGE ligands, which results in the absence of RAGE/ligand complex formation and RAGE activation. Recently, the group of Fritz has proposed a second mechanism of action for sRAGE: Fritz et al. suggest that sRAGE could form a complex with the extracellular part of another full-length receptor and that this receptor complex would not be functional because it possesses only one intracellular domain [63]. According to this hypothesis, RAGE can only transmit a signal if two intracellular domains form a dimer [63].

The role of sRAGE as biomarker has also been investigated in many diseases but has resulted in contradictory data for certain pathologies. In Alzheimer's disease patients, the circulating plasma levels of sRAGE have been shown to be significantly reduced compared to healthy individuals [64]. A more detailed immunohistological examination of AD brain showed that the reduction in sRAGE was more pronounced in the hippocampus of AD brains than normal brains [65]. Systemic low levels of sRAGE have also been found in patients with emphysema, a form of chronic obstructive pulmonary disease (COPD) and sRAGE is suggested to be a biomarker for this lung disease [66, 67]. However, in diabetes, the situation is more complex and in different studies the levels of sRAGE have been either positively or negatively correlated with the disease (reviewed and discussed in [68])

In cancer, an association between sRAGE and the progression of cancer has also been shown. Significantly lower levels of sRAGE have been found in lung, breast, liver or pancreatic cancer patients than in normal individuals [69-72]. Our study of 40 melanoma human samples also showed significantly lower transcript levels of the spliced form of RAGE in 90% of melanoma stage III and stage IV tissue samples compared to normal samples [73].

2.2. RAGE structure and signaling

RAGE is a single transmembrane receptor with a large extracellular part comprising of three domains that share structural features with immunoglobulin domains: a variable type (V) domain (residues 23-119), and two constant type domains (C1: residues 120-233, and C2: residues 234-325) (Figure 1) [74]. The V and C1 domains form a structural and functional unit and are the site of binding of most ligands [26].

Recent studies have suggested that RAGE structure is as complex as RAGE signaling is, and multiple conformational forms of RAGE in complex with its ligands have been proposed [75]. Recent evidence suggests that RAGE exists as a dimer on the surface of cells, in the absence of ligand [76, 77]. It has been suggested that the interaction of RAGE with its ligands occurs mainly through electrostatic interactions between the positive charges present on the V and C1 domains of RAGE and the negative charges present on RAGE ligands [39, 63]. Because both RAGE and its ligands can form oligomers, several oligomeric models of RAGE in complex with its ligands have been proposed to reflect the possible RAGE/ligand interactions [39, 63, 75-79]. RAGE oligomerization could occur through contacts between the V domain [80], C1 domain [80], [77] or C2 domain, [75, 79], in a ligand dependent manner [79].

RAGE signaling is complex and RAGE/ligand interaction results in the activation of multiple signaling pathways that are ligand and tissue specific (Figure 1) [34, 81-84]. In general, RAGE engagement by its ligand leads to the activation of key elements of the PI3K/Akt pathways or the mitogen-activated protein (MAP) kinase signaling pathways which include ERK1/2, p38 and JNK. Small GTPases such as p21-Ras, Rac-1 or cdc42 can also be activated as a result of RAGE activation [28, 81, 85-87]. In many cases, RAGE activation by its ligands leads to the initiation of, and sustained inflammation through the activation of the transcription factor NF-κB, but also AP-1, STAT-3 and CREB (Figure 1) [36-38, 68, 88].

2.3. RAGE in melanoma

A role of RAGE in melanoma progression was first suggested by Huttunen et al [19]. In their study, the authors generated tumors in mice using the mouse melanoma B16F10 cell-line expressing either full-length RAGE or a form of RAGE lacking the cytoplasmic domain [19]. Comparison of the number of metastases formed in the two groups of mice revealed that mice that were implanted with cells expressing the mutant form of RAGE generated significantly less tumors than mice implanted with cells expressing full-length RAGE. In a different study, Abe et al. showed that the growth of xenograft tumor in mice could be reduced using anti-RAGE antibodies [21]. We showed that RAGE overexpression in the WM115 human melanoma cell line resulted in a significant decrease in cell proliferation, but also in a significant increase in cell migration and invasion suggesting that RAGE can modulate different aspects of cancer [24]. We demonstrated that the decrease in cell proliferation was accompanied with a decrease in the activity of ERK1/2 [24] and p38 (Meghnani et al. 2014, International Journal of Biochemistry and Cell Biology, in press). The recent report of Popa et al. also suggests the presence of different oligomeric forms of RAGE with different roles and subcellular location during melanoma progression [25].

Studies in human melanoma tissue samples have shown that RAGE was not present in all melanoma samples but rather in a subset of samples. Hsieh et al. showed that only 20% tissue samples showed RAGE staining [20]. Our analysis of 40 samples of human melanoma tissue samples also showed large variations in RAGE transcripts levels, with up to 50-fold differences between samples [22].

Other studies have identified RAGE ligands as important elements in melanoma development. S100B has been studied in details and its role as a diagnostic marker for melanoma patients is well established (see section 3.1.1 on S100B). Abe et al. showed that AGEs could promote the proliferation of melanoma cells in culture [21]. Saha et al. showed that S100A8/A9 could attract B16F10 melanoma cells to a metastatic site, in a RAGE dependent manner [23]. In addition, our recent study showed a strong correlation between the expression of RAGE and that of its S100 protein ligands, in mouse xenograft melanoma tumors (Meghnani et al. 2014, International Journal of Biochemistry and Cell Biology, in press).

3. RAGE ligands

Since the identification of AGEs as ligands of RAGE, the list of RAGE ligands has grown to more than ten ligands or groups of ligands (Table 1). In this section, we will discuss the current knowledge on ligands that have been shown to play a role in melanoma progression, with a focus on S100 proteins.

RAGE ligand	Examples of disease where the ligand is involved	References
Advanced glycation end products	Inflammation, cancer, Alzheimer's disease, atherosclerosis, aging	[74, 89-92]
S100 proteins	Inflammation, cancer, aging, neurodegenerative disorders	[82, 93-95]
High mobility group box 1 (HMGB-1)	Cancer, inflammation, aging	[34, 96-99]
Alzheimer's β-peptide	Alzheimer's disease	[32, 60]
Transthyretin	Transthyretin amyloidosis	[100]
Prion	Prion's disease	[101, 102]
Mac-1	Diseases of the immune system	[40, 103]
Complement proteins C3a and C1q	Diseases of the immune system	[104, 105]
Phophatidylserine	Diseases of apoptosis	[106, 107]
Heparan sulfate	Cancer, inflammation, developmental disorder	[78, 108, 109]
DNA, RNA	Infectious diseases, autoimmune disorders	[110]

Table 1. Non-exhaustive list of the different ligands of RAGE. The S100 proteins that are ligands of RAGE will be described in details in section 3.1

3.1. S100 proteins

Members of the S100 protein family have amino-acid sequence and structure similarities [111, 112]. They are small calcium binding proteins and belong to the superfamily of EF-hand proteins [111]. Restricted to vertebrates, S100 proteins show strong tissue and cell specificity [111, 113]. Most S100 genes (S100A1 to S100A16) are located on chromosome 1 in a region that is prone to chromosomal rearrangement, linking these S100 proteins to cancer [113]. The presence of EF-hands within the structure of S100 proteins enable them to bind calcium with moderate micromolar affinity [111, 112, 114, 115]. In addition to calcium, S100 proteins can also bind zinc and copper [116, 117]. For most S100 proteins, binding to calcium results in conformational rearrangements that allow the S100 proteins to interact with their targets [115, 117, 118]. Certain target proteins are S100 specific whereas others are shared among multiple S100s (Reviewed in [119]).

Most S100 target proteins are intracellular [111, 112, 120]. An example of such target that plays a role in cancer is the tumor suppressor p53 protein [121-126]. Several members of the S100 protein family (S100B, S100A1, S100A2, S100A4, S100A6 and S100A10] bind to p53 but the outcome of this interaction differs depending of the S100 [121-126]. S100 proteins can also be secreted into the extracellular space through mechanisms that are not clearly understood [127, 128]. When secreted, many S100 proteins have been shown to interact with RAGE [82, 93, 129].

Many S100 proteins are found in cells constituting the epidermis [130]. S100B and S100A6 have been found in both melanocytes and Langerhan's cells [131-133]. S100A2, A7, A10, A11, A12 and S100A15 have been described in normal keratinocytes [131-138]. In pathophysiological conditions, such as in inflamed keratinocytes and melanoma, many S100 proteins have been found overexpressed [130, 136]. The next section will describe the role of these S100 proteins in melanoma.

3.1.1. S100B

S100B is used as a prognostic marker for stage IV malignant melanoma patients [139-141]. Serum concentration of S100B increases during the disease and high levels of S100B in the serum is indicative of a poor prognosis [139-141]. In melanoma tumors, melanoma cells are the main cells responsible for secreting S100B [141]. Within the cells, the role of S100B is not clearly understood but the main target of S100B appears to be the tumor suppressor p53 protein. Indeed, several studies from the group of Weber have shown that S100B interacts with p53 in melanoma cells and tumors, resulting in p53 inhibition and increased expression of S100B, in a negative feedback loop [142-144]. His group is currently investigating small interfering antisense RNA inhibitors of S100B as inhibitors of melanoma tumor growth [145].

Other intracellular target proteins of S100B could also contribute to increases in cellular proliferation and tumor growth in melanoma. For example, S100B interacts with and activates the glycolytic enzyme fructose-1,6-biphosphate aldolase, [146]. Consequences of this activation could be an increase in melanoma cell metabolism and glycolysis. Inhibiting melanoma cell metabolism and glycolysis is currently been considered in clinical trials [147, 148]. Inhibiting S100B/ fructose-1,6-biphosphate aldolase could be an approach to further reduce glycolytic activity in melanoma cells. S100B also interacts with many components of the cytoskeleton such as tubulin [149, 150], the actin binding protein caldesmon [151] or the small GTPase Rac1 and the cdc42 effector IQGAP1 [152]. All these proteins play important function in malignant melanoma [153-155] and increases in S100B levels could therefore favor increases in cell proliferation, migration and invasion through their modulation. S100B could also play a role in melanoma cell growth through the activation of the Nuclear Dbf2 related (ndr) kinase [156-158] and the interaction with the phosphoprotein AHNAK/desmoyokin [159-161].

As mentioned earlier, S100B is secreted from melanoma cells. The mechanisms of S100B secretion are still poorly understood but recent studies have suggested that RAGE participates in the translocation and secretion of several S100s including S100B [127, 128]. Similarly, the role of RAGE/S100B in melanoma is slowly being unraveled. S100B has been shown to signal through RAGE in a large number of diseases (reviewed in [162]) and we studied in details the *in vitro* interaction of RAGE with S100B [26, 81, 163]. For example, we showed that not only dimeric S100B but also tetrameric and hexameric S100B could interact with RAGE and signal in cells [163]. In addition, we recently showed that overexpression of RAGE, in human WM115 melanoma cells, was accompanied by the up-regulation of S100B in these cells [24], suggesting a strong association between RAGE and S100B in melanoma. When the RAGE transfected WM115 cells were implanted in mice as xenografts, we also observed higher levels of S100B in the serum of these animals, compared to animals implanted with control WM115 cells (Meghnani et al. 2014, International Journal of Biochemistry and Cell Biology, in press).

3.1.2. S100A2

S100A2 is mainly located in the nuclei of cells [164]. The function of S100A2 in cancer is not clear. In certain cancers such as prostate, oral, lung and breast cancers, S100A2 has been shown to play the role of tumor suppressor [22, 165-169], whereas in other cancers such as esophageal squamous carcinoma, gastric, and ovarian cancer, studies indicate that it acts as tumor promoter [170-172]. In addition, in certain cancers, such as in non-small cell lung cancer (NSCLC), studies are contradictory since both down-and up-regulation of S100A2 have been reported [173-175].

In melanoma, most studies reported that S100A2 plays the role of tumor suppressor [130, 132, 165, 176]. We also showed a significant reduction in S100A2 mRNA level in both stage III and stage IV melanoma patients samples compared to control samples [22]. Additional evidences of a tumor suppressor effect of S100A2 comes from several studies that show positive correlations between the levels of S100A2 and anti-proliferative effects of chemotherapeutic agents in melanoma cells [177, 178]. However, our most recent study shows that xenograft melanoma tumors overexpressing RAGE, presented a growth advantage over control tumors, and exhibited significant higher levels of S100A2 than control tumors (Meghnani et al. 2014, International Journal of Biochemistry and Cell Biology, in press). We observed that S100A2 was up-regulated, both at the transcript and protein levels, in the RAGE overexpressing tumors (Meghnani et al. unpublished results). These data suggest a complex role of S100A2 in promoting or suppressing melanoma tumor growth.

As mentioned above, S100A2 is located in the nuclei of cells and has been shown to interact with the tumor suppressor p53, in two oral cancer cell lines (FADU and SCC-25), thereby modulating the transcriptional activity of p53 [123]. *In vitro* binding studies have confirmed the interaction between S100A2 and p53 and has shown differences in binding of p53 to S100B and S100A2; for example, although both S100B and S100A2 could bind to the monomeric form of p53, only S100B was able to disrupt the oligomerization of p53, suggesting different mode of transcriptional modulation of p53 by the S100 proteins [124, 126]. In addition to interacting with p53, S100A2 transcriptional activity is regulated by other members of the large p53 family, such as p63 and p73, suggesting an additional level of complexity of the S100A2/p53 regulation [179-181]. In breast cancer tissues and cells, it was shown that both the p53 homologue Np63, and BRCA1 were important for the transcriptional activity of S100A2 [182]. These recent data could have a large impact in understanding the molecular mechanism of melanoma because positive correlations have been found between the BRCA1 associated protein (BAP1) and malignant uveal and cutaneous melanoma [183-185].

We recently demonstrated that *in vitro*, S100A2 could interact with RAGE [22] and our recent study showed an association between RAGE overexpression and the levels of S100A2 in melanoma xenograft tumors (Meghnani et al. 2014, International Journal of Biochemistry and

Cell Biology, in press). However, a direct interaction of S100A2/RAGE in melanoma cells and tissue has yet to be demonstrated.

3.1.3. S100A4

S100A4 was initially identified from metastatic cells and was hence named metastasin [186]. Overexpression of S100A4 in multiple cell lines has been shown to increase cancer cell invasiveness and motility [187, 188]. The role of S100A4 in cancer was further demonstrated in S100A4-/-mice that showed delayed tumor growth, compared to control mice, when implanted with highly metastatic mammary carcinoma cells [189, 190].

In melanoma, the role of S100A4 is complex and appears to vary during the progression of the disease. An early study showed no significant differences in S100A4 mRNA levels between melanoma tissue samples and control samples [165]. Our analysis of 40 samples of stage III and stage IV melanoma tissue samples showed a significantly reduction of S100A4 mRNA in stage IV compared to control samples [22]. Another study also reported different correlation between the levels of S100A4 and patient survival rates during the progression of melanoma: high levels of S100A4 in primary melanoma tumors were associated with low patient survival rates whereas high S100A4 levels in metastatic tumors were not associated with differences in patient survival rates, suggesting a role of S100A4 at a early stage of the disease [191].

S100A4 exerts both intra-and extracellular functions (reviewed in [192]). Inside the cells, S100A4 can be found in the nuclei and cytoplasm [192]. S100A4 has been shown to interact with p53 and, as described for S100B, to disrupt p53 oligomerization [193, 194]. *In vivo*, interaction of S100A4 with p53 has been shown to promote degradation of p53, resulting in increases in tumor growth [195]. In the cytoplasm, S100A4 interacts with a large number of proteins of the cytoskeleton such as non-muscle myosin II [196] and tropomyosin [197], resulting in cytoskeletal reorganization, which occurs during cell migration and invasion [198, 199].

An important property of S100A4 is that it has been found secreted in the extracellular medium of cells and is present in the milieu of many tumor types such as breast cancer [200], ovarian carcinoma [201], osteosarcoma [202] or adenocarcinoma tumors [203]. Many cells from normal tissues and from tumors have been shown to release S100A4. These cells include fibroblasts, leukocytes, and endothelial cells [192, 204]. Extracellular S100A4 has been shown to promote tumor growth and metastasis [192], neovascularization and angiogenesis [205-207].

Two main targets of extracellular S100A4 with relevance to tumor growth and metastasis have been identified: Annexin II and RAGE [208, 209]. Interaction of S100A4 with annexin II has been associated with increased mechanisms of angiogenesis such as the formation of capillary-like tubes by endothelial cells [208]. S100A4 has been shown to enhance motility of pulmonary artery smooth muscle cells in a RAGE dependent manner [210]. Similarly, S100A4 was shown to promote prostate and colorectal cancer tumorigenesis and metastasis in a RAGE dependent manner [211, 212]. In melanoma, a recent study has demonstrated that S100A4 derived from macrophages could promote lung colonization of B16F10 melanoma cells in mice, in a RAGE dependent manner as well [213]. We have also observed that RAGE overexpression in the

WM115 melanoma cells resulted in the up-regulation of S100A4, by the melanoma cells, in xenograft tumors implanted in mice (Meghnani et al. 2014, International Journal of Biochemistry and Cell Biology, in press).

3.1.4. S100A6

S100A6 is another member of the S100 family with a link to cancer. S100A6 was identified from melanoma tissue samples by comparing melanocytic lesions from normal nevi [214]. S100A6 is most abundant in epithelial cells and fibroblasts but is also found, in smaller amounts, in other cell-types such as neurons, glial cells, smooth muscle cells, cardiac myocytes, platelets and lymphocytes [215, 216](reviewed in [217]). S100A6 has been found elevated in a large number of cancer types which include colorectal cancer, pancreatic, hepato-cellular carcinoma, melanoma, lung cancer and gastric cancer [165, 218-224](reviewed in [217]). In melanoma tumor samples, a positive correlation was found between the levels of S100A6 transcripts and the severity of the disease [165]. In animal models, S100A6 was found to correlate with the metastatic behavior of the melanoma cells [214, 225]. We also observed higher levels of S1006, at the transcript level, in 43% of stage III melanoma samples examined, compared to control samples [22]. In agreement with our study, examination of another set of melanoma tissue samples showed that 33% of the samples stained positive for S100A6 [133]. However, examination of melanoma tumor biopsies by immunohistochemistry often shows that the expression of S100A6 is weak and patchy, and that other non-melanoma cutaneous lesions also stain positive for S100A6, making it difficult to use S100A6 as a diagnostic marker for melanoma [176, 226, 227].

S100A6 has been shown to interact with both nuclear and cytoplasmic proteins. S100A6 interacts with the tumor suppressor p53 but this interaction is different than the interaction of p53 with S100B, suggesting different regulation of the transcriptional activity of p53 by the two S100 proteins [124, 228]. S100A6 was shown to interact with a peptide derived from cell membrane associated annexin I, but the physiological relevance of this interaction has yet to be demonstrated [229]. We showed that S100A6 could interact with both the VC1 and the C2 domain of RAGE, but that in human neuroblastoma, signaling was transduced through the C2 domain [81]. The interaction of the C3S mutant form of S100A6 with the V domain of RAGE has recently been studied in details [230]. Similarly to what we observed with S100B, S100A2 and S100A4, RAGE overexpression in the WM115 melanoma cells resulted in the up-regulation of S100A6, by the melanoma cells, when the cells were forming xenograft tumors in nude mice, compared to control tumors (Meghnani et al. 2014, International Journal of Biochemistry and Cell Biology, in press).

3.1.5. S100A8/A9

S100A8 and S100A9 are mainly expressed by cells of myeloid origin such as monocytes and macrophages, and were first described as cytokine-like proteins for their up-regulation in inflamed tissues and inflammatory disorders [231]. Recent studies have also shown that they play significant roles in cancer where they promote tumor growth and metastasis in a large number of cancers such as in breast, prostate and pancreatic cancer [232-238]. In tumors, recent studies have shown that S100A8/A9 regulates the accumulation of myeloid-derived suppressor cells (MDSC), and also promote the expansion of these cells, resulting in increased tumor growth [239-243].

Neither S100A8 nor S100A9 is present in significant amounts in the cells of a normal epidermis, including melanocytes [130, 244]. Although a study described that S100A8/A9 was absent from melanocytic lesions [244], other studies have suggested that they participate in melanoma progression. S100A9 has been shown to promote melanoma metastases formation in a mouse model [245]. In a different mouse model of melanoma, the levels of MDSCs correlated with the levels of S100A9, [246]. In addition, Saha et al. recently demonstrated that tail-vein injected B16F10 melanoma cells, that do not express S100A8 or S100A9, could migrate to S100A8/A9-abondant lungs of uteroglobin-knockout mice [23]. The migration of the B16F10 cells occurred along a concentration gradient of S100A8/A9, and resulted in the formation of secondary tumors in the lungs [23].

S100A8/A9 mediates their effect through the interaction with cell surface receptors or molecules. The two pattern recognition receptors, toll-like receptor 4 (TLR-4) and RAGE, have been shown to transmit RAGE signaling [23, 247, 248]. In certain conditions, signaling through RAGE has been shown to require carboxylated glycans that are covalently attached to RAGE [249, 250]. The importance of RAGE glycosylation for RAGE signaling has also been demonstrated for another member of the S100 protein family, S100A12 [251]. S100A8/A9 has been shown to interact with other glycans, such as heparin or heparin sulfate glycosaminoglycans [137]. In addition, S100A9 has also been shown to interact with and transmit signal through EMMPIRIN [245].

3.1.6. Other S100 proteins

Other S100 proteins are found in cells of the epidermis (reviewed by [130]), and their association with melanoma will be briefly described in this paragraph.

S100A7 or "psoriasin" has been linked to psoriasis because of its up-regulation in this disease [252, 253]. Although no direct role of S100A7 in melanoma has been described yet, in one study, significantly higher levels of S100A7 were found in the urine of melanoma patients compared to that of healthy patients [254].

S100A10 has been found expressed at various levels in melanoma tumor samples and melanocytes [22, 244]. Our recent study where we compared the levels of S100 proteins in WM115 xenografts, generated from either control WM115 cells or from RAGE overexpressing WM115 cells, showed that S100A10 was up-regulated in the RAGE overexpressing tumors (unpublished data). Comparison of the WM115-RAGE cells with control cells did not reveal any difference in S100A10 levels between the two cell lines, suggesting that RAGE overexpression was responsible for the up-regulation of S100A10 in the tumors. S100A10 could therefore play a role in melanoma progression.

S100A11 can either promote tumor growth or play the role of tumor suppressor, depending of the type of cancer (reviewed in [255]). S100A11 has been suggested to play a role in uveal melanoma, but has not yet been linked to cutaneous melanoma [256].

3.2. Other ligands of RAGE

3.2.1. Advanced Glycation End products (AGEs)

Among RAGE ligands, AGEs were the first group of ligands to be identified [89]. AGEs form a group of very heterogeneous compounds since they are the result of condensation and oxidation reactions between proteins and sugars [257]. Although the term AGE was initially reserved for brown, fluorescent and cross-linked structures that were produced during the Maillard reaction, such as those found in glycated collagen, it is now used to describe other types of modifications and AGEs now include proteins containing carboxymethyllysine, carboxymethyl hydroxylysine or pyrraline [257]. Since many types of sugars (glucose, ribose…) can modify many proteins, the number of different structures produced by glycation is very large. The large heterogeneity in AGE compounds renders the comparison among studies also very difficult. When comparing the results of studies involving AGEs, it is therefore important to know the type of AGEs used in the study.

Melanoma cells have been shown to produce high levels of reactive carbonyl species such as glyoxal, methylglyoxal and malondialdehyde, which all can lead to the glycation of proteins, and which have been implicated in melanoma cell proliferation and formation of metastases [258-260]. Abe et al. investigated the effects of different AGEs (glucose-derived AGE, glyceraldehyde-derived AGE, glycoaldehyde AGE, methylglyoxal-AGE, glyoxal-AGE and carboxymethyllysine-AGE) on melanoma cell proliferation, migration and invasion, and showed that all these AGEs were strongly present in human melanoma specimen whereas they were hardly detected in melanocytes [21]. However, the same authors showed that only certain types of AGE compounds (glyceraldehyde-derived AGE and glycoaldehyde AGE) could stimulate the proliferation, migration and invasion of G361 metastatic human melanoma cells *in vitro*. The role of RAGE in the *in vitro* AGE-dependent proliferation was demonstrated with anti-RAGE antibodies [21]. In addition, the authors showed that treatment of mice carrying G361 melanoma tumors, with anti-RAGE antibodies, resulted in reduced tumor growth and formation of lungs metastases [21]. These results strongly suggested a role of AGE/RAGE in the development of melanoma tumors by the G361 human melanoma cell line [21]. Our detailed study on melanoma cell proliferation of a panel of 20 glycated proteins showed that many factors influenced the proliferation, such as the extent of lysine modification, the percentage of β-sheet and the oligomerization state of the glycated proteins [261]. We showed that glycated proteins that demonstrated higher percentage of oligomeric forms, β-sheet content and modification of lysine, promoted stronger cell proliferation that proteins that contained lower levels of oligomers, β-sheet or lysine modification.

3.2.2. High Mobility Group Box 1 protein (HMGB1)

HMGB-1 is present in most eukaryotic cells (reviewed by [97]). It functions both as a nuclear protein, where it binds to DNA and assists in the transcription of multiple genes, and as an extracellular protein, where it binds to the pattern recognition receptors TLR-2, TLR-4 and TLR-9 as well as to RAGE, thereby promoting inflammation, mediating response to infection and injury as well as promoting cell proliferation, migration or invasion [98, 262-266]. HMGB-1 is also described as an alarmin or damage-associated molecular pattern [267]. HMGB-1 interacts directly with a large number of transcription factors that are relevant in cancer, and include the tumor suppressor p53, p73, the retinoblastoma protein (RB), the p50 subunit of NF-κB and the estrogen receptor (reviewed by [268]). The release of HMGB-1 has been shown to be triggered by necrosis or apoptosis, such as following treatment of tumors with a chemotherapeutic agent [264, 266, 267].

HMGB-1 has also been shown to be released from necrotic or apoptotic melanoma cells [269]. A recent study showed that HMGB-1 could be released from keratinocytes in culture, or from murine skin, following exposure to UV light [270]. Using a genetically engineered mouse model of melanoma, Bald et al. showed that UV exposure also promoted metastasis and angiogenesis, through HMGB-1, and TLR-4 signaling [271]. In a different mouse model, Tang et al. showed the role of the HMGB-1/RAGE axis in promoting melanoma tumor growth [272]. In melanoma patients, HMGB-1 levels have also been shown to predict patient survival rates [273].

3.2.3. Glycosaminoglycans, β2 integrin Mac-1 and phosphatidylserine

RAGE has been shown to interact with various glycosaminoglycans such as chondroitin sulfate, dermatan sulfate and heparin sulfate [108]. Many of these glycosaminoglycans are abundantly present in tumor stroma and have been shown to be key players of melanoma progression and metastasis formation [274, 275]. RAGE also interacts with β2 integrin Mac-1 on leukocytes and has been shown to promote leukocyte recruitment at the site of inflammation [40]. The interaction between RAGE and Mac-1 is dependent of the presence of cations, and has been shown to be significantly augmented by the presence of S100B. In a different study, S100A9 has also been shown to activate β2 integrin Mac-1 on neutrophils suggesting that other S100 proteins could also participate to the complex between Mac-1 and RAGE [276]. Leukocyte recruitment at tumor sites is an important process that allows cytotoxic T-cells to infiltrate tumors and to help in the elimination of cancer cells [277]. In melanoma, success of the therapy with interleukin-2 (IL-2) is based on the infiltration of cytotoxic T-cells to the interior of the tumor [277]. The involvement of S100 proteins and RAGE in leukocyte recruitment suggests that therapeutic approaches targeting RAGE should be carefully evaluated to avoid inhibiting the recruitment of cytotoxic T-cells at the site of melanoma tumors. On the other hand, targeting RAGE could also result in suppressing the recruitment of MDSCs, another form of leukocyte expressing β2 integrin Mac-1 [278], at the tumor site, which would be beneficial for patients [279, 280].

RAGE has also been shown to interact with the negatively charged phospholipid phosphatidylserine (PS) [106]. This interaction has direct relevance in melanoma because PS has been shown to be exposed to the outer leaflet of the plasma membrane of cells forming melanoma metastases [281]. An association between malignancy of melanoma and PS exposure has also been described [281]. Further studies would be necessary to determine whether RAGE/PS could be targeted in melanoma.

4. Conclusion and therapeutic approaches

In the last two decades, RAGE has emerged as a new therapeutic target in a large number of diseases. Because of the large number of ligands of RAGE that are relevant in melanoma, targeting RAGE/ligand appears to be a promising approach. Several molecules could be used as inhibitors and include the soluble form of the receptor (sRAGE), antibodies against RAGE or small molecules. Both soluble RAGE and anti-RAGE antibodies have been used to demonstrate the role of RAGE in experimental models of a large number of diseases such as atherosclerosis, Alzheimer's disease or melanoma [21, 60, 282-286]. Two small molecule inhibitors of RAGE are currently available. One compound PFS-ZM1 has been recently used in an experimental model of Alzheimer's disease [287]. This inhibitor interacts with the V domain of RAGE and blocks the interaction of amyloid β-peptide with the receptor. The second compound (TPP488) has been evaluated for safety and efficacy, in a phase 2 study, in mild to moderate Alzheimer's disease patients. However, because of the large variation in the levels of RAGE observed in melanoma tumor samples, it is currently not known whether targeting RAGE would be efficacious in all melanoma tumors or only in the subset of tumors where it is overexpressed. Additional studies would be necessary to answer this important question.

Acknowledgements

The author was supported by the NDSU College of Pharmacy, Nursing and Allied Sciences and in part by the NDSU Advance FORWARD program sponsored by NSF HRD-0811239 and ND EPSCoR through grant #EPS-0814442.

Author details

Estelle Leclerc*

Address all correspondence to: Estelle.Leclerc@ndsu.edu

North Dakota State University/Department of Pharmaceutical Sciences, USA

References

[1] Howell PM, Jr., Liu S, Ren S, Behlen C, Fodstad O, Riker AI. Epigenetics in human melanoma. Cancer Control. 2009;16(3):200-18.

[2] Patino WD, Susa J. Epigenetics of cutaneous melanoma. Adv Dermatol. 2008;24:59-70.

[3] Palmieri G, Capone M, Ascierto ML, Gentilcore G, Stroncek DF, Casula M, et al. Main roads to melanoma. J Transl Med. 2009;7:86.

[4] Bhatia S, Tykodi SS, Thompson JA. Treatment of metastatic melanoma: an overview. Oncology (Williston Park). 2009;23(6):488-96.

[5] Eggermont AM, Robert C. Melanoma in 2011: A new paradigm tumor for drug development. Nat Rev Clin Oncol. 2012.

[6] Hodi FS, Oble DA, Drappatz J, Velazquez EF, Ramaiya N, Ramakrishna N, et al. CTLA-4 blockade with ipilimumab induces significant clinical benefit in a female with melanoma metastases to the CNS. Nat Clin Pract Oncol. 2008;5(9):557-61.

[7] Nelson AL, Dhimolea E, Reichert JM. Development trends for human monoclonal antibody therapeutics. Nat Rev Drug Discov. 2010;9(10):767-74.

[8] Robert C, Mateus C. [Anti-CTLA-4 monoclonal antibody: a major step in the treatment of metastatic melanoma]. Med Sci (Paris). 2011;27(10):850-8.

[9] Trinh VA, Hagen B. Ipilimumab for advanced melanoma: A pharmacologic perspective. J Oncol Pharm Pract. 2012.

[10] Wang T, Somasundaram R, Herlyn M. Combination therapy of immunocytokines with ipilimumab: a cure for melanoma? J Invest Dermatol. 2013;133(3):595-6.

[11] Chapman PB, Hauschild A, Robert C, Haanen JB, Ascierto P, Larkin J, et al. Improved survival with vemurafenib in melanoma with BRAF V600E mutation. N Engl J Med. 2011;364(26):2507-16.

[12] Luke JJ, Hodi FS. Vemurafenib and BRAF inhibition: a new class of treatment for metastatic melanoma. Clin Cancer Res. 2012;18(1):9-14.

[13] Flaherty KT, Puzanov I, Kim KB, Ribas A, McArthur GA, Sosman JA, et al. Inhibition of mutated, activated BRAF in metastatic melanoma. N Engl J Med. 2010;363(9): 809-19.

[14] Nazarian R, Shi H, Wang Q, Kong X, Koya RC, Lee H, et al. Melanomas acquire resistance to B-RAF(V600E) inhibition by RTK or N-RAS upregulation. Nature. 2010;468(7326):973-7.

[15] Wagle N, Emery C, Berger MF, Davis MJ, Sawyer A, Pochanard P, et al. Dissecting therapeutic resistance to RAF inhibition in melanoma by tumor genomic profiling. J Clin Oncol. 2011;29(22):3085-96.

[16] Poulikakos PI, Persaud Y, Janakiraman M, Kong X, Ng C, Moriceau G, et al. RAF inhibitor resistance is mediated by dimerization of aberrantly spliced BRAF(V600E). Nature. 2011;480(7377):387-90.

[17] Wolchok JD, Neyns B, Linette G, Negrier S, Lutzky J, Thomas L, et al. Ipilimumab monotherapy in patients with pretreated advanced melanoma: a randomised, double-blind, multicentre, phase 2, dose-ranging study. Lancet Oncol. 2010;11(2):155-64.

[18] Quail DF, Joyce JA. Microenvironmental regulation of tumor progression and metastasis. Nat Med. 2013;19(11):1423-37.

[19] Huttunen HJ, Fages C, Kuja-Panula J, Ridley AJ, Rauvala H. Receptor for advanced glycation end products-binding COOH-terminal motif of amphoterin inhibits invasive migration and metastasis. Cancer Res. 2002;62(16):4805-11.

[20] Hsieh HL, Schafer BW, Sasaki N, Heizmann CW. Expression analysis of S100 proteins and RAGE in human tumors using tissue microarrays. Biochem Biophys Res Commun. 2003;307(2):375-81.

[21] Abe R, Shimizu T, Sugawara H, Watanabe H, Nakamura H, Choei H, et al. Regulation of human melanoma growth and metastasis by AGE-AGE receptor interactions. J Invest Dermatol. 2004;122(2):461-7.

[22] Leclerc E, Heizmann CW, Vetter SW. RAGE and S100 protein transcription levels are highly variable in human melanoma tumors and cells. Gen Physiol Biophys. 2009;28 Spec No Focus:F65-75.

[23] Saha A, Lee YC, Zhang ZJ, Chandra G, Su SB, Mukherjee AB. Lack of an Endogenous Anti-inflammatory Protein in Mice Enhances Colonization of B16F10 Melanoma Cells in the Lungs. Journal of Biological Chemistry. 2010;285(14):10822-31.

[24] Meghnani V, Vetter SW, Leclerc E. RAGE overexpression confers a metastatic phenotype to the WM115 human primary melanoma cell line. Biochim Biophys Acta. 2014;1842(7):1017-27.

[25] Popa I, Ganea E, Petrescu SM. Expression and subcellular localization of RAGE in melanoma cells. Biochem Cell Biol. 2014;92(2):127-36.

[26] Dattilo BM, Fritz G, Leclerc E, Kooi CW, Heizmann CW, Chazin WJ. The extracellular region of the receptor for advanced glycation end products is composed of two independent structural units. Biochemistry. 2007;46(23):6957-70.

[27] Ishihara K, Tsutsumi K, Kawane S, Nakajima M, Kasaoka T. The receptor for advanced glycation end-products (RAGE) directly binds to ERK by a D-domain-like docking site. FEBS Lett. 2003;550(1-3):107-13.

[28] Hudson BI, Kalea AZ, Del Mar Arriero M, Harja E, Boulanger E, D'Agati V, et al. Interaction of the RAGE cytoplasmic domain with diaphanous-1 is required for ligand-stimulated cellular migration through activation of Rac1 and Cdc42. J Biol Chem. 2008;283(49):34457-68.

[29] Sakaguchi M, Murata H, Yamamoto K, Ono T, Sakaguchi Y, Motoyama A, et al. TI-RAP, an adaptor protein for TLR2/4, transduces a signal from RAGE phosphorylated upon ligand binding. PLoS One. 2011;6(8):e23132.

[30] Schmidt AM, Yan SD, Yan SF, Stern DM. The multiligand receptor RAGE as a progression factor amplifying immune and inflammatory responses. J Clin Invest. 2001;108(7):949-55.

[31] Schmidt AM, Yan SD, Yan SF, Stern DM. The biology of the receptor for advanced glycation end products and its ligands. Biochim Biophys Acta. 2000;1498(2-3):99-111.

[32] Yan SD, Bierhaus A, Nawroth PP, Stern DM. RAGE and Alzheimer's disease: a progression factor for amyloid-beta-induced cellular perturbation? J Alzheimers Dis. 2009;16(4):833-43.

[33] Bierhaus A, Nawroth PP. Multiple levels of regulation determine the role of the receptor for AGE (RAGE) as common soil in inflammation, immune responses and diabetes mellitus and its complications. Diabetologia. 2009;52(11):2251-63.

[34] Sparvero LJ, Asafu-Adjei D, Kang R, Tang D, Amin N, Im J, et al. RAGE (Receptor for Advanced Glycation Endproducts), RAGE ligands, and their role in cancer and inflammation. J Transl Med. 2009;7:17.

[35] van Zoelen MA, Achouiti A, van der Poll T. RAGE during infectious diseases. Front Biosci (Schol Ed). 2011;3:1119-32.

[36] Sims GP, Rowe DC, Rietdijk ST, Herbst R, Coyle AJ. HMGB1 and RAGE in Inflammation and Cancer. Annual Review of Immunology. 2010;28:367-88.

[37] Ramasamy R, Yan SF, Schmidt AM. Receptor for AGE (RAGE): signaling mechanisms in the pathogenesis of diabetes and its complications. Ann N Y Acad Sci. 2011;1243:88-102.

[38] Park S, Yoon SJ, Tae HJ, Shim CY. RAGE and cardiovascular disease. Front Biosci. 2011;16:486-97.

[39] Fritz G. RAGE: a single receptor fits multiple ligands. Trends Biochem Sci. 2011;36(12):625-32.

[40] Chavakis T, Bierhaus A, Al-Fakhri N, Schneider D, Witte S, Linn T, et al. The pattern recognition receptor (RAGE) is a counterreceptor for leukocyte integrins: a novel pathway for inflammatory cell recruitment. J Exp Med. 2003;198(10):1507-15.

[41] Lin L. RAGE on the Toll Road? Cellular & molecular immunology. 2006;3(5):351-8.

[42] Liliensiek B, Weigand MA, Bierhaus A, Nicklas W, Kasper M, Hofer S, et al. Receptor for advanced glycation end products (RAGE) regulates sepsis but not the adaptive immune response. J Clin Invest. 2004;113(11):1641-50.

[43] Rong LL, Trojaborg W, Qu W, Kostov K, Yan SD, Gooch C, et al. Antagonism of RAGE suppresses peripheral nerve regeneration. Faseb J. 2004;18(15):1812-7.

[44] Rong LL, Yan SF, Wendt T, Hans D, Pachydaki S, Bucciarelli LG, et al. RAGE modulates peripheral nerve regeneration via recruitment of both inflammatory and axonal outgrowth pathways. Faseb J. 2004;18(15):1818-25.

[45] Brett J, Schmidt AM, Yan SD, Zou YS, Weidman E, Pinsky D, et al. Survey of the distribution of a newly characterized receptor for advanced glycation end products in tissues. Am J Pathol. 1993;143(6):1699-712.

[46] Queisser MA, Kouri FM, Konigshoff M, Wygrecka M, Schubert U, Eickelberg O, et al. Loss of RAGE in pulmonary fibrosis: molecular relations to functional changes in pulmonary cell types. Am J Respir Cell Mol Biol. 2008;39(3):337-45.

[47] Ramsgaard L, Englert JM, Tobolewski J, Tomai L, Fattman CL, Leme AS, et al. The role of the receptor for advanced glycation end-products in a murine model of silicosis. PLoS One. 2010;5(3):e9604.

[48] Buckley ST, Ehrhardt C. The receptor for advanced glycation end products (RAGE) and the lung. J Biomed Biotechnol. 2010:in press.

[49] Sakatani S, Yamada K, Homma C, Munesue S, Yamamoto Y, Yamamoto H, et al. Deletion of RAGE causes hyperactivity and increased sensitivity to auditory stimuli in mice. PLoS One. 2009;4(12):e8309.

[50] Ohe K, Watanabe T, Harada S, Munesue S, Yamamoto Y, Yonekura H, et al. Regulation of alternative splicing of the receptor for advanced glycation endproducts (RAGE) through G-rich cis-elements and heterogenous nuclear ribonucleoprotein H. J Biochem. 2010;147(5):651-9.

[51] Hudson BI, Carter AM, Harja E, Kalea AZ, Arriero M, Yang H, et al. Identification, classification, and expression of RAGE gene splice variants. Faseb J. 2008;22(5): 1572-80.

[52] Galichet A, Weibel M, Heizmann CW. Calcium-regulated intramembrane proteolysis of the RAGE receptor. Biochem Biophys Res Commun. 2008;370(1):1-5.

[53] Raucci A, Cugusi S, Antonelli A, Barabino SM, Monti L, Bierhaus A, et al. A soluble form of the receptor for advanced glycation endproducts (RAGE) is produced by proteolytic cleavage of the membrane-bound form by the sheddase a disintegrin and metalloprotease 10 (ADAM10). Faseb J. 2008;22(10):3716-27.

[54] Zhang L, Bukulin M, Kojro E, Roth A, Metz VV, Fahrenholz F, et al. Receptor for advanced glycation end products is subjected to protein ectodomain shedding by metalloproteinases. J Biol Chem. 2008;283(51):35507-16.

[55] Ding Q, Keller JN. Splice variants of the receptor for advanced glycosylation end products (RAGE) in human brain. Neurosci Lett. 2005;373(1):67-72.

[56] Yonekura H, Yamamoto Y, Sakurai S, Petrova RG, Abedin MJ, Li H, et al. Novel splice variants of the receptor for advanced glycation end-products expressed in human vascular endothelial cells and pericytes, and their putative roles in diabetes-induced vascular injury. Biochem J. 2003;370(Pt 3):1097-109.

[57] Park IH, Yeon SI, Youn JH, Choi JE, Sasaki N, Choi IH, et al. Expression of a novel secreted splice variant of the receptor for advanced glycation end products (RAGE) in human brain astrocytes and peripheral blood mononuclear cells. Mol Immunol. 2004;40(16):1203-11.

[58] Kalea AZ, Reiniger N, Yang H, Arriero M, Schmidt AM, Hudson BI. Alternative splicing of the murine receptor for advanced glycation end-products (RAGE) gene. FASEB J. 2009;23(6):1766-74.

[59] Jules J, Maiguel D, Hudson BI. Alternative splicing of the RAGE cytoplasmic domain regulates cell signaling and function. PLoS One. 2013;8(11):e78267.

[60] Deane R, Du Yan S, Submamaryan RK, LaRue B, Jovanovic S, Hogg E, et al. RAGE mediates amyloid-beta peptide transport across the blood-brain barrier and accumulation in brain. Nat Med. 2003;9(7):907-13.

[61] Park L, Raman KG, Lee KJ, Lu Y, Ferran LJ, Jr., Chow WS, et al. Suppression of accelerated diabetic atherosclerosis by the soluble receptor for advanced glycation end-products. Nat Med. 1998;4(9):1025-31.

[62] Yan SS, Wu ZY, Zhang HP, Furtado G, Chen X, Yan SF, et al. Suppression of experimental autoimmune encephalomyelitis by selective blockade of encephalitogenic T-cell infiltration of the central nervous system. Nat Med. 2003;9(3):287-93.

[63] Koch M, Chitayat S, Dattilo BM, Schiefner A, Diez J, Chazin WJ, et al. Structural basis for ligand recognition and activation of RAGE. Structure. 2010;18(10):1342-52.

[64] Emanuele E, D'Angelo A, Tomaino C, Binetti G, Ghidoni R, Politi P, et al. Circulating levels of soluble receptor for advanced glycation end products in Alzheimer disease and vascular dementia. Arch Neurol. 2005;62(11):1734-6.

[65] Nozaki I, Watanabe T, Kawaguchi M, Akatsu H, Tsuneyama K, Yamamoto Y, et al. Reduced expression of endogenous secretory receptor for advanced glycation end-products in hippocampal neurons of Alzheimer's disease brains. Arch Histol Cytol. 2007;70(5):279-90.

[66] Cheng DT, Kim DK, Cockayne DA, Belousov A, Bitter H, Cho MH, et al. Systemic soluble receptor for advanced glycation endproducts is a biomarker of emphysema and associated with AGER genetic variants in patients with chronic obstructive pulmonary disease. Am J Respir Crit Care Med. 2013;188(8):948-57.

[67] Miniati M, Calugi S, Rucci P, Shear MK, Benvenuti A, Santoro D, et al. Predictors of response among patients with panic disorder treated with medications in a naturalistic follow-up: the role of adult separation anxiety. J Affect Disord. 2012;136(3):675-9.

[68] Yan SF, Ramasamy R, Schmidt AM. Soluble RAGE: therapy and biomarker in unraveling the RAGE axis in chronic disease and aging. Biochem Pharmacol. 2010;79(10): 1379-86.

[69] Jing R, Cui M, Wang J, Wang H. Receptor for advanced glycation end products (RAGE) soluble form (sRAGE): a new biomarker for lung cancer. Neoplasma. 2010;57(1):55-61.

[70] Tesarova P, Kalousova M, Jachymova M, Mestek O, Petruzelka L, Zima T. Receptor for advanced glycation end products (RAGE)--soluble form (sRAGE) and gene polymorphisms in patients with breast cancer. Cancer Invest. 2007;25(8):720-5.

[71] Moy KA, Jiao L, Freedman ND, Weinstein SJ, Sinha R, Virtamo J, et al. Soluble receptor for advanced glycation end products and risk of liver cancer. Hepatology. 2013;57(6):2338-45.

[72] Jiao L, Weinstein SJ, Albanes D, Taylor PR, Graubard BI, Virtamo J, et al. Evidence that serum levels of the soluble receptor for advanced glycation end products are inversely associated with pancreatic cancer risk: a prospective study. Cancer Res. 2011;71(10):3582-9.

[73] Leclerc E, Heizmann CW, Vetter SW. RAGE and S100 protein transcription levels are highly variable in human melanoma tumors and cells. General Physiology and Biophysics. 2009;28(Focus Issue):F65-F75.

[74] Neeper M, Schmidt AM, Brett J, Yan SD, Wang F, Pan YC, et al. Cloning and expression of a cell surface receptor for advanced glycosylation end products of proteins. J Biol Chem. 1992;267(21):14998-5004.

[75] Yatime L, Andersen GR. Structural insights into the oligomerization mode of the human receptor for advanced glycation end-products. FEBS J. 2013;280(24):6556-68.

[76] Zong H, Madden A, Ward M, Mooney MH, Elliott CT, Stitt AW. Homodimerization is essential for the receptor for advanced glycation end products (RAGE)-mediated signal transduction. J Biol Chem. 2010;285(30):23137-46.

[77] Xie J, Reverdatto S, Frolov A, Hoffmann R, Burz DS, Shekhtman A. Structural basis for pattern recognition by the receptor for advanced glycation end products (RAGE). J Biol Chem. 2008;283:27255-69.

[78] Xu D, Young JH, Krahn JM, Song D, Corbett KD, Chazin WJ, et al. Stable RAGE-Heparan Sulfate Complexes Are Essential for Signal Transduction. ACS Chem Biol. 2013;8(7):1611-20.

[79] Wei W, Lampe L, Park S, Vangara BS, Waldo GS, Cabantous S, et al. Disulfide bonds within the C2 domain of RAGE play key roles in its dimerization and biogenesis. PLoS One. 2012;7(12):e50736.

[80] Xu D, Young J, Song D, Esko JD. Heparan sulfate is essential for high mobility group protein 1 (HMGB1) signaling by the receptor for advanced glycation end products (RAGE). J Biol Chem. 2011;286(48):41736-44.

[81] Leclerc E, Fritz G, Weibel M, Heizmann CW, Galichet A. S100B and S100A6 differentially modulate cell survival by interacting with distinct RAGE (receptor for advanced glycation end products) immunoglobulin domains. J Biol Chem. 2007;282(43): 31317-31.

[82] Donato R. RAGE: a single receptor for several ligands and different cellular responses: the case of certain S100 proteins. Curr Mol Med. 2007;7(8):711-24.

[83] Logsdon CD, Fuentes MK, Huang EH, Arumugam T. RAGE and RAGE ligands in cancer. Curr Mol Med. 2007;7(8):777-89.

[84] Soman S, Raju R, Sandhya VK, Advani J, Khan AA, Harsha HC, et al. A multicellular signal transduction network of AGE/RAGE signaling. J Cell Commun Signal. 2013;7(1):19-23.

[85] Lander HM, Tauras JM, Ogiste JS, Hori O, Moss RA, Schmidt AM. Activation of the receptor for advanced glycation end products triggers a p21(ras)-dependent mitogen-activated protein kinase pathway regulated by oxidant stress. J Biol Chem. 1997;272(28):17810-4.

[86] Huttunen HJ, Fages C, Rauvala H. Receptor for advanced glycation end products (RAGE)-mediated neurite outgrowth and activation of NF-kappaB require the cytoplasmic domain of the receptor but different downstream signaling pathways. J Biol Chem. 1999;274(28):19919-24.

[87] Brozzi F, Arcuri C, Giambanco I, Donato R. S100B Protein Regulates Astrocyte Shape and Migration via Interaction with Src Kinase: IMPLICATIONS FOR ASTROCYTE DEVELOPMENT, ACTIVATION, AND TUMOR GROWTH. J Biol Chem. 2009;284(13):8797-811.

[88] Bierhaus A, Stern DM, Nawroth PP. RAGE in inflammation: a new therapeutic target? Curr Opin Investig Drugs. 2006;7(11):985-91.

[89] Schmidt AM, Vianna M, Gerlach M, Brett J, Ryan J, Kao J, et al. Isolation and characterization of two binding proteins for advanced glycosylation end products from bovine lung which are present on the endothelial cell surface. J Biol Chem. 1992;267(21): 14987-97.

[90] Basta G, Schmidt AM, De Caterina R. Advanced glycation end products and vascular inflammation: implications for accelerated atherosclerosis in diabetes. Cardiovasc Res. 2004;63(4):582-92.

[91] Yan SF, Ramasamy R, Schmidt AM. The receptor for advanced glycation endproducts (RAGE) and cardiovascular disease. Expert Rev Mol Med. 2009;11:e9.

[92] Srikanth V, Maczurek A, Phan T, Steele M, Westcott B, Juskiw D, et al. Advanced glycation endproducts and their receptor RAGE in Alzheimer's disease. Neurobiol Aging. 2011;32(5):763-77.

[93] Hofmann MA, Drury S, Fu C, Qu W, Taguchi A, Lu Y, et al. RAGE mediates a novel proinflammatory axis: a central cell surface receptor for S100/calgranulin polypeptides. Cell. 1999;97(7):889-901.

[94] Donato R, Cannon BR, Sorci G, Riuzzi F, Hsu K, Weber DJ, et al. Functions of S100 proteins. Curr Mol Med. 2013;13(1):24-57.

[95] Chen H, Xu C, Jin Q, Liu Z. S100 protein family in human cancer. Am J Cancer Res. 2014;4(2):89-115.

[96] Hori O, Brett J, Slattery T, Cao R, Zhang J, Chen JX, et al. The receptor for advanced glycation end products (RAGE) is a cellular binding site for amphoterin. Mediation of neurite outgrowth and co-expression of rage and amphoterin in the developing nervous system. J Biol Chem. 1995;270(43):25752-61.

[97] Huttunen HJ, Rauvala H. Amphoterin as an extracellular regulator of cell motility: from discovery to disease. J Intern Med. 2004;255(3):351-66.

[98] Lotze MT, Tracey KJ. High-mobility group box 1 protein (HMGB1): nuclear weapon in the immune arsenal. Nat Rev Immunol. 2005;5(4):331-42.

[99] Enokido Y, Yoshitake A, Ito H, Okazawa H. Age-dependent change of HMGB1 and DNA double-strand break accumulation in mouse brain. Biochem Biophys Res Commun. 2008;376(1):128-33.

[100] Sousa MM, Yan SD, Stern D, Saraiva MJ. Interaction of the receptor for advanced glycation end products (RAGE) with transthyretin triggers nuclear transcription factor kB (NF-kB) activation. Lab Invest. 2000;80(7):1101-10.

[101] Sasaki N, Takeuchi M, Chowei H, Kikuchi S, Hayashi Y, Nakano N, et al. Advanced glycation end products (AGE) and their receptor (RAGE) in the brain of patients with Creutzfeldt-Jakob disease with prion plaques. Neurosci Lett. 2002;326(2):117-20.

[102] Natale G, Ferrucci M, Lazzeri G, Paparelli A, Fornai F. Transmission of prions within the gut and towards the central nervous system. Prion. 2011;5(3):142-9.

[103] Bullard DC, Hu X, Schoeb TR, Axtell RC, Raman C, Barnum SR. Critical requirement of CD11b (Mac-1) on T cells and accessory cells for development of experimental autoimmune encephalomyelitis. J Immunol. 2005;175(10):6327-33.

[104] Ruan BH, Li X, Winkler AR, Cunningham KM, Kuai J, Greco RM, et al. Complement C3a, CpG oligos, and DNA/C3a complex stimulate IFN-alpha production in a receptor for advanced glycation end product-dependent manner. J Immunol. 2010;185(7): 4213-22.

[105] Ma W, Rai V, Hudson BI, Song F, Schmidt AM, Barile GR. RAGE binds C1q and enhances C1q-mediated phagocytosis. Cell Immunol. 2012;274(1-2):72-82.

[106] He M, Kubo H, Morimoto K, Fujino N, Suzuki T, Takahasi T, et al. Receptor for advanced glycation end products binds to phosphatidylserine and assists in the clearance of apoptotic cells. EMBO Rep. 2011;12(4):358-64.

[107] Fischer U, Schulze-Osthoff K. New approaches and therapeutics targeting apoptosis in disease. Pharmacol Rev. 2005;57(2):187-215.

[108] Mizumoto S, Sugahara K. Glycosaminoglycans are functional ligands for receptor for advanced glycation end-products in tumors. FEBS J. 2013;280(10):2462-70.

[109] Lindahl U, Kjellen L. Pathophysiology of heparan sulphate: many diseases, few drugs. J Intern Med. 2013;273(6):555-71.

[110] Sirois CM, Jin T, Miller AL, Bertheloot D, Nakamura H, Horvath GL, et al. RAGE is a nucleic acid receptor that promotes inflammatory responses to DNA. J Exp Med. 2013;210(11):2447-63.

[111] Heizmann CW, Fritz G, Schäfer BW. S100 proteins: structure, functions and pathology. Front Biosci. 2002;7:d1356-68.

[112] Donato R. Intracellular and extracellular roles of S100 proteins. Microsc Res Tech. 2003;60(6):540-51.

[113] Marenholz I, Lovering RC, Heizmann CW. An update of the S100 nomenclature. Biochim Biophys Acta. 2006;1763(11):1282-3.

[114] Heizmann CW, Ackermann GE, Galichet A. Pathologies involving the S100 proteins and RAGE. Subcell Biochem. 2007;45:93-138.

[115] Zimmer DB, Weber DJ. The Calcium-Dependent Interaction of S100B with Its Protein Targets. Cardiovasc Psychiatry Neurol. 2010;2010.

[116] Moroz OV, Wilson KS, Bronstein IB. The role of zinc in the S100 proteins: insights from the X-ray structures. Amino Acids 2010:in press.

[117] Fritz G, Heizmann CW. 3D Structures of the Calcium and Zinc Binding S100 Proteins. In: Sons JW, editor. Encyclopedia of Inorganic and Bioinorganic Chemistry: Wiley Online Library; 2011.

[118] Nelson MR, Thulin E, Fagan PA, Forsen S, Chazin WJ. The EF-hand domain: a globally cooperative structural unit. Protein Sci. 2002;11(2):198-205.

[119] Leclerc E, Heizmann CW. The importance of Ca2+/Zn2+signaling S100 proteins and RAGE in translational medicine. Frontiers in Biosciences. 2011;S3:1232-62.

[120] Santamaria-Kisiel L, Rintala-Dempsey AC, Shaw GS. Calcium-dependent and-independent interactions of the S100 protein family. Biochem J. 2006;396(2):201-14.

[121] Baudier J, Delphin C, Grunwald D, Khochbin S, Lawrence JJ. Characterization of the tumor suppressor protein p53 as a protein kinase C substrate and a S100b-binding protein. Proc Natl Acad Sci U S A. 1992;89(23):11627-31.

[122] Wilder PT, Lin J, Bair CL, Charpentier TH, Yang D, Liriano M, et al. Recognition of the tumor suppressor protein p53 and other protein targets by the calcium-binding protein S100B. Biochim Biophys Acta. 2006;1763(11):1284-97.

[123] Mueller A, Schäfer BW, Ferrari S, Weibel M, Makek M, Hochli M, et al. The calcium-binding protein S100A2 interacts with p53 and modulates its transcriptional activity. J Biol Chem. 2005;280(32):29186-93.

[124] Fernandez-Fernandez MR, Rutherford TJ, Fersht AR. Members of the S100 family bind p53 in two distinct ways. Protein Sci. 2008;17(10):1663-70.

[125] van Dieck J, Teufel DP, Jaulent AM, Fernandez-Fernandez MR, Rutherford TJ, Wyslouch-Cieszynska A, et al. Posttranslational modifications affect the interaction of S100 proteins with tumor suppressor p53. J Mol Biol. 2009;394(5):922-30.

[126] van Dieck J, Fernandez-Fernandez MR, Veprintsev DB, Fersht AR. Modulation of the oligomerization state of p53 by differential binding of proteins of the S100 family to p53 monomers and tetramers. J Biol Chem. 2009;284(20):13804-11.

[127] Hsieh HL, Schäfer BW, Weigle B, Heizmann CW. S100 protein translocation in response to extracellular S100 is mediated by receptor for advanced glycation endproducts in human endothelial cells. Biochem Biophys Res Commun. 2004;316(3):949-59.

[128] Perrone L, Peluso G, Melone MA. RAGE recycles at the plasma membrane in S100B secretory vesicles and promotes Schwann cells morphological changes. J Cell Physiol. 2008;217(1):60-71.

[129] Leclerc E, Fritz G, Vetter SW, Heizmann CW. Binding of S100 proteins to RAGE: an update. Biochim Biophys Acta. 2009;1793(6):993-1007.

[130] Eckert RL, Broome AM, Ruse M, Robinson N, Ryan D, Lee K. S100 proteins in the epidermis. Journal of Investigative Dermatology. 2004;123(1):23-33.

[131] Ito M, Kizawa K. Expression of calcium-binding S100 proteins A4 and A6 in regions of the epithelial sac associated with the onset of hair follicle regeneration. J Invest Dermatol. 2001;116(6):956-63.

[132] Boni R, Burg G, Doguoglu A, Ilg EC, Schafer BW, Muller B, et al. Immunohistochemical localization of the Ca2+binding S100 proteins in normal human skin and melanocytic lesions. Br J Dermatol. 1997;137(1):39-43.

[133] Ribe A, McNutt NS. S100A6 protein expression is different in Spitz nevi and melanomas. Mod Pathol. 2003;16(5):505-11.

[134] Zhang T, Woods TL, Elder JT. Differential responses of S100A2 to oxidative stress and increased intracellular calcium in normal, immortalized, and malignant human keratinocytes. J Invest Dermatol. 2002;119(5):1196-201.

[135] Deshpande R, Woods TL, Fu J, Zhang T, Stoll SW, Elder JT. Biochemical characterization of S100A2 in human keratinocytes: subcellular localization, dimerization, and oxidative cross-linking. J Invest Dermatol. 2000;115(3):477-85.

[136] Broome AM, Ryan D, Eckert RL. S100 protein subcellular localization during epidermal differentiation and psoriasis. Journal of Histochemistry & Cytochemistry. 2003;51(5):675-85.

[137] Robinson MJ, Tessier P, Poulsom R, Hogg N. The S100 family heterodimer, MRP-8/14, binds with high affinity to heparin and heparan sulfate glycosaminoglycans on endothelial cells. J Biol Chem. 2002;277(5):3658-65.

[138] Mirmohammadsadegh A, Tschakarjan E, Ljoljic A, Bohner K, Michel G, Ruzicka T, et al. Calgranulin C is overexpressed in lesional psoriasis. Journal of Investigative Dermatology. 2000;114(6):1207-8.

[139] Balch CM, Gershenwald JE, Soong SJ, Thompson JF, Atkins MB, Byrd DR, et al. Final version of 2009 AJCC melanoma staging and classification. J Clin Oncol. 2009;27(36): 6199-206.

[140] Ghanem G, Loir B, Morandini R, Sales F, Lienard D, Eggermont A, et al. On the release and half-life of S100B protein in the peripheral blood of melanoma patients. Int J Cancer. 2001;94(4):586-90.

[141] Harpio R, Einarsson R. S100 proteins as cancer biomarkers with focus on S100B in malignant melanoma. Clin Biochem. 2004;37(7):512-8.

[142] Lin J, Blake M, Tang C, Zimmer D, Rustandi RR, Weber DJ, et al. Inhibition of p53 transcriptional activity by the S100B calcium-binding protein. J Biol Chem. 2001;276(37):35037-41.

[143] Lin J, Yang Q, Wilder PT, Carrier F, Weber DJ. The calcium-binding protein S100B down-regulates p53 and apoptosis in malignant melanoma. J Biol Chem. 2010;285(35):27487-98.

[144] Lin J, Yang Q, Yan Z, Markowitz J, Wilder PT, Carrier F, et al. Inhibiting S100B restores p53 levels in primary malignant melanoma cancer cells. J Biol Chem. 2004;279(32):34071-7.

[145] Cavalier M, Wilder PT, Coop A, MacKerell A, Weber DJ, editors. Inhibitors of S100B (SBiXs) in malignant melanoma. AACR-NCI-EORTC International Conference: Molecular Targets and Cancer Therapeutics; 2013; Boston, MA: Mol Cancer Ther.

[146] Zimmer DB, Van Eldik LJ. Identification of a molecular target for the calcium-modulated protein S100. Fructose-1,6-bisphosphate aldolase. J Biol Chem. 1986;261(24): 11424-8.

[147] Hersey P, Watts RN, Zhang XD, Hackett J. Metabolic approaches to treatment of melanoma. Clin Cancer Res. 2009;15(21):6490-4.

[148] Xu RH, Pelicano H, Zhou Y, Carew JS, Feng L, Bhalla KN, et al. Inhibition of glycolysis in cancer cells: a novel strategy to overcome drug resistance associated with mitochondrial respiratory defect and hypoxia. Cancer Res. 2005;65(2):613-21.

[149] Donato R. Calcium-independent, pH-regulated effects of S-100 proteins on assembly-disassembly of brain microtubule protein in vitro. J Biol Chem. 1988;263(1):106-10.

[150] Ferguson PL, Shaw GS. Human S100B protein interacts with the Escherichia coli division protein FtsZ in a calcium-sensitive manner. J Biol Chem. 2004;279(18):18806-13.

[151] Skripnikova EV, Gusev NB. Interaction of smooth muscle caldesmon with S-100 protein. FEBS Lett. 1989;257(2):380-2.

[152] Mbele GO, Deloulme JC, Gentil BJ, Delphin C, Ferro M, Garin J, et al. The zinc-and calcium-binding S100B interacts and co-localizes with IQGAP1 during dynamic rearrangement of cell membranes. J Biol Chem. 2002;277(51):49998-50007.

[153] Koganehira Y, Takeoka M, Ehara T, Sasaki K, Murata H, Saida T, et al. Reduced expression of actin-binding proteins, h-caldesmon and calponin h1, in the vascular smooth muscle inside melanoma lesions: an adverse prognostic factor for malignant melanoma. Br J Dermatol. 2003;148(5):971-80.

[154] Wang Z, Chen J, Wang J, Ahn S, Li CM, Lu Y, et al. Novel tubulin polymerization inhibitors overcome multidrug resistance and reduce melanoma lung metastasis. Pharm Res. 2012;29(11):3040-52.

[155] Jameson KL, Mazur PK, Zehnder AM, Zhang J, Zarnegar B, Sage J, et al. IQGAP1 scaffold-kinase interaction blockade selectively targets RAS-MAP kinase-driven tumors. Nat Med. 2013;19(5):626-30.

[156] Bhattacharya S, Large E, Heizmann CW, Hemmings B, Chazin WJ. Structure of the Ca2+/S100B/NDR kinase peptide complex: insights into S100 target specificity and activation of the kinase. Biochemistry. 2003;42(49):14416-26.

[157] Bichsel SJ, Tamaskovic R, Stegert MR, Hemmings BA. Mechanism of activation of NDR (nuclear Dbf2-related) protein kinase by the hMOB1 protein. J Biol Chem. 2004;279(34):35228-35.

[158] Millward TA, Heizmann CW, Schafer BW, Hemmings BA. Calcium regulation of Ndr protein kinase mediated by S100 calcium-binding proteins. Embo J. 1998;17(20): 5913-22.

[159] Gentil BJ, Delphin C, Mbele GO, Deloulme JC, Ferro M, Garin J, et al. The giant protein AHNAK is a specific target for the calcium-and zinc-binding S100B protein: po-

tential implications for Ca2+homeostasis regulation by S100B. J Biol Chem. 2001;276(26):23253-61.

[160] Shtivelman E, Bishop JM. The human gene AHNAK encodes a large phosphoprotein located primarily in the nucleus. J Cell Biol. 1993;120(3):625-30.

[161] Fedida-Metula S, Elhyany S, Tsory S, Segal S, Hershfinkel M, Sekler I, et al. Targeting lipid rafts inhibits protein kinase B by disrupting calcium homeostasis and attenuates malignant properties of melanoma cells. Carcinogenesis. 2008;29(8):1546-54.

[162] Donato R, Sorci G, Riuzzi F, Arcuri C, Bianchi R, Brozzi F, et al. S100B's double life: intracellular regulator and extracellular signal. Biochim Biophys Acta. 2009;1793(6): 1008-22.

[163] Ostendorp T, Leclerc E, Galichet A, Koch M, Demling N, Weigle B, et al. Structural and functional insights into RAGE activation by multimeric S100B. Embo J. 2007;26(16):3868-78.

[164] Glenney JR, Jr., Kindy MS, Zokas L. Isolation of a new member of the S100 protein family: amino acid sequence, tissue, and subcellular distribution. J Cell Biol. 1989;108(2):569-78.

[165] Maelandsmo GM, Florenes VA, Mellingsaeter T, Hovig E, Kerbel RS, Fodstad O. Differential expression patterns of S100A2, S100A4 and S100A6 during progression of human malignant melanoma. Int J Cancer. 1997;74(4):464-9.

[166] Gupta S, Hussain T, MacLennan GT, Fu P, Patel J, Mukhtar H. Differential expression of S100A2 and S100A4 during progression of human prostate adenocarcinoma. J Clin Oncol. 2003;21(1):106-12.

[167] Suzuki F, Oridate N, Homma A, Nakamaru Y, Nagahashi T, Yagi K, et al. S100A2 expression as a predictive marker for late cervical metastasis in stage I and II invasive squamous cell carcinoma of the oral cavity. Oncol Rep. 2005;14(6):1493-8.

[168] Feng G, Xu X, Youssef EM, Lotan R. Diminished expression of S100A2, a putative tumor suppressor, at early stage of human lung carcinogenesis. Cancer Res. 2001;61(21):7999-8004.

[169] Lee SW, Tomasetto C, Swisshelm K, Keyomarsi K, Sager R. Down-regulation of a member of the S100 gene family in mammary carcinoma cells and reexpression by azadeoxycytidine treatment. Proc Natl Acad Sci U S A. 1992;89(6):2504-8.

[170] Imazawa M, Hibi K, Fujitake S, Kodera Y, Ito K, Akiyama S, et al. S100A2 overexpression is frequently observed in esophageal squamous cell carcinoma. Anticancer Res. 2005;25:1247-50.

[171] El-Rifai W, Moskaluk CA, Abdrabbo MK, Harper J, Yoshida C, Riggins GJ, et al. Gastric cancers overexpress S100A calcium-binding proteins. Cancer Res. 2002;62(23): 6823-6.

[172] Hough CD, Cho KR, Zonderman AB, Schwartz DR, Morin PJ. Coordinately up-regulated genes in ovarian cancer. Cancer Res. 2001;61(10):3869-76.

[173] Smith SL, Gugger M, Hoban P, Ratschiller D, Watson SG, Field JK, et al. S100A2 is strongly expressed in airway basal cells, preneoplastic bronchial lesions and primary non-small cell lung carcinomas. Br J Cancer. 2004;91(8):1515-24.

[174] Strazisar M, Mlakar V, Glavac D. The expression of COX-2, hTERT, MDM2, LATS2 and S100A2 in different types of non-small cell lung cancer (NSCLC). Cell Mol Biol Lett. 2009;14(3):442-56.

[175] Bulk E, Sargin B, Krug U, Hascher A, Jun Y, Knop M, et al. S100A2 induces metastasis in non-small cell lung cancer. Clin Cancer Res. 2009;15(1):22-9.

[176] Nonaka D, Chiriboga L, Rubin BP. Differential expression of S100 protein subtypes in malignant melanoma, and benign and malignant peripheral nerve sheath tumors. J Cutan Pathol. 2008;35(11):1014-9.

[177] Gollob JA, Sciambi CJ. Decitabine up-regulates S100A2 expression and synergizes with IFN-gamma to kill uveal melanoma cells. Clin Cancer Res. 2007;13(17):5219-25.

[178] Klopper JP, Sharma V, Bissonnette R, Haugen BR. Combination PPARgamma and RXR Agonist Treatment in Melanoma Cells: Functional Importance of S100A2. PPAR Res. 2010;2010:729876.

[179] Tan M, Heizmann CW, Guan K, Schafer BW, Sun Y. Transcriptional activation of the human S100A2 promoter by wild-type p53. FEBS Lett. 1999;445(2-3):265-8.

[180] Lapi E, Iovino A, Fontemaggi G, Soliera AR, Iacovelli S, Sacchi A, et al. S100A2 gene is a direct transcriptional target of p53 homologues during keratinocyte differentiation. Oncogene. 2006;25(26):3628-37.

[181] Kirschner RD, Sanger K, Muller GA, Engeland K. Transcriptional activation of the tumor suppressor and differentiation gene S100A2 by a novel p63-binding site. Nucleic Acids Res. 2008;36(9):2969-80.

[182] Buckley NE, D'Costa Z, Kaminska M, Mullan PB. S100A2 is a BRCA1/p63 coregulated tumour suppressor gene with roles in the regulation of mutant p53 stability. Cell death & disease. 2014;5:e1070.

[183] Harbour JW, Onken MD, Roberson ED, Duan S, Cao L, Worley LA, et al. Frequent mutation of BAP1 in metastasizing uveal melanomas. Science. 2010;330(6009):1410-3.

[184] Carbone M, Ferris LK, Baumann F, Napolitano A, Lum CA, Flores EG, et al. BAP1 cancer syndrome: malignant mesothelioma, uveal and cutaneous melanoma, and MBAITs. J Transl Med. 2012;10:179.

[185] Njauw CN, Kim I, Piris A, Gabree M, Taylor M, Lane AM, et al. Germline BAP1 inactivation is preferentially associated with metastatic ocular melanoma and cutaneous-ocular melanoma families. PLoS One. 2012;7(4):e35295.

[186] Ebralidze A, Tulchinsky E, Grigorian M, Afanasyeva A, Senin V, Revazova E, et al. Isolation and characterization of a gene specifically expressed in different metastatic cells and whose deduced gene product has a high degree of homology to a Ca^{2+}-binding protein family. Genes Dev. 1989;3(7):1086-93.

[187] Takenaga K, Nakamura Y, Endo H, Sakiyama S. Involvement of S100-related calcium-binding protein pEL98 (or mts1) in cell motility and tumor cell invasion. Japanese journal of cancer research : Gann. 1994;85(8):831-9.

[188] Jenkinson SR, Barraclough R, West CR, Rudland PS. S100A4 regulates cell motility and invasion in an in vitro model for breast cancer metastasis. Br J Cancer. 2004;90(1): 253-62.

[189] Grum-Schwensen B, Klingelhofer J, Berg CH, El-Naaman C, Grigorian M, Lukanidin E, et al. Suppression of tumor development and metastasis formation in mice lacking the S100A4(mts1) gene. Cancer Res. 2005;65(9):3772-80.

[190] Ambartsumian N, Grigorian M, Lukanidin E. Genetically modified mouse models to study the role of metastasis-promoting S100A4(mts1) protein in metastatic mammary cancer. J Dairy Res. 2005;72 Spec No:27-33.

[191] Andersen K, Nesland JM, Holm R, Florenes VA, Fodstad O, Maelandsmo GM. Expression of S100A4 combined with reduced E-cadherin expression predicts patient outcome in malignant melanoma. Mod Pathol. 2004;17(8):990-7.

[192] Boye K, Maelandsmo GM. S100A4 and metastasis: a small actor playing many roles. Am J Pathol. 2010;176(2):528-35.

[193] Fernandez-Fernandez MR, Veprintsev DB, Fersht AR. Proteins of the S100 family regulate the oligomerization of p53 tumor suppressor. Proc Natl Acad Sci U S A. 2005;102(13):4735-40.

[194] Berge G, Maelandsmo GM. Evaluation of potential interactions between the metastasis-associated protein S100A4 and the tumor suppressor protein p53. Amino Acids. 2010:in press.

[195] Orre LM, Panizza E, Kaminskyy VO, Vernet E, Graslund T, Zhivotovsky B, et al. S100A4 interacts with p53 in the nucleus and promotes p53 degradation. Oncogene. 2013;32(49):5531-40.

[196] Ford HL, Zain SB. Interaction of metastasis associated Mts1 protein with nonmuscle myosin. Oncogene. 1995;10(8):1597-605.

[197] Takenaga K, Nakamura Y, Sakiyama S, Hasegawa Y, Sato K, Endo H. Binding of pEL98 protein, an S100-related calcium-binding protein, to nonmuscle tropomyosin. J Cell Biol. 1994;124(5):757-68.

[198] Li ZH, Bresnick AR. The S100A4 metastasis factor regulates cellular motility via a direct interaction with myosin-IIA. Cancer Res. 2006;66(10):5173-80.

[199] Kriajevska M, Bronstein IB, Scott DJ, Tarabykina S, Fischer-Larsen M, Issinger O, et al. Metastasis-associated protein Mts1 (S100A4) inhibits CK2-mediated phosphorylation and self-assembly of the heavy chain of nonmuscle myosin. Biochim Biophys Acta. 2000;1498(2-3):252-63.

[200] Cabezon T, Celis JE, Skibshoj I, Klingelhofer J, Grigorian M, Gromov P, et al. Expression of S100A4 by a variety of cell types present in the tumor microenvironment of human breast cancer. Int J Cancer. 2007;121(7):1433-44.

[201] Kikuchi N, Horiuchi A, Osada R, Imai T, Wang C, Chen X, et al. Nuclear expression of S100A4 is associated with aggressive behavior of epithelial ovarian carcinoma: an important autocrine/paracrine factor in tumor progression. Cancer Sci. 2006;97(10): 1061-9.

[202] Pedersen KB, Andersen K, Fodstad O, Maelandsmo GM. Sensitization of interferon-gamma induced apoptosis in human osteosarcoma cells by extracellular S100A4. BMC Cancer. 2004;4:52.

[203] Schmidt-Hansen B, Klingelhofer J, Grum-Schwensen B, Christensen A, Andresen S, Kruse C, et al. Functional significance of metastasis-inducing S100A4(Mts1) in tumor-stroma interplay. J Biol Chem. 2004;279(23):24498-504.

[204] Gibbs FE, Barraclough R, Platt-Higgins A, Rudland PS, Wilkinson MC, Parry EW. Immunocytochemical distribution of the calcium-binding protein p9Ka in normal rat tissues: variation in the cellular location in different tissues. J Histochem Cytochem. 1995;43(2):169-80.

[205] Ambartsumian N, Klingelhofer J, Grigorian M, Christensen C, Kriajevska M, Tulchinsky E, et al. The metastasis-associated Mts1(S100A4) protein could act as an angiogenic factor. Oncogene. 2001;20(34):4685-95.

[206] Ochiya T, Takenaga K, Endo H. Silencing of S100A4, a metastasis-associated protein, in endothelial cells inhibits tumor angiogenesis and growth. Angiogenesis. 2014;17(1):17-26.

[207] Schmidt-Hansen B, Ornas D, Grigorian M, Klingelhofer J, Tulchinsky E, Lukanidin E, et al. Extracellular S100A4(mts1) stimulates invasive growth of mouse endothelial cells and modulates MMP-13 matrix metalloproteinase activity. Oncogene. 2004;23(32):5487-95.

[208] Semov A, Moreno MJ, Onichtchenko A, Abulrob A, Ball M, Ekiel I, et al. Metastasis-associated protein S100A4 induces angiogenesis through interaction with Annexin II and accelerated plasmin formation. J Biol Chem. 2005;280(21):20833-41.

[209] Kiryushko D, Novitskaya V, Soroka V, Klingelhofer J, Lukanidin E, Berezin V, et al. Molecular mechanisms of Ca^{2+}signaling in neurons induced by the S100A4 protein. Mol Cell Biol. 2006;26(9):3625-38.

[210] Spiekerkoetter E, Guignabert C, de Jesus Perez V, Alastalo TP, Powers JM, Wang L, et al. S100A4 and bone morphogenetic protein-2 codependently induce vascular

smooth muscle cell migration via phospho-extracellular signal-regulated kinase and chloride intracellular channel 4. Circ Res. 2009;105(7):639-47, 13 p following 47.

[211] Dahlmann M, Okhrimenko A, Marcinkowski P, Osterland M, Herrmann P, Smith J, et al. RAGE mediates S100A4-induced cell motility via MAPK/ERK and hypoxia signaling and is a prognostic biomarker for human colorectal cancer metastasis. Oncotarget. 2014;5(10):3220-33.

[212] Siddique HR, Adhami VM, Parray A, Johnson JJ, Siddiqui IA, Shekhani MT, et al. The S100A4 Oncoprotein Promotes Prostate Tumorigenesis in a Transgenic Mouse Model: Regulating NFkappaB through the RAGE Receptor. Genes & cancer. 2013;4(5-6):224-34.

[213] Haase-Kohn C, Wolf S, Herwig N, Mosch B, Pietzsch J. Metastatic potential of B16-F10 melanoma cells is enhanced by extracellular S100A4 derived from RAW264.7 macrophages. Biochem Biophys Res Commun. 2014;446(1):143-8.

[214] Weterman MA, van Muijen GN, Bloemers HP, Ruiter DJ. Expression of calcyclin in human melanocytic lesions. Cancer Res. 1993;53(24):6061-6.

[215] Kuznicki J, Kordowska J, Puzianowska M, Wozniewicz BM. Calcyclin as a marker of human epithelial cells and fibroblasts. Exp Cell Res. 1992;200(2):425-30.

[216] Kuznicki J, Filipek A, Heimann P, Kaczmarek L, Kaminska B. Tissue specific distribution of calcyclin--10.5 kDa Ca2+-binding protein. FEBS Lett. 1989;254(1-2):141-4.

[217] Lesniak W, Slomnicki LP, Filipek A. S100A6-new facts and features. Biochem Biophys Res Commun. 2009;390(4):1087-92.

[218] Komatsu K, Andoh A, Ishiguro S, Suzuki N, Hunai H, Kobune-Fujiwara Y, et al. Increased expression of S100A6 (Calcyclin), a calcium-binding protein of the S100 family, in human colorectal adenocarcinomas. Clin Cancer Res. 2000;6(1):172-7.

[219] Nedjadi T, Kitteringham N, Campbell F, Jenkins RE, Park BK, Navarro P, et al. S100A6 binds to annexin 2 in pancreatic cancer cells and promotes pancreatic cancer cell motility. Br J Cancer. 2009;101(7):1145-54.

[220] De Petris L, Orre LM, Kanter L, Pernemalm M, Koyi H, Lewensohn R, et al. Tumor expression of S100A6 correlates with survival of patients with stage I non-small-cell lung cancer. Lung Cancer. 2009;63:410-7.

[221] Ohuchida K, Mizumoto K, Yu J, Yamaguchi H, Konomi H, Nagai E, et al. S100A6 is increased in a stepwise manner during pancreatic carcinogenesis: clinical value of expression analysis in 98 pancreatic juice samples. Cancer Epidemiol Biomarkers Prev. 2007;16(4):649-54.

[222] Yang YQ, Zhang LJ, Dong H, Jiang CL, Zhu ZG, Wu JX, et al. Upregulated expression of S100A6 in human gastric cancer. J Dig Dis. 2007;8(4):186-93.

[223] Vimalachandran D, Greenhalf W, Thompson C, Luttges J, Prime W, Campbell F, et al. High nuclear S100A6 (Calcyclin) is significantly associated with poor survival in pancreatic cancer patients. Cancer Res. 2005;65(8):3218-25.

[224] Li Z, Tang M, Ling B, Liu S, Zheng Y, Nie C, et al. Increased expression of S100A6 promotes cell proliferation and migration in human hepatocellular carcinoma. Journal of molecular medicine. 2014;92(3):291-303.

[225] Weterman MA, Stoopen GM, van Muijen GN, Kuznicki J, Ruiter DJ, Bloemers HP. Expression of calcyclin in human melanoma cell lines correlates with metastatic behavior in nude mice. Cancer Res. 1992;52(5):1291-6.

[226] Fullen DR, Garrisi AJ, Sanders D, Thomas D. Expression of S100A6 protein in a broad spectrum of cutaneous tumors using tissue microarrays. J Cutan Pathol. 2008;35 Suppl 2:28-34.

[227] Puri PK, Elston CA, Tyler WB, Ferringer TC, Elston DM. The staining pattern of pigmented spindle cell nevi with S100A6 protein. J Cutan Pathol. 2011;38(1):14-7.

[228] Slomnicki LP, Nawrot B, Lesniak W. S100A6 binds p53 and affects its activity. Int J Biochem Cell Biol. 2009;41(4):784-90.

[229] Streicher WW, Lopez MM, Makhatadze GI. Annexin I and annexin II N-terminal peptides binding to S100 protein family members: specificity and thermodynamic characterization. Biochemistry. 2009;48(12):2788-98.

[230] Mohan SK, Gupta AA, Yu C. Interaction of the S100A6 mutant (C3S) with the V domain of the receptor for advanced glycation end products (RAGE). Biochem Biophys Res Commun. 2013;434(2):328-33.

[231] Roth J, Vogl T, Sorg C, Sunderkotter C. Phagocyte-specific S100 proteins: a novel group of proinflammatory molecules. Trends Immunol. 2003;24(4):155-8.

[232] Yin C, Li H, Zhang B, Liu Y, Lu G, Lu S, et al. RAGE-binding S100A8/A9 promotes the migration and invasion of human breast cancer cells through actin polymerization and epithelial-mesenchymal transition. Breast Cancer Res Treat. 2013;142(2): 297-309.

[233] Grebhardt S, Muller-Decker K, Bestvater F, Hershfinkel M, Mayer D. Impact of S100A8/A9 expression on prostate cancer progression in vitro and in vivo. J Cell Physiol. 2014;229(5):661-71.

[234] Khammanivong A, Wang C, Sorenson BS, Ross KF, Herzberg MC. S100A8/A9 (calprotectin) negatively regulates G2/M cell cycle progression and growth of squamous cell carcinoma. PLoS One. 2013;8(7):e69395.

[235] Kwon CH, Moon HJ, Park HJ, Choi JH, Park do Y. S100A8 and S100A9 promotes invasion and migration through p38 mitogen-activated protein kinase-dependent NF-kappaB activation in gastric cancer cells. Mol Cells. 2013;35(3):226-34.

[236] Ehrchen JM, Sunderkotter C, Foell D, Vogl T, Roth J. The endogenous Toll-like receptor 4 agonist S100A8/S100A9 (calprotectin) as innate amplifier of infection, autoimmunity, and cancer. J Leukoc Biol. 2009;86(3):557-66.

[237] Ghavami S, Chitayat S, Hashemi M, Eshraghi M, Chazin WJ, Halayko AJ, et al. S100A8/A9: a Janus-faced molecule in cancer therapy and tumorgenesis. Eur J Pharmacol. 2009;625(1-3):73-83.

[238] Ang CW, Nedjadi T, Sheikh AA, Tweedle EM, Tonack S, Honap S, et al. Smad4 loss is associated with fewer S100A8-positive monocytes in colorectal tumors and attenuated response to S100A8 in colorectal and pancreatic cancer cells. Carcinogenesis. 2010;31(9):1541-51.

[239] Sinha P, Okoro C, Foell D, Freeze HH, Ostrand-Rosenberg S, Srikrishna G. Proinflammatory S100 proteins regulate the accumulation of myeloid-derived suppressor cells. J Immunol. 2008;181(7):4666-75.

[240] Srikrishna G. S100A8 and S100A9: new insights into their roles in malignancy. Journal of innate immunity. 2012;4(1):31-40.

[241] Wang L, Chang EW, Wong SC, Ong SM, Chong DQ, Ling KL. Increased myeloid-derived suppressor cells in gastric cancer correlate with cancer stage and plasma S100A8/A9 proinflammatory proteins. J Immunol. 2013;190(2):794-804.

[242] Basso D, Fogar P, Plebani M. The S100A8/A9 complex reduces CTLA4 expression by immature myeloid cells: Implications for pancreatic cancer-driven immunosuppression. Oncoimmunology. 2013;2(6):e24441.

[243] Burke M, Choksawangkarn W, Edwards N, Ostrand-Rosenberg S, Fenselau C. Exosomes from myeloid-derived suppressor cells carry biologically active proteins. J Proteome Res. 2014;13(2):836-43.

[244] Petersson S, Shubbar E, Enerback L, Enerback C. Expression patterns of S100 proteins in melanocytes and melanocytic lesions. Melanoma Res. 2009;19(4):215-25.

[245] Hibino T, Sakaguchi M, Miyamoto S, Yamamoto M, Motoyama A, Hosoi J, et al. S100A9 is a novel ligand of EMMPRIN that promotes melanoma metastasis. Cancer Res. 2013;73(1):172-83.

[246] Meyer C, Sevko A, Ramacher M, Bazhin AV, Falk CS, Osen W, et al. Chronic inflammation promotes myeloid-derived suppressor cell activation blocking antitumor immunity in transgenic mouse melanoma model. Proc Natl Acad Sci U S A. 2011;108(41):17111-6.

[247] Vogl T, Tenbrock K, Ludwig S, Leukert N, Ehrhardt C, van Zoelen MA, et al. MRP8 and MRP14 are endogenous activators of Toll-like receptor 4, promoting lethal, endotoxin-induced shock. Nat Med. 2007;13(9):1042-9.

[248] Ghavami S, Rashedi I, Dattilo BM, Eshraghi M, Chazin WJ, Hashemi M, et al. S100A8/A9 at low concentration promotes tumor cell growth via RAGE ligation and MAP kinase-dependent pathway. J Leukoc Biol. 2008;83(6):1484-92.

[249] Turovskaya O, Foell D, Sinha P, Vogl T, Newlin R, Nayak J, et al. RAGE, carboxylated glycans and S100A8/A9 play essential roles in colitis-associated carcinogenesis. Carcinogenesis. 2008;29:2035-43.

[250] Srikrishna G, Panneerselvam K, Westphal V, Abraham V, Varki A, Freeze HH. Two proteins modulating transendothelial migration of leukocytes recognize novel carboxylated glycans on endothelial cells. J Immunol. 2001;166(7):4678-88.

[251] Srikrishna G, Nayak J, Weigle B, Temme A, Foell D, Hazelwood L, et al. Carboxylated N-glycans on RAGE promote S100A12 binding and signaling. J Cell Biochem. 2010;110(3):645-59.

[252] Hagens G, Masouye I, Augsburger E, Hotz R, Saurat JH, Siegenthaler G. Calcium-binding protein S100A7 and epidermal-type fatty acid-binding protein are associated in the cytosol of human keratinocytes. Biochemical Journal. 1999;339:419-27.

[253] Semprini S, Capon F, Tacconelli A, Giardina E, Orecchia A, Mingarelli R, et al. Evidence for differential S100 gene over-expression in psoriatic patients from genetically heterogeneous pedigrees. Hum Genet. 2002;111(4-5):310-3.

[254] Brouard MC, Saurat JH, Ghanem G, Siegenthaler G. Urinary excretion of epidermal-type fatty acid-binding protein and S100A7 protein in patients with cutaneous melanoma. Melanoma Res. 2002;12(6):627-31.

[255] He H, Li J, Weng S, Li M, Yu Y. S100A11: diverse function and pathology corresponding to different target proteins. Cell Biochem Biophys. 2009;55(3):117-26.

[256] Van Ginkel PR, Gee RL, Walker TM, Hu DN, Heizmann CW, Polans AS. The identification and differential expression of calcium-binding proteins associated with ocular melanoma. Biochim Biophys Acta. 1998;1448(2):290-7.

[257] Reddy S, Bichler J, Wells-Knecht KJ, Thorpe SR, Baynes JW. N epsilon-(carboxymethyl)lysine is a dominant advanced glycation end product (AGE) antigen in tissue proteins. Biochemistry. 1995;34(34):10872-8.

[258] Thornalley PJ. Advances in glyoxalase research. Glyoxalase expression in malignancy, anti-proliferative effects of methylglyoxal, glyoxalase I inhibitor diesters and S-D-lactoylglutathione, and methylglyoxal-modified protein binding and endocytosis by the advanced glycation endproduct receptor. Crit Rev Oncol Hematol. 1995;20(1-2): 99-128.

[259] Wondrak GT, Jacobson MK, Jacobson EL. Antimelanoma activity of apoptogenic carbonyl scavengers. J Pharmacol Exp Ther. 2006;316(2):805-14.

[260] Sander CS, Hamm F, Elsner P, Thiele JJ. Oxidative stress in malignant melanoma and non-melanoma skin cancer. Br J Dermatol. 2003;148(5):913-22.

[261] Indurthi VS, Leclerc E, Vetter SW. Interaction between glycated serum albumin and AGE-receptors depends on structural changes and the glycation reagent. Arch Biochem Biophys. 2012;528(2):185-96.

[262] Bianchi ME, Beltrame M, Paonessa G. Specific recognition of cruciform DNA by nuclear protein HMG1. Science. 1989;243(4894 Pt 1):1056-9.

[263] Wang H, Bloom O, Zhang M, Vishnubhakat JM, Ombrellino M, Che J, et al. HMG-1 as a late mediator of endotoxin lethality in mice. Science. 1999;285(5425):248-51.

[264] Scaffidi P, Misteli T, Bianchi ME. Release of chromatin protein HMGB1 by necrotic cells triggers inflammation. Nature. 2002;418(6894):191-5.

[265] Tian J, Avalos AM, Mao SY, Chen B, Senthil K, Wu H, et al. Toll-like receptor 9-dependent activation by DNA-containing immune complexes is mediated by HMGB1 and RAGE. Nat Immunol. 2007;8(5):487-96.

[266] Dong Xda E, Ito N, Lotze MT, Demarco RA, Popovic P, Shand SH, et al. High mobility group box I (HMGB1) release from tumor cells after treatment: implications for development of targeted chemoimmunotherapy. J Immunother. 2007;30(6):596-606.

[267] Bianchi ME. DAMPs, PAMPs and alarmins: all we need to know about danger. J Leukoc Biol. 2007;81(1):1-5.

[268] Tang D, Kang R, Zeh HJ, 3rd, Lotze MT. High-mobility group box 1 and cancer. Biochim Biophys Acta. 2010;1799(1-2):131-40.

[269] Ito N, DeMarco RA, Mailliard RB, Han J, Rabinowich H, Kalinski P, et al. Cytolytic cells induce HMGB1 release from melanoma cell lines. J Leukoc Biol. 2007;81(1): 75-83.

[270] Johnson KE, Wulff BC, Oberyszyn TM, Wilgus TA. Ultraviolet light exposure stimulates HMGB1 release by keratinocytes. Archives of dermatological research. 2013;305(9):805-15.

[271] Bald T, Quast T, Landsberg J, Rogava M, Glodde N, Lopez-Ramos D, et al. Ultraviolet-radiation-induced inflammation promotes angiotropism and metastasis in melanoma. Nature. 2014;507(7490):109-13.

[272] Tang Q, Li J, Zhu H, Li P, Zou Z, Xiao Y. Hmgb1-IL-23-IL-17-IL-6-Stat3 axis promotes tumor growth in murine models of melanoma. Mediators of inflammation. 2013;2013:713859.

[273] Li Q, Li J, Wen T, Zeng W, Peng C, Yan S, et al. Overexpression of HMGB1 in melanoma predicts patient survival and suppression of HMGB1 induces cell cycle arrest and senescence in association with p21 (Waf1/Cip1) up-regulation via a p53-independent, Sp1-dependent pathway. Oncotarget. 2014;5(15):6387-403.

[274] O'Connell MP, Weeraratna AT. A spoonful of sugar makes the melanoma go: the role of heparan sulfate proteoglycans in melanoma metastasis. Pigment Cell Melanoma Res. 2011;24(6):1133-47.

[275] Nikitovic D, Mytilinaiou M, Berdiaki A, Karamanos NK, Tzanakakis GN. Heparan sulfate proteoglycans and heparin regulate melanoma cell functions. Biochim Biophys Acta. 2014;1840(8):2471-81.

[276] Newton RA, Hogg N. The human S100 protein MRP-14 is a novel activator of the beta 2 integrin Mac-1 on neutrophils. J Immunol. 1998;160(3):1427-35.

[277] Carlos TM. Leukocyte recruitment at sites of tumor: dissonant orchestration. J Leukoc Biol. 2001;70(2):171-84.

[278] Gabrilovich DI, Nagaraj S. Myeloid-derived suppressor cells as regulators of the immune system. Nat Rev Immunol. 2009;9(3):162-74.

[279] Mahnke K, Skorokhod A, Grabbe S, Enk AH. Opening a niche for therapy: local lymphodepletion helps the immune system to fight melanoma. J Invest Dermatol. 2014;134(7):1794-6.

[280] Najjar YG, Finke JH. Clinical perspectives on targeting of myeloid derived suppressor cells in the treatment of cancer. Frontiers in oncology. 2013;3:49.

[281] Riedl S, Rinner B, Asslaber M, Schaider H, Walzer S, Novak A, et al. In search of a novel target-phosphatidylserine exposed by non-apoptotic tumor cells and metastases of malignancies with poor treatment efficacy. Biochim Biophys Acta. 2011;1808(11):2638-45.

[282] Bro S, Flyvbjerg A, Binder CJ, Bang CA, Denner L, Olgaard K, et al. A neutralizing antibody against receptor for advanced glycation end products (RAGE) reduces atherosclerosis in uremic mice. Atherosclerosis. 2008;201(2):274-80.

[283] Taguchi A, Blood DC, del Toro G, Canet A, Lee DC, Qu W, et al. Blockade of RAGE-amphoterin signalling suppresses tumour growth and metastases. Nature. 2000;405(6784):354-60.

[284] Bierhaus A, Humpert PM, Morcos M, Wendt T, Chavakis T, Arnold B, et al. Understanding RAGE, the receptor for advanced glycation end products. J Mol Med. 2005;83(11):876-86.

[285] Hudson BI, Bucciarelli LG, Wendt T, Sakaguchi T, Lalla E, Qu W, et al. Blockade of receptor for advanced glycation endproducts: a new target for therapeutic intervention in diabetic complications and inflammatory disorders. Arch Biochem Biophys. 2003;419(1):80-8.

[286] Oldfield MD, Bach LA, Forbes JM, Nikolic-Paterson D, McRobert A, Thallas V, et al. Advanced glycation end products cause epithelial-myofibroblast transdifferentiation

via the receptor for advanced glycation end products (RAGE). J Clin Invest. 2001;108(12):1853-63.

[287] Deane R, Singh I, Sagare AP, Bell RD, Ross NT, LaRue B, et al. A multimodal RAGE-specific inhibitor reduces amyloid beta-mediated brain disorder in a mouse model of Alzheimer disease. J Clin Invest. 2012;122(4):1377-92.

4

Can Redirected T Cells Outsmart Aggressive Melanoma?The Promise and Challenge of Adoptive Cell Therapy

Jennifer Makalowski and Hinrich Abken

1. Introduction

1.1. The challenge to induce lasting remission in late stage melanoma

In early stages of the disease surgical resection of melanoma lesions is a curative option; a 10-year-survival rate of 75-85% can be achieved in stage I or II of the disease. However, stage III or IV melanoma is associated with low survival rates of less than 1 year upon diagnosis [1]. The poor prognosis in advanced stages of the disease is thought to be particularly due to the properties of melanoma cells to systemically spread into various organs, to form micro-metastases beyond the detection limit of current imaging procedures [2, 3] and to give rise to relapse of the disease. This is even the case after initially complete response to therapy and after more than a decade from initial treatment. Durable remission is so far only achieved in pre-defined patient subsets despite the development of novel drugs and major improvements in therapeutic regimens [4-6]. This unsatisfactory situation is thought to be due to the extra-ordinary property of melanoma cells to persist in "dormancy" for long periods of time which is associated with their resistance to chemo-and radiotherapy [7-10]. Taken together, durable cure from melanoma requires eliminating single melanoma cells in a highly specific and efficient fashion even in dormant micro-metastatic lesions.

In this situation recruiting the cellular immune defense machinery to detect and destroy individual melanoma cells is a powerful alternative to conventional therapeutic regimens. The hope is sustained by the supportive effect of high dose interleukin-2 (IL-2) [11] and anti-cytotoxic T-lymphocyte-associated antigen-4 (CTLA-4) antibody [12] as well as interferon (IFN) α-2b to prolong the disease-free survival even in late stages of the disease. However, the response rate is quite low and frequently not curative over time [13, 14].

A number of strategies for sharpening the immune cell response against melanoma are currently explored, some of these with remarkable success. In particular, the adoptive transfer of tumor infiltrating lymphocytes (TILs), isolated from melanoma biopsies and amplified to therapeutic relevant numbers ex vivo, produced encouraging phase II results [15, 16]. In a further development, patients' blood T cells are genetically engineered with pre-defined specificity for melanoma-associated antigens making adoptive cell therapy with melanoma specific T cells possible. In this contribution we will discuss the rationale for adoptive cell therapy of melanoma, evidence for efficacy and current challenges to achieve long-term remission. Upcoming strategies in melanoma stem cell targeting are also discussed.

2. Adoptive therapy with ex vivo amplified TILs can induce regression of melanoma

An effective immune response can control melanoma. This notion is supported by the observation that spontaneous and complete melanoma regressions can occur and that immune compromised patients suffer from a higher frequency of melanoma [17, 18]. The conclusion is moreover sustained by the clinical observation that treatment with high dose IL-2 produces an objective response even in late stage melanoma, some patients with long-term complete response for years [11, 19]. Although about 16%, the response rate is remarkable compared to the low and short-lived response rates of classical therapeutic regimens.

First described in 1969 [20], melanoma is infiltrated by T cells of both effector and helper cell origin which can be expanded to high numbers ex vivo in the presence of IL-2. Pioneered by the NCI-Surgery Branch, such tumor infiltrating T cells (TILs) were selected for melanoma reactivity by incubation on feeder cells expressing melanoma-associated antigens [21] and re-administered in substantial numbers together with high dose IL-2 to the patient (Figure 1). Initial trials produced an objective response rate of 11/20 patients [22] which is remarkable since TILs are obviously capable to fight melanoma even in late stage patients who experienced multiple lines of therapy. Responses, however, were of short duration and TILs did not persist for longer period in the peripheral blood after administration. Subsequent trials identified that the key to successful TIL therapy was the number of TILs administered to the patient, the activity of those cells against melanoma and the rapidity of T cell amplification ex vivo [23, 24]. During the subsequent years the initial protocols were optimized with respect to these and other issues and adopted according to GMP standards [25]; a number of trials are currently open in various centers (Table 1).

Persistence of administered TILs in circulation was substantially improved by depletion of the lymphoid compartment of the patient prior to adoptive cell therapy [26-28]. Such pre-conditioning by non-myeloablative chemotherapy had the effect that cytokines sustaining lymphocyte amplification including IL-7 and IL-15 were present in augmented levels ("cyto-kine sink"). Moreover, space for transferred lymphocytes was created and suppressor cells including regulatory T cells were depleted which additionally helped to improve engraftment of adoptively transferred T cells.

Target antigen	Adoptively transferred T cells and additional treatment	NCT ID	Center
	TILs, IL-2 in variable doses	NCT00001832	NIH
	TILs vs. lymphokine-activated killer (LAK) cells	NCT00002535	StLMC
	TILs, high dose IL-2	NCT00096382	NIH
	TILs, low dose IL-2 s.c.	NCT00200577	NUH
	TILs with vs. without IL-2	NCT00314106	NIH
	TILs, high dose IL-2 with or without dendritic cell immunization	NCT00338377	MDACC
	TILs, high dose IL-2	NCT00604136	HMC
	TILs, high dose IL-2	NCT00863330	AHC
	TILs, high dose IL-2	NCT00937625	HUH
	TILs, high dose IL-2	NCT01005745	MOFFITT
	TILs, low dose IL-2 and intra-tumoral injection of IFN-γ producing adenovirus	NCT01082887	NUH
	TILs, high dose IL-2	NCT01659151	MOFFITT
	TILs, high dose IL-2	NCT01701674	MOFFITT
	TILs, high dose IL-2	NCT01807182	FHCRC
	"re-stimulated"(autologous DCs &anti-CD3 antibody) TILs, low dose IL-2	NCT01883297	UHN
	TILs, low dose IL-2	NCT01883323	UHN
	TILs, dendritic cell vaccination with NY-ESO-1	NCT01946373	KUH
	TILs, high vs. low dose IL-2	NCT01995344	CHNHSFT
	4-1BB selected TILs	NCT02111863	NIH
	"young" TILs, high dose IL-2	NCT00287131	SMC
	"young" TILs with or without CD4+ T cell depletion, high dose IL-2	NCT00513604	NIH
	"young" CD8+ TILs, high dose IL-2	NCT01118091	NIH
	"young" TILs, high dose IL-2	NCT01319565	NIH
	"young" TILs, high dose IL-2	NCT01369875	NIH
	"young" TILs, IL-15	NCT01369888	NIH
	"young" TILs	NCT01468818	NIH
	"young" TILs, high dose IL-2, BRAF kinase inhibitor	NCT01585415	NIH
	"young" TILs, with or without high dose IL-2	NCT01814046	NIH
	"young" TILs, anti-CTLA-4 antibody	NCT01988077	SMC
	"young" TILs, high dose IL-2 with standard vs. low dose chemotherapy	NCT01993719	NIH

Aurora Health Care; **CHNHSFT**, Christie Hospital NHS Foundation Trust; **FHCRC**, Fred Hutchinson Cancer Research Center; **HMC**, Hadassah Medical Center; **HUH**, Herlev University Hospital (Copenhagen); **KUH,** Karolinska University Hospital; **MDACC**, M.D. Anderson Cancer Center; **MOFFITT**, H. Lee Moffitt Cancer Center and Research Institute; **MUH**, Mie University Hospital; **NIH**, National Institutes of Health; **NUH**, Nantes University Hospital; **SMC**, Sheba Medical Center; **StLMC**, St. Luke's Medical Center; **UC**, University of California; **UHN**, University Health Network (Toronto)

Table 1. Adoptive cell therapy with tumor infiltrating lymphocytes (TILs) in patients with melanoma

There are still some issues to be addressed, for instance whether clinically most potent TILs can be defined by phenotype and whether these cells can be selectively expanded. There is a common sense that for therapeutic efficacy in the long-term the functional activity of T cells needs to be preserved without signs of exhaustion which is particularly crucial when T cells experienced extensive amplification ex vivo. In the further development of the procedure, TILs were only selected with respect to their proliferative capacities which is independent of their antigen specificity and represents a furthermore simplification of the standard protocol (Figure 1) [29-31]. Those so-called "young TILs" after short-term ex vivo expansions passed through fewer cell division cycles prior to infusion and are thereby in a maturation stage less prone to terminal differentiation and senescence [32]. Those protocols do not further select TILs for their melanoma reactivity based on the observation that infusion of ex vivo activated, IFN-γ^+TILs produced no superior therapeutic efficacy compared to non-responding TILs [16]. These modifications in the protocol resulted in improved persistence of young TILs [33] and about 50% response rates [27, 29, 34], so far in non-randomized trials (Table 1). A series of recent clinical trials with TILs following different lympho-conditioning regimes resulted in objective responses in 56% and complete responses in 22% of patients at the Surgery Branch [35]. Current TIL trials at various centers reproduced objective response rates of 40-50% in melanoma patients, a significant portion of patients free of disease 3-5 years after treatment [36, 37]. Of note, TILs can have anti-tumor activity also towards brain metastases as shown in a NCI trial with 7/17 complete and 6/17 partial remissions [38] sustaining the hope that adoptive cell therapy may be effective towards metastases which are otherwise not accessible.

While most trials apply non-separated TILs, administration of isolated CD8$^+$T cell clones with specificity for Melan-A and gp100 mediated only moderate benefit, required IL-2 and did not persist for longer times [39]. Those CD8$^+$T cells which persisted long-term acquired a phenotype of central memory-type T cells in vivo [40]. It is therefore assumed that CD8$^+$TILs require help of CD4$^+$cells for prolonged persistence making application of non-separated T cell populations more suitable.

Not only the stage of maturation but also the recruitment of T cells through chemokine gradients is crucial for therapeutic success. A recent prospective-retrospective hypothesis-driven analysis revealed that coordinate over-expression of CXCL9, CXCL10, CXCL11, CCL5 in melanoma is associated with responsiveness to treatment after TIL therapy [41].

Melanoma-reactive T cells need to persist in circulation to ensure therapeutic success of TIL therapy [42, 43]. This is reflected by the median survival of patients treated with Melan-A specific TILs of 53.5 months compared to 3.5 months for patients who received TILs of unknown specificity [44]. Some trials are initiated using melanoma specific patient's T cells from the peripheral blood for adoptive cell therapy of melanoma (Table 2). MART-1 or gp100 specific T cell clones isolated and amplified ex vivo produced a 50% response rate [45], however, technical difficulties limit a broad application of such specific T cells since melanoma reactive T cells in the peripheral blood of melanoma patients are extremely rare.

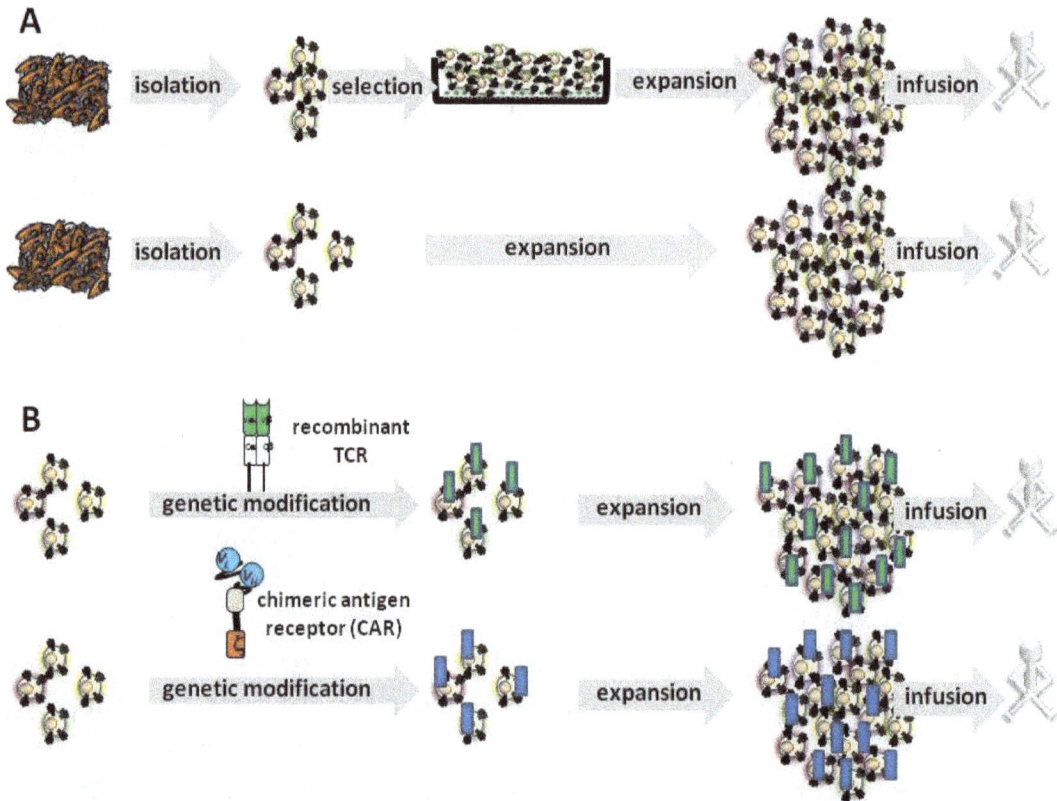

Figure 1. T cells used in adoptive cell therapy of melanoma. (A) Tumor infiltrating T cells (TILs) are isolated from melanoma biopsies, selected for reactivity towards melanoma cells, amplified in the presence of IL-2 to clinically relevant numbers and infused to the patient. Alternatively, TILs are expanded without prior selection for melanoma reactivity using a short-term amplification protocol ("young TILs"). (B) T cells from the peripheral blood of melanoma patients are genetically modified by retro- or lentivirus transduction to express a recombinant T cell receptor (TCR) or a chimeric antigen receptor (CAR), specific for a melanoma associated antigen, amplified and administered to the patient.

Target antigen	Adoptively transferred T cells	NCT ID	Center
MAGE-1 or MAGE-3	melanoma specific CD8+ T cells	NCT00045149	FHCRC
Tyrosinase	tyrosinase specific CD8+ T cells	NCT00002786	FHCRC
MART-1	MART-1 specific CD8+ T cells with or without high dose IL-2	NCT01495572	NIH
MART-1	MART-1 specific CD8+ T cells	NCT00512889	DFCI
MART-1	MART-1 specific T cells	NCT00720031	NUH
MART-1	MART-1 specific CD8+ T cells	NCT00324623	CHUV
MART-1	MART-1 specific TILs, high dose IL-2	NCT00924001	NIH
MART-1	MART-1 specific CD8+ T cells, low dose IL-2	NCT01106235	FHCRC
NY-ESO-1	NY-ESO-1 specific CD8+ T cells, low dose IL-2, anti-CTLA-4 antibody	NCT00871481	FHCRC

CHUV, Centre Hospitalier Universitaire Vaudois; **DFCI**, Dana-Farber Cancer Institute; **FHCRC**, Fred Hutchinson Cancer Research Center; **NIH**, National Institutes of Health; **NUH**, Nantes University Hospital

Table 2. Adoptive cell therapy with autologous, antigen specific T cells in patients with melanoma

3. T cells with engineered anti-melanoma specificity

The success of melanoma antigen specific T cells from peripheral blood strengthened efforts to obtain melanoma-specific T cell clones by genetic engineering of patient's T cells from the peripheral blood. In particular, the molecular cloning of the TCR from melanoma-reactive T cells enabled the engraftment of melanoma specificity to any T cell (Figure 1) [46-49]. A TCR with specificity for gp100 was cloned from melanoma reactive TILs and transferred by retrovirus-mediated gene transfer into blood T cells which thus obtained redirected specificity for gp100+cells in addition to their parental specificity. TCR engineered T cells recognized gp100+melanoma cells, secreted pro-inflammatory cytokines including IFN-γ and lysed gp100+melanoma cells [50, 51]. By the same strategy, blood T cells were modified with the TCR specific for other melanoma associated antigens (Table 3). Using T cells modified with a gp100 specific TCR objective response was induced in 19% of patients, most responses were persistent [49]. Melanoma regression was also obtained in 5/11 melanoma patients after transfer of T cells modified with a TCR that recognizes NY-ESO-1, a protein encoded by a member of the cancer/germline family of genes [52, 53].

Melanoma regression was obtained in about 30% of patients after cell therapy with MART-1 specific T cells [49, 52, 54-56]. As a side effect, patients suffered from vitiligo and destruction of melanocytes in the eye and ear indicating that T cells with engineered specificity can target rare and healthy cells even with the cognate antigen at low levels. In a recent trial, patients were treated with T cells engineered with an anti-MAGE-A3 TCR [57]. While 5/9 patients experienced melanoma regression, three of them had mental status changes and two lapsed into coma and died. Histology revealed necrotizing leukoencephalopathy which is likely due to the recognition of previously unknown epitopes of MAGE-A9/A12, the latter expressed in the brain.

Prolonged clinical remission was observed when engineered T cells persisted in the circulation for longer times; TCR modified T cells were recorded in the blood for more than a year after initiation of treatment [56, 58]. Moreover, TCR engineered T cells were capable to penetrate the blood-brain barrier and to induce regression of brain metastases [57] giving hope that patients with metastases at otherwise incurable sites may benefit from adoptive cell therapy. However, tumor cells may become invisible to TCR modified T cells due to repression of the MHC complex [60], β2 microglobulin mutation [61], and deficiencies in the antigen processing machinery [60, 62], all of them resulting in diminished antigen presentation and less TCR-mediated T cell activation.

Engineering T cells with a recombinant TCR may produce a safety hazard when the transgenic αβ TCR forms hetero-dimers with the respective α and β TCR chains of the endogenous TCR. Such mis-pairing of TCR chains can induce severe auto-reactivity as a result in gain of an unpredictable specificity [63, 64]. The situation was technically solved by different means including replacing the human by the homologous murine constant moieties of the TCR [65] and by inserting additional cysteine bridges [66] to facilitate preferential pairing of the recombinant TCR αβ chains in the presence of the physiologic αβ TCR. These and other technical difficulties of the TCR strategy promoted the development of an artificial "all-in-one" receptor molecule to redirect T cells in an antigen-restricted fashion as summarized below.

Target antigen	Adoptively transferred T cells	NCT ID	Center
	IL-12 engineered TILs	NCT01236573	NIH
	IL-2 engineered TILs	NCT00062036	NIH
	CXCR2 and NGFR transduced TILs, high dose IL-2	NCT01740557	MDACC
	TGF-Beta resistant (DNRII) and NGFR transduced TILs, high dose IL-2	NCT01955460	MDACC
gp-100	anti-gp-100 TCR engineered CD8+ cells, anti-gp-100 TCR engineered TILs, high dose IL-2	NCT00085462	NIH
gp-100	anti-gp-100 TCR engineered T cells, high dose IL-2 plus gp-100 vaccination	NCT00610311	NIH
gp-100 & MART-1	anti-gp-100 TCR & anti-MART-1 TCR engineered T cells high dose IL-2 Peptide Immunization	NCT00923195	NIH
MAGE-A3	anti-MAGE-A3/12 TCR engineered T cells, high dose IL-2	NCT01273181	NIH
MAGE-A3	anti-MAGE-A3 TCR engineered T cells, high dose IL-2	NCT02153905	NIH
MAGE-A3	anti-MAGE-A3-DP4 TCR engineered CD4+ cells, high dose IL-2	NCT02111850	NIH
MAGE-A4	anti-MAGE-A4 TCR engineered T cells	NCT02096614	MUH
MAGE-A4	anti-MAGE-A4 TCR engineered T cells	NCT01694472	TMUCIH
MART-1	anti-MART-1 TCR engineered T cells, IL-2, peptide immunization	NCT00091104	NIH
MART-1	anti-MART-1 TCR engineered T cells, IL-2, MART-1 peptide pulsed dendritic cells	NCT00910650	UC
MART-1	anti-MART-1 TCR engineered T cells, high dose IL-2, peptide immunization	NCT00612222	NIH
MART-1	anti-MART-1 TCR T cells vs. anti-MART-1 TCR TILs, high dose IL-2	NCT00509288	NIH
MART-1	anti-MART-1 TCR engineered T cells, low dose IL-2, peptide immunization	NCT00706992	NIH
NY-ESO-1	anti-NY-ESO-1 TCR engineered T cells, high dose IL-2	NCT00670748	NIH
NY-ESO-1	anti-NY ESO-1 mTCR engineered T cells, high dose IL-2	NCT01967823	NIH
NY-ESO-1	anti-NY ESO-1 TCR CD62L+ T cells, high dose IL-2	NCT02062359	NIH
NY-ESO-1	anti-NY-ESO-1 TCR engineered T cells	NCT01350401	Adaptimmune
NY-ESO-1	anti-NY-ESO-1 TCR engineered T cells, cotransduced with IL-12 cDNA	NCT01457131	NIH
p53	anti-p53 TCR engineered T cells, high dose IL-2, p53 peptide pulsed dendritic cells	NCT00704938	NIH
p53	anti-p53 TCR engineered T cells, high dose IL-2	NCT00393029	NIH
tyrosinase	anti-tyrosinase(368-376) TCR engineered T cells	NCT01586403	LU
GD2	3rd generation anti-GD2 CAR engineered T cells	NCT02107963	NIH
VEGFR2	anti-VEGFR2 CAR engineered CD8+ T cells, low dose IL-2	NCT01218867	NIH

LU, Loyola University (Chicago); MDACC, M.D. Anderson Cancer Center; MUH, Mie University Hospital; NIH, National Institutes of Health; TMUCIH, Tianjin Medical University Cancer Institute and Hospital; UC, University of California;

Table 3. Adoptive cell therapy with engineered antigen specific T cells in patients with melanoma

4. CAR T cells with engineered specificity for melanoma

In order to link antigen recognition with the downstream signaling machinery of the TCR, Zelig Eshhar (Weizmann Institute of Science) reported a chimeric antigen receptor (CAR) molecule, also named immunoreceptor, which is composed in the extracellular moiety of a single chain fragment of variable region (scFv) antibody for binding and in the intracellular moiety of the CD3ζ endodomain to initiate T cell activation [67]. The coding sequence of such recombinant receptor molecule is transferred by retro- or lentiviral transduction into T cells in vitro (Figure 1) [68]. CAR engineered T cells, also nick-named "T-bodies", recognize their new target by CAR binding and become activated to secrete pro-inflammatory cytokines, to amplify and to lyse the cognate target cells. Since the binding domain is derived from an antibody the CAR recognizes the target in a MHC-independent fashion which makes major differences to TCR mediated T cell recognition. For instance, the CAR recognizes its target independently of the individual HLA subtype and CAR T cells are not affected by MHC repression and loss of HLA molecules on target cells which frequently occurs during tumor progression. However, recognition by CARs is restricted to target antigens on the cell surface; intracellular antigens like transcription factors are not visible to CAR T cells. Despite that limitation, a nearly infinite variety of targets can be recognized including those which are not classical T cell targets like carbohydrates and gangliosides [69].

Full and lasting T cell activation requires two complementary signals, one provided by the TCR/CD3 and the other by co-receptors the prototype of which is CD28. Prolonged T cell activation, however, requires costimulation and autocrine factors, in particular IL-2 which is only secreted upon TCR and simultaneous CD28 signaling. The lack of appropriate costimu-lation in the tumor lesion provides the rationale for combining the intracellular CD3ζ with the CD28 signaling domain in one polypeptide chain of a "second generation" CAR (Figure 2). A CAR with combined CD28-CD3ζ signaling domain provides both the primary CD3ζ and the required costimlatory signal when engaging the cognate target. CARs with a costimulatory domain clearly provide clinical benefit and improved T cell persistence compared to CARs with the CD3ζ domain only [70-72]. Other costimulatory moieties, such as 4-1BB (CD137) and OX40 (CD134), also provide full T cell activation when linked to CD3ζ in a CAR; the individual costimulory domains have different impact on T cell effector functions [73]. These and other costimulatory domains were furthermore combined in so-called "3rd generation" CARs which provide advantage for matured effector T cells in terminal differentiation but less in younger stages of T cell development [74]. A number of additional modifications of the CAR design were explored in order to improve T cell persistence and activation and finally the anti-tumor response [75, 76].

While the antibody domain defines the target specificity of the CAR, a plethora of antigens can potentially be used as target for the adoptive cell therapy of melanoma. T cells engineered for targeting melanoma-associated antigens include CARs with specificity for HMW-MAA, also known as MCSP [77, 78], melanotransferrin [79], and the gangliosides GD2 [80] and GD3 [81]. Trials are currently recruiting; to our best knowledge no published data are so far available.

During the last years spectacular efficacy was achieved with CAR T cells in phase I trials for the treatment of lymphoma/leukemia [82, 83]. Clinical response and prolonged T cell activation was accompanied by a "cytokine storm", which occurred even weeks after initial T cell administration; the side effect can clinically be managed by treatment with a neutralizing anti-IL-6 antibody without affecting the anti-tumor efficacy.

The enthusiasm in CAR T cell therapy, however, was dampened by reports on serious adverse events and fatalities after CAR T cell administration [84, 85]. Targeting ErbB2 produced respiratory failure which is thought to be due to low levels of antigen on a number of healthy cells which are sufficient to trigger "on-target-off-organ" T cell activation [86]. This and other serious adverse events emphasize a careful evaluation of potential targets and the necessity for T cell dose escalation studies to balance anti-tumor efficacy and auto-immunity [75, 87, 88].

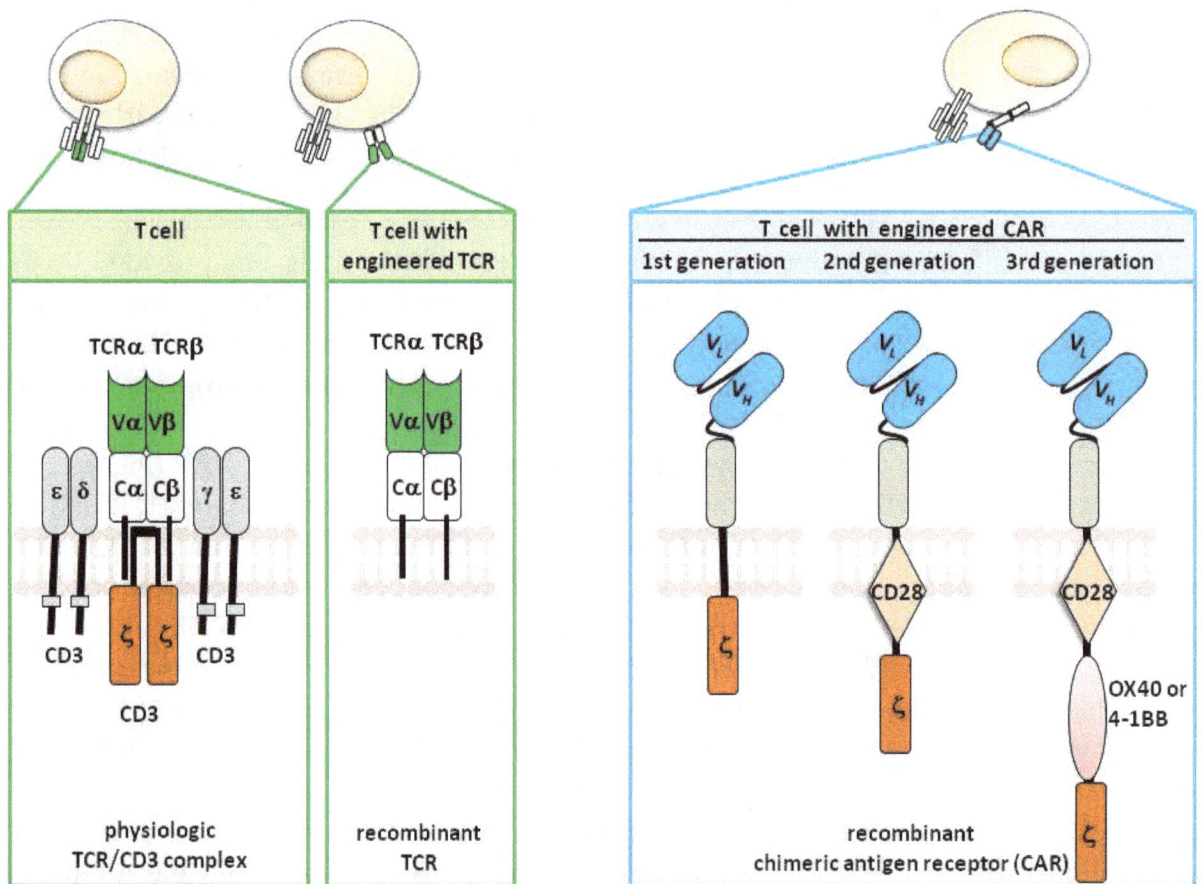

Figure 2. T cells with engineered specificity. T cells physiologically recognize their target by the T cell receptor (TCR) complex which is composed of the TCR α and β chain for recognition and the CD3 chains for signaling. The variable regions of each TCR chain (Vα and Vβ) together bind to the MHC presented antigen, Cα and Cβ represent the constant domains. T cells can be genetically engineered with defined specificity by expression of recombinant TCR αβ chains of known specificity. In contrast to the TCR, the chimeric antigen receptor (CAR) is one polypeptide chain composed of a single chain fragment of variable region (scFv) antibody for antigen recognition, the extracellular spacer domain, a trans-membrane domain and the intracellular CD3ζ ("first generation" CAR), the CD28-CD3ζ ("second generation" CAR), or the CD28-OX40-CD3ζ ("third generation" CAR) signaling chain.

5. "Melanoma stem cells": Target cells to achieve long-term remission?

Despite the tremendous cellular and phenotypic heterogeneity in tumor lesions, cancer is thought to be initiated and maintained by so-called cancer stem cells (CSCs). Such pluripotent stem cells are of low abundance, induce tumors upon transplantation under limiting dilution conditions, resist radiation and chemotherapy, and drive self-renewal and a-symmetric differentiation into a variety of cell types. Residual CSCs are thought to initiate cancer relapse even after years of "dormancy", which can be more than a decade after surgical treatment of the primary lesion [89]. While the concept of the hierarchical organization in driving tumor progression was initially drawn upon deciphering hematological malignancies, basically the same organization was subsequently reported for other solid cancers including mammary, prostate, pancreatic, colon carcinoma and glioma [90-94].

Transplantation of melanoma cell subsets into recipient mice under limiting dilution conditions also revealed that a defined subset of cancer cells, and not every cell from the same biopsy, can induce tumors of same histology as the parental tumor [90, 95-97]. One conclusion is that melanoma is organized in a hierarchical manner originating from a particular initiator cell, the cancer stem cell, which gives rise to the described diversity of cells in an established lesion. Melanoma initiating cells were described by various, but not common markers, including the transporter protein ABCB5 [95], CD20 [97], or the nerve growth factor receptor CD271 [98]. While CD271+melanoma cells are present in a frequency of approximately 1/2000 cells [98], transplantation under more rigorous conditions, i.e., ideally of one single melanoma cell, revealed that nearly every fourth randomly taken melanoma cell (1/2-1/15) can induce tumors in the host animal. This observation, however, questioned the validity of the stem cell paradigm for melanoma [99, 100]. Subsequent studies made clear that the potential to induce melanoma is not closely associated with a particular phenotype and that the number of potential CSCs in melanoma may not necessarily be low. If nearly every melanoma cell is capable to re-program to a tumor initiating cell under certain conditions, blocking stem cell properties in melanoma will reduce tumor initiation and growth in a transplantation model finally resulting in melanoma ablation [101].

Once the tumor lesion is established, a minor subset of cancer cells seems to take over to control malignant progression. Evidence for this hypothesis was provided from a pre-clinical model [79] which asked whether all or a defined subset of melanoma cells in an established xeno-transplanted lesion need to be eliminated to cause tumor regression. Such melanoma sustaining cell may be, but not must be identical to melanoma stem cells identified by transplantation assays.

Evidence for a particular targetable melanoma cell subset which sustains tumor progression was provided by the observation that elimination of CD20+melanoma cells by adoptive transfer of CAR T cells completely eradicated xeno-transplanted melanoma. Those human melanoma biopsies contained a subset of CD20+melanoma cells which constituted about 1-2% of melanoma cells and which are present in different histological melanoma types and tumor stages. A caveat is that in approximately 20% of melanoma samples analyzed so far, no CD20+melanoma cells were detected by histological screening; CD20-specific CAR T cells did not induce regression of those transplanted tumor lesions. Interestingly, CD20 re-expression in a random subpopulation of those tumor cells by genetic modification did not render the tumor lesion sensitive for eradication indicating that CD20 expression per se is not sufficient but requires additional capabilities to sustain melanoma progression [79].

There are additionally clinical observations that sustain the notion of CD20$^+$cells in promoting melanoma progression. Firstly, a patient with stage III/IV metastatic, refractory melanoma and 2% CD20$^+$melanoma cells who received intra-lesional injections of the anti-CD20 therapeutic antibody rituximab experienced lasting remission accompanied by a decline of the melanoma serum marker S-100 to physiological levels and a switch of a T helper-2 to a more pro-inflammatory T helper-1 response [102]. Although anecdotic, data provide the first clinical evidence that targeted elimination of CD20$^+$melanoma cells can produce regression of chemotherapy-refractory melanoma. Secondly, in a small pilot trial, stage IV melanoma patients without evidence of disease by way of surgery, chemo-and/or radiation therapy received the anti-CD20 antibody systemically for a 2 year period [103]. Data suggest a benefit of anti-CD20 therapy in overall and recurrence-free survival; a caveat being that the number of patients is still small for definitive conclusions.

Currently, the hierarchical stem cell model in the maintenance of an established melanoma is supported by some experimental evidence [79], whereas a body of information on melanoma initiation by transplantation of single melanoma cells sustains the stochastic model [99, 100], although not confirmed by others [98]. The most determining proof of the stem cell hypothesis, however, will be the successful melanoma elimination by targeting stem cells or stem cell properties. For the development of such therapeutic strategies several aspects need to be taken into account.

First, standard therapy will rapidly de-bulk the tumor lesion and the remaining melanoma stem cells, which are more chemo-and radiation resistant, will drive relapse of the disease. Since those melanoma initiating cells are merely in a "dormant" state and replicate less frequently than the majority of melanoma cells in the same lesion, anti-proliferative strategies by classical chemotherapeutic drugs are unlikely efficient. Transporter systems including ABCB5, which is highly expressed by melanoma stem cells [95], additionally contribute to chemotherapy resistance; the chemotherapy and/or radiation itself may promote expression of those transporter systems and survival of those resistant cells which finally contributes to relapse of the disease.

Second, if clinical progression correlates with the prevalence of CD20$^+$melanoma cells, targeted elimination of those melanoma cells requires to meet the fact that those target cells are a small minority. Targeted elimination, e.g., by CD20 redirected cytotoxic T cells or by CD20-specific therapeutic antibodies like Rituxan™ (rituximab) or Arzerra™ (ofatumumab), will be required to obtain substantial efficacy.

Third, the extraordinary functional and phenotypic plasticity of melanoma cells may make it necessary to have the therapeutic agent in place for a longer time. In their pre-clinical model, Schmidt and colleagues [79] used CAR T cells which persist for long-term acting as an antigen-specific guardian as long as target cells are present. Since repetitive re-stimulation sustains the persistence and amplification of CAR T cells, cellular therapy has a major advantage compared to pharmaceutical drugs with a comparable short half-life. CAR T cells can moreover provide antigen-specific memory with defined specificity [104], potentially contributing to control melanoma in the long-term.

6. Production of engineered T cells for clinical application

Application of adoptive cell therapy to clinical use requires efficient production of cells according to good manufacturing practice (GMP). This particularly applies to patient's T cells which are ex vivo genetically modified. The vector used for T cell modification is of major relevance with respect to the efficiency and stability in modification. Crucial steps in this process are the stable integration of the genetic vector, the site of integration to avoid insertion mutagenesis, and the resistance of the vector to genetic repression. To date, most clinical trials were performed employing retroviral or lentiviral vectors which fulfill some but not all of these requirements. Recently, other vector systems including RNA modification are alternatively utilized and it is expected that these systems will be explored in parallel in the near future.

The way of stimulating the T cells ex vivo for genetic modification and subsequent amplification is crucial for both the success in transduction and the functional capacities of modified cells. T cells are commonly activated by TCR/CD3 stimulation in addition to IL-2 [105]; most protocols use anti-CD3 and anti-CD28 magnetic beads [83, 106] which can be easily eliminated during the production process. IL-2 is replaced by other cytokines such as IL-7 and IL-15 to obtain a T cell population with a more naive and central memory phenotype [107]. Alternatively, cell lines were engineered, so-called "artificial APCs", which are modified with the various co-stimulating molecules to mimic the physiological stimulation and to provide the required signals [108]. However, difficulties in adopting those cells to GMP standard prevent their broad application in large scale production processes.

For the production itself, static culture systems in flasks or gas permeable bags are traditionally used. Due to their amplification at low cell densities (0.25-1×10^6 cells per ml), high culture volumes are required to obtain clinically relevant T cell numbers which is more easily achieved by non-static systems including the WAVE-Bioreactor or the G-Rex100 device [83, 106, 109]. In order to produce engineered T cells for a large number of patients it will be required to manufacture cells in a closed system and to produce multiple batches in parallel in the same clean room facility without the risk of batch contamination.

7. Challenges and promise in the adoptive cell therapy of melanoma

To date, approximately half of the melanoma patients benefit from adoptive cell therapy with TILs. Specifically targeted T cells may further improve the therapeutic response. Despite substantial success, the strategy still has major challenges which need to be addressed in the near future.

Significant numbers of effector T cells have to accumulate in the targeted tumor lesion which is mediated by a network of chemokines. Adoptively transferred T cells use these networks to accumulate at the tumor site; melanoma cells secrete a number of chemokines including CXCL1 to attract lymphocytes. However, early imaging studies revealed that melanoma-specific T cells massively infiltrate the lungs, spleen and liver with only some accumulation at the tumor site before the cells decline to undetectable levels in circulation [110-112]. To improve tumor targeting TILs were engineered with CXCR2, the receptor for melanoma secreted CXCL1, which resulted in improved anti-tumor activity in a mouse model [113]. The strategy is currently being explored in an early phase I trial (Table 3) [113].

Since tumor eradication requires a beneficial T cell-to-target cell ratio, higher numbers of tumor-specific T cells applied per dose likely increase the clinical efficacy. The optimal dose of T cells, however, is still a matter of discussion and requires empiric evaluation. A number of trials, in particular applying TILs, administered up to 10^{10} cells per dose [27]. Such high doses in turn require extended expansions of T cells ex vivo with the risk of loss of the "young" phenotype and gain of more matured T cells. Highly expanded T cells become hypo-responsive to CD28 costimulation and rapidly enter activation induced cell death, in particular upon IL-2 driven expansion [114]. With respect to more potent effector functions short-term amplification protocols are envisioned for both TILs and engineered T cells. This may be achieved by T cell amplification in the presence of IL-15 and IL-21 and/or by 4-1BB co-stimulation [115].

On the other hand, administration of about 10^5 engineered T cells induced remarkable therapeutic efficacy in recent trials targeting CD19+ leukemia [83]. Since the T cells substantially amplify in vivo upon antigen encounter, the capacity of cells to amplify under appropriate conditions is more relevant than the applied cell number.

Once targeted in sufficient numbers to the tumor tissue, a major challenge is the tumor selectivity of redirected T cells. While the TCR and the CAR is specific for a particular target, in most cases the targeted antigen is not exclusively expressed by cancer but also by healthy cells, although sometimes at lower levels [116, 117]. MART-1, frequently expressed by the majority of melanoma cells, is also expressed by melanocytes. Targeting such type of antigen frequently produces vitiligo, sometimes also inner ear toxicity with a certain degree of deafness [49]. Since nearly all "tumor-associated antigens" which are frequently used as targets for adoptive cell therapy are self-antigens, strategies are needed to minimize such off-target toxicities. Among these, low-avidity TCRs or CARs or combinatorial antigen recognition by two CARs are currently explored.

Melanoma cells may become invisible to TILs or TCR modified T cells due to down-regulation of their MHC components or due to deficiencies in antigen processing. However, melanoma cells may still be visible to CAR T cells which recognized their target by their antibody-derived binding domain in a MHC independent fashion. On the other hand, TCR T cells are capable to recognize cross-presented antigen, for instance tumor antigen presented by stroma cells, which is invisible to CAR T cells but helps to destroy the tumor lesion in the long-term [118, 119].

Consequently, a TCR-like CAR aims at combining the benefits of TCR and CAR redirected T cells. This is performed by using a single chain antibody with TCR-like specificity for recognizing MHC presented antigen. T cells with such a TCR-like CAR were successfully redirected in a MHC restricted fashion towards NY-ESO-1 and MAGE-A1, respectively [120, 121].

The redirected T cell activation depends on the amount of target antigen and binding affinity. Compared to TILs and TCR modified T cells, CAR T cells bind with extraordinary high affinity by their antibody-derived CAR binding domain. A furthermore increase in affinity by affinity maturation does not necessarily improve CAR redirected T cell activation [120, 122]; CD28 costimulation does not add to the affinity dependent activation threshold, however, prolongs T cell persistence and resistance to apoptosis [123]. Targeting cancer cells also depends on the amount of target antigen in addition to the binding affinity. Low affinity CARs require abundant antigen levels for efficient activation of engineered T cells while high affinity CARs are likewise effective against low antigen levels on target cells. In this context, the selectivity in targeting melanoma cells versus healthy cells needs to be discussed not only with respect to the targeted antigen itself but also to antigen amount and binding affinity.

Amplification and persistence of adoptively transferred cells correlates with clinical outcome in some trials [124]. T cells will persist in detectable numbers as long as targeted antigen is present, however, will contract to undetectable levels and disappear from circulation when no target is furthermore present. To enable survival of CAR T cells in the long-term, Epstein-Barr virus (EBV)-specific T cells were used as effector cells and modified with a tumor-specific CAR. The rationale is that EBV specific T cells are maintained in a sizable population in circulation by recognizing EBV antigens by their physiological TCR. The strategy is sustained by the first clinical observation that EBV-specific T cells engineered with an anti-GD2 CAR showed benefit over non-virus-specific, CAR engineered T cells in the treatment of neuroblastoma (NCT00085930) [124]. Other trials use EBV or CMV specific, autologous T cells engineered with a first or second generation CAR, for instance directed against HER2/neu (ErbB2) (NCT01109095), CD30 (NCT01192464), or CD19 (NCT00709033; NCT01475058; NCT01430390; NCT00840853; NCT01195480).

The T cell subset matters, adoptively transferred CD8+T cell clones poorly persist [125] and need help of CD4+cells. Prolonged T cell anti-tumor response also requires resistance to repression in the tumor tissue. A number of efforts are currently undertaken to counteract tumor associated T cell repression, in particular mediated by Treg cells and checkpoint mediators. In animal models, CD28 costimulation without induction of IL-2 secretion protects a CAR redirected T cell response from Treg cell repression [126]. On the other hand, repetitive T cell stimulation upregulates CTLA-4 which acts as negative regulator to return the T cell to a resting stage. Administration of a CTLA-4 blocker, e.g., ipilimumab antibody, may prolong the anti-tumor activation of transferred T cells, although it is not locally restricted and will likewise affect all T cells [127, 128]. Expression profiling of TCR-engineered T cells demonstrates overexpression of multiple inhibitory receptors in persisting lymphocytes, including PD-1 and CD160, the latter associated with decreased reactivity of TCR T cells in a ligand independent manner [129]. Essentially the same was observed for CAR T cells [130]. These analyses point to a multi-factorial T cell repression in the tumor tissue; there is more than one uni-directional strategy needed to sustain the T cell anti-tumor response in the long-term.

A major hurdle of specific immunotherapy in general is the tremendous heterogeneity of cancer cells within the same lesion. Low or loss of target antigen expression negatively affects the long-term therapeutic efficacy of an antigen-redirected approach. This is supported by several reports which document a relapse of antigen-loss tumor metastases after adoptive therapy with melanoma-reactive T cell clones [39,131, 132]. A solution may be the use of polyclonal T cells with specificities for various melanoma antigens or T cells modified with different CARs recognizing different antigens; however, target-negative tumor cells will not be recognized. On the other hand, pro-inflammatory cytokines secreted by redirected T cells upon activation can attract a second wave of innate immune cells which in turn may eradiate the antigen-negative tumor cells. At least in an animal model, antigen-negative melanoma cells are indeed eliminated when co-inoculated with antibody-targeted cytokines [133]. T cells engineered with induced expression of transgenic IL-12 can attract innate immune cells including macrophages into the tumor tissue which eliminate antigen-negative tumor cells in the same lesion, at least in an immune competent animal model [134]. Such "TRUCK" cells ("T cells redirected for unrestricted cytokine killing") may pave a novel way to deliver transgenic cell products to pre-defined, target lesions.

Combination of adoptive cell therapy with pathway inhibitors may improve the efficacy in melanoma cell elimination, in particular in disseminated stages of the disease. Metastatic melanoma patients with the B-raf activating mutation V600E benefit from a small molecule drug, PLX4032 or vemurafenib, which inhibits the mitogen-activated protein kinase (MAPK) pathway. Treatment with vemurafenib is accompanied by increased T cell infiltrations in the melanoma lesions [135, 136] which may contribute to the therapeutic effect and may be improved by co-administration of melanoma-specific T cells.

While adoptive cell therapy is mostly performed with modified or non-modified T cells, other cells like monocytes, macrophages as well as NK cells can also be redirected by CARs in an antigen-specific fashion [137-141, 144]. In contrast to T cells, NK cells can be rapidly activated and exhibit high cytotoxic potential and continuously growing NK cell lines such as NK-92 can be used for adoptive cancer immunotherapy [142]. CD3ζ chain CARs trigger cytolytic activities of NK cells which has been shown for CARs with various specificities [138, 141, 143-147]. Similar to T cells, the anti-tumor activity was improved by adding 4-1BB or 2B4 (CD244) costimulatory domains [148, 149]. Since NK cells cannot provide IL-2 or IL-15 required for amplification, CAR modified NK cells were additionally engineered to release IL-15 which sustains NK cell expansion and CAR-mediated cytotoxicity in the absence of IL-2 [150]. Despite these and other advances during the last years, experience with CAR engineered primary NK cells in clinical trials is still limited; whether redirected cells of the innate immune system are more advantageous in melanoma elimination than modified T cells has moreover to be explored in clinical trials.

Acknowledgements

Work in the author's laboratory was supported by the Deutsche Forschungsgemeinschaft, Bonn, Deutsche Krebshilfe, Bonn, Else Kröner-Fresenius-Stiftung, Bad Homburg v.d.H., Wilhelm Sander-Stiftung, München, the European Union (European Regional Development Fund-Investing in your future), the German federal state North Rhine-Westphalia (NRW), and the Fortune program of the Medical Faculty of the University of Cologne.

Author details

Jennifer Makalowski[1,2] and Hinrich Abken[1,2*]

*Address all correspondence to: hinrich.abken@uk-koeln.de

1 Center for Molecular Medicine Cologne (CMMC), University of Cologne, Germany

2 Dept. I Internal Medicine, University Hospital Cologne, Cologne, Germany

References

[1] Garbe C, Peris K, Hauschild A, Saiag P, Middleton M, Spatz A, Grob J-J, Malvehy J, Newton-Bishop J, Stratigos A, Pehamberger H, Eggermont A. Diagnosis and treatment of melanoma: European consensus-based interdisciplinary guideline. European Journal of Cancer 2010;46(2) 270-283.

[2] Denninghoff VC, Kahn AG, Falco J, Curutchet HP, Elsner B. Sentinel lymph node: detection of micrometastases of melanoma in a molecular study. Molecular Diagnosis 2004;8(4) 253-258.

[3] Bedikian AY, Wei C, Detry M, Kim KB, Papadopoulos NE, Hwu WJ, Homsi J, Davies M, McIntyre S, Hwu P. Predictive Factors for the Development of Brain Metastasis in Advanced Unresectable Metastatic Melanoma. American Journal of Clinical Oncology 2010;34(6) 603-610.

[4] Chapman PB, Hauschild A, Robert C, Haanen JB, Ascierto P, Larkin J, Dummer R, Garbe C, Testori A, Maio M, Hogg D, Lorigan P, Lebbe C, Jouary T, Schadendorf D, Ribas A, O'Day SJ, Sosman JA, Kirkwood JM, Eggermont AM, Dreno B, Nolop K, Li J, Nelson B, Hou J, Lee RJ, Flaherty KT. Improved survival with vemurafenib in melanoma with BRAF V600E mutation. The New England Journal of Medicine 2011;364 (26) 2507-2516.

[5] Carter RD, Krementz ET, Hill GJ 2nd, Metter GE, Fletcher WS, Golomb FM, Grage TB, Minton JP, Sparks FC. DTIC (nsc-45388) and combination therapy for melanoma.

I. Studies with DTIC, BCNU (NSC-409962), CCNU (NSC-79037), vincristine (NSC-67574), and hydroxyurea (NSC-32065). Cancer Treat Rep. 1976;60(5) 601-609.

[6] Flaherty KT, Puzanov I, Kim KB, Ribas A, McArthur GA, Sosman JA, O'Dwyer PJ, Lee RJ, Grippo JF, Nolop K, Chapman PB. Inhibition of mutated, activated BRAF in metastatic melanoma. The New England Journal of Medicine 2010;363(9) 809-819.

[7] Leiter U, Eigentler TK, Forschner A, Pflugfelder A, Weide B, Held L, Meier F, Garbe C. Excision guidelines and follow-up strategies in cutaneous melanoma: Facts and controversies. Clinics in Dermatology 2010;28(3) 311-315.

[8] Bradbury PA, Middleton MR. DNA repair pathways in drug resistance in melanoma. Anti-cancer Drugs 2004;15(5) 421-426.

[9] Pak BJ, Chu W, Lu SJ, Kerbel RS, Ben-David Y. Lineage-specific mechanism of drug and radiation resistance in melanoma mediated by tyrosinase-related protein 2. Cancer Metastasis Reviews 2001;20(1-2) 27-32.

[10] Pak BJ, Lee J, Thai BL, Fuchs SY, Shaked Y, Ronai Z, Kerbel RS, Ben-David Y. Radiation resistance of human melanoma analysed by retroviral insertional mutagenesis reveals a possible role for dopachrome tautomerase. Oncogene 2004;23(1) 30-38.

[11] Atkins MB, Lotze MT, Dutcher JP, Fisher RI, Weiss G, Margolin K, Abrams J, Sznol M, Parkinson D, Hawkins M, Paradise C, Kunkel L, Rosenberg SA. High-dose recombinant interleukin 2 therapy for patients with metastatic melanoma: analysis of 270 patients treated between 1985 and 1993. Journal of Clinical Oncology 1999;17(7) 2105-2116.

[12] Hodi FS, O'Day SJ, McDermott DF, Weber RW, Sosman JA, Haanen JB, Gonzalez R, Robert C, Schadendorf D, Hassel JC, Akerley W, van den Eertwegh AJ, Lutzky J, Lorigan P, Vaubel JM, Linette GP, Hogg D, Ottensmeier CH, Lebbé C, Peschel C, Quirt I, Clark JI, Wolchok JD, Weber JS, Tian J, Yellin MJ, Nichol GM, Hoos A, Urba WJ. Improved survival with ipilimumab in patients with metastatic melanoma. The New England Journal of Medicine 2010;363(8) 711-723.

[13] Kirkwood JM, Ibrahim JG, Sondak VK, Richards J, Flaherty LE, Ernstoff MS, Smith TJ, Rao U, Steele M, Blum RH. High-and low-dose interferon alfa-2b in high-risk melanoma: first analysis of intergroup trial E1690/S9111/C9190. Journal of Clinical Oncology 2000;18(12) 2444-2458.

[14] Kirkwood JM, Strawderman MH, Ernstoff MS, Smith TJ, Borden EC, Blum RH. Interferon alfa-2b adjuvant therapy of high-risk resected cutaneous melanoma: the Eastern Cooperative Oncology Group Trial EST 1684. Journal of Clinical Oncology 1996;14(1) 7-17.

[15] Galluzzi L, Vacchelli E, Eggermont A, Fridman WH, Galon J, Sautès-Fridman C, Tartour E, Zitvogel L, Kroemer G. Trial Watch: Adoptive cell transfer immunotherapy. Oncoimmunology 2012;1(3) 306-315.

[16] Bernatchez C, Radvanyi LG, Hwu P. Advances in the treatment of metastatic melanoma: adoptive T-cell therapy. Seminars in Oncology 2012;39(2) 215-226.

[17] Grulich AE, van Leeuwen MT, Falster MO, Vajdic CM. Incidence of cancers in people with HIV/AIDS compared with immunosuppressed transplant recipients: a meta-analysis. Lancet 2007;370(9581) 59-67.

[18] Nathanson. Spontaneous regression of malignant melanoma: a review of the literature on incidence, clinical features, and possible mechanisms. National Cancer Institute Monograph 1976;44 67-76.

[19] Rosenberg SA, Yang JC, Topalian SL, Schwartzentruber DJ, Weber JS, Parkinson DR, Seipp CA, Einhorn JH, White DE. Treatment of 283 consecutive patients with metastatic melanoma or renal cell cancer using high-dose bolus interleukin 2. The journal of the American Medical Association 1994;271(12) 907-913.

[20] Clark WH Jr, From L, Bernardino EA, Mihm MC. The histogenesis and biologic behavior of primary human malignant melanomas of the skin. Cancer Research 1969;29(3) 705-727.

[21] Vignard V, Lemercier B, Lim A, Pandolfino MC, Guilloux Y, Khammari A, Rabu C, Echasserieau K, Lang F, Gougeon ML, Dreno B, Jotereau F, Labarriere N. Adoptive transfer of tumor-reactive Melan-A-specific CTL clones in melanoma patients is followed by increased frequencies of additional Melan-A-specific T cells. Journal of Immunology 2005;175(7) 4797-4805.

[22] Rosenberg SA, Packard BS, Aebersold PM, Solomon D, Topalian SL, Toy ST, Simon P, Lotze MT, Yang JC, Seipp CA, et al. Use of tumor-infiltrating lymphocytes and interleukin-2 in the immunotherapy of patients with metastatic melanoma. N. Engl. J. Med. 1988;319(25), 1676–1680.

[23] Clemente CG, Mihm MC Jr, Bufalino R, Zurrida S, Collini P, Cascinelli N. Prognostic value of tumor infiltrating lymphocytes in the vertical growth phase of primary cutaneous melanoma. Cancer 1996;77(7) 1303-1310.

[24] Burton AL, Roach BA, Mays MP, Chen AF, Ginter BA, Vierling AM, Scoggins CR, Martin RC, Stromberg AJ, Hagendoorn L, McMasters KM. Prognostic significance of tumor infiltrating lymphocytes in melanoma. The American Surgeon 2011;77(2) 188-192.

[25] Hinrichs CS, Rosenberg SA. Exploiting the curative potential of adoptive T-cell therapy for cancer. Immunological Reviews Adoptive Immunotherapy for Cancer 2014; 257(1) 56–71.

[26] Dudley ME, Wunderlich JR, Robbins PF, Yang JC, Hwu P, Schwartzentruber DJ, Topalian SL, Sherry R, Restifo NP, Hubicki AM, Robinson MR, Raffeld M, Duray P, Seipp CA, Rogers-Freezer L, Morton KE, Mavroukakis SA, White DE, Rosenberg SA.

Cancer regression and autoimmunity in patients after clonal repopulation with anti-tumor lymphocytes. *Science* 2002;298(5594) 850–854.

[27] Dudley ME, Wunderlich JR, Yang JC, Sherry RM, Topalian SL, Restifo NP, Royal RE, Kammula U, White DE, Mavroukakis SA, Rogers LJ, Gracia GJ, Jones SA, Mangiameli DP, Pelletier MM, Gea-Banacloche J, Robinson MR, Berman DM, Filie AC, Abati A, Rosenberg SA. Adoptive cell transfer therapy following non-myeloablative but lymphodepleting chemotherapy for the treatment of patients with refractory metastatic melanoma. Journal of Clinical Oncology 2005;23(10) 2346-2357.

[28] Dudley ME, Yang JC, Sherry R, Hughes MS, Royal R, Kammula U, Robbins PF, Huang J, Citrin DE, Leitman SF, Wunderlich J, Restifo NP, Thomasian A, Downey SG, Smith FO, Klapper J, Morton K, Laurencot C, White DE, Rosenberg SA. Adoptive cell therapy for patients with metastatic melanoma: evaluation of intensive myeloablative chemoradiation preparative regimens. Journal of Clinical Oncology 2008;26(32) 5233-5239.

[29] Besser MJ, Shapira-Frommer R, Treves AJ, Zippel D, Itzhaki O, Hershkovitz L, Levy D, Kubi A, Hovav E, Chermoshniuk N, Shalmon B, Hardan I, Catane R, Markel G, Apter S, Ben-Nun A, Kuchuk I, Shimoni A, Nagler A, Schachter J. Clinical responses in a phase II study using adoptive transfer of short-term cultured tumor infiltration lymphocytes in metastatic melanoma patients. Clinical Cancer Research 2010;16(9) 2646-2655.

[30] Tran KQ, Zhou J, Durflinger KH, Langhan MM, Shelton TE, Wunderlich JR, Robbins PF, Rosenberg SA, Dudley ME. Minimally cultured tumor-infiltrating lymphocytes display optimal characteristics for adoptive cell therapy. J. Immunother 2008;31(8) 742–751.

[31] Dudley ME, Gross CA, Langhan MM, Garcia MR, Sherry RM, Yang JC, Phan GQ, Kammula US, Hughes MS, Citrin DE, Restifo NP, Wunderlich JR, Prieto PA, Hong JJ, Langan RC, Zlott DA, Morton KE, White DE, Laurencot CM, Rosenberg SA. CD8+enriched "young" tumor infiltrating lymphocytes can mediate regression of metastatic melanoma. Clinical Cancer Research 2010;16(24) 6122-6131.

[32] Itzhaki O, Hovav E, Ziporen Y, Levy D, Kubi A, Zikich D, Hershkovitz L, Treves AJ, Shalmon B, Zippel D, Markel G, Shapira-Frommer R, Schachter J, Besser MJ. Establishment and large-scale expansion of minimally cultured "young" tumor infiltrating lymphocytes for adoptive transfer therapy. Journal of Immunology 2011;34(2) 212-220.

[33] Shen X, Zhou J, Hathcock KS, Robbins P, Powell DJ Jr, Rosenberg SA, Hodes RJ. Persistence of tumor infiltrating lymphocytes in adoptive immunotherapy correlates with telomere length. Journal of Immunology 2007;30(1) 123-129.

[34] Besser MJ, Shapira-Frommer R, Treves AJ, Zippel D, Itzhaki O, Schallmach E, Kubi A, Shalmon B, Hardan I, Catane R, Segal E, Markel G, Apter S, Nun AB, Kuchuk I, Shimoni A, Nagler A, Schachter J. Minimally cultured or selected autologous tumor-

infiltrating lymphocytes after a lympho-depleting chemotherapy regimen in metastatic melanoma patients. Journal of Immunotherapy 2009;32(4) 415-423.

[35]   Rosenberg SA, Yang JC, Sherry RM, Kammula US, Hughes MS, Phan GQ, Citrin DE, Restifo NP, Robbins PF, Wunderlich JR, Morton KE, Laurencot CM, Steinberg SM, White DE, Dudley ME. Durable complete responses in heavily pretreated patients with metastatic melanoma using T-cell transfer immunotherapy. Clin Cancer Res 2011;17(13) 4550–4557.

[36]   Radvanyi LG, Bernatchez C, Zhang M, Fox PS, Miller P, Chacon J, Wu R, Lizee G, Mahoney S, Alvarado G, Glass M, Johnson VE, McMannis JD, Shpall E, Prieto V, Papadopoulos N, Kim K, Homsi J, Bedikian A, Hwu WJ, Patel S, Ross MI, Lee JE, Gershenwald JE, Lucci A, Royal R, Cormier JN, Davies MA, Mansaray R, Fulbright OJ, Toth C, Ramachandran R, Wardell S, Gonzalez A, Hwu P. Specific lymphocyte subsets predict response to adoptive cell therapy using expanded autologous tumor-infiltrating lymphocytes in metastatic melanoma patients. Clin Cancer Res 2012;18 (24) 6758–6770.

[37]   Itzhaki O, Hovav E, Ziporen Y, Levy D, Kubi A, Zikich D, Hershkovitz L, Treves AJ, Shalmon B, Zippel D, Markel G, Shapira-Frommer R, Schachter J, Besser MJ. Establishment and large-scale expansion of minimally cultured "young" tumor infiltrating lymphocytes for adoptive transfer therapy. J Immunother 2011;34(2) 212–220.

[38]   Hong JJ, Rosenberg SA, Dudley ME, Yang JC, White DE, Butman JA, Sherry RM. Successful treatment of melanoma brain metastases with adoptive cell therapy. Clin Cancer Res 2006;16(19), 4892–4898.

[39]   Yee C, Thompson JA, Byrd D, Riddell SR, Roche P, Celis E, Greenberg PD. Adoptive T cell therapy using antigen-specific CD8+T cell clones for the treatment of patients with metastatic melanoma: in vivo persistence, migration, and antitumor effect of transferred T cells. Proc Natl Acad Sci USA (2002);99(25) 16168–16173.

[40]   Inozume T, Hanada K, Wang QJ, Ahmadzadeh M, Wunderlich JR, Rosenberg SA, Yang JC. (2010) Selection of CD8+PD-1+lymphocytes in fresh human melanomas enriches for tumor-reactive T cells. J Immunother(2010); 33(9) 956–964.

[41]   Bedognetti D, Spivey TL, Zhao Y, Uccellini L, Tomei S, Dudley ME, Ascierto ML, De Giorgi V, Liu Q, Delogu LG, Sommariva M, Sertoli MR, Simon R, Wang E, Rosenberg SA, Marincola FM. CXCR3/CCR5 pathways in metastatic melanoma patients treated with adoptive therapy and interleukin-2. British Journal of Cancer 2013;109(9) 2412–2423.

[42]   Vignard V, Lemercier B, Lim A, Pandolfino MC, Guilloux Y, Khammari A, Rabu C, Echasserieau K, Lang F, Gougeon ML, Dreno B, Jotereau F, Labarriere N. Adoptive transfer of tumor-reactive Melan-A-specific CTL clones in melanoma patients is followed by increased frequencies of additional Melan-A-specific T cells. Journal of Immunology 2005;175(7) 4797-4805.

[43] Kawakami Y, Eliyahu S, Jennings C, Sakaguchi K, Kang X, Southwood S, Robbins PF, Sette A, Appella E, Rosenberg SA. Recognition of multiple epitopes in the human melanoma antigen gp100 by tumor-infiltrating T lymphocytes associated with in vivo tumor regression. Journal of Immunology 1995;154(8) 3961-39618.

[44] Benlalam H, Vignard V, Khammari A, Bonnin A, Godet Y, Pandolfino MC, Jotereau F, Dreno B, Labarrière N. Infusion of Melan-A/Mart-1 specific tumor-infiltrating lymphocytes enhanced relapse-free survival of melanoma patients. Cancer Immunology Immunotherapy 2007;56(4) 515-526.

[45] Khammari A, Labarrière N, Vignard V, Nguyen JM, Pandolfino MC, Knol AC, Quéreux G, Saiagh S, Brocard A, Jotereau F, Dreno B. Treatment of metastatic melanoma with autologous Melan-A/MART-1-specific cytotoxic T lymphocyte clones. The Journal of Investigative Dermatology 2009;129(12) 2835-2842.

[46] Johnson LA, Heemskerk B, Powell DJ Jr, Cohen CJ, Morgan RA, Dudley ME, Robbins PF, Rosenberg SA. Gene transfer of tumor-reactive TCR confers both high avidity and tumor reactivity to nonreactive peripheral blood mononuclear cells and tumor-infiltrating lymphocytes. Journal of Immunology 2006;177(9) 6548-6559.

[47] Zhao Y, Zheng Z, Khong HT, Rosenberg SA, Morgan RA. Transduction of an HLA-DP4-restricted NY-ESO-1-specific TCR into primary human CD4+lymphocytes. Journal of Immunology 2006;29(4) 398-406.

[48] Frankel TL, Burns WR, Peng PD, Yu Z, Chinnasamy D, Wargo JA, Zheng Z, Restifo NP, Rosenberg SA, Morgan RA. Both CD4 and CD8 T cells mediate equally effective in vivo tumor treatment when engineered with a highly avid TCR targeting tyrosinase. Journal of Immunology 2010;184(11) 5988-5998.

[49] Johnson LA, Morgan RA, Dudley ME, Cassard L, Yang JC, Hughes MS, Kammula US, Royal RE, Sherry RM, Wunderlich JR, Lee CC, Restifo NP, Schwarz SL, Cogdill AP, Bishop RJ, Kim H, Brewer CC, Rudy SF, VanWaes C, Davis JL, Mathur A, Ripley RT, Nathan DA, Laurencot CM, Rosenberg SA. Gene therapy with human and mouse T-cell receptors mediates cancer regression and targets normal tissues expressing cognate antigen. Blood 2009;114(3) 535-546.

[50] Schaft N, Willemsen RA, de Vries J, Lankiewicz B, Essers BW, Gratama JW, Figdor CG, Bolhuis RL, Debets R, Adema GJ. Peptide fine specificity of anti-glycoprotein 100 CTL is preserved following transfer of engineered TCR alpha beta genes into primary human T lymphocytes. Journal of Immunology 2003;170(4) 2186-2194.

[51] Morgan RA, Dudley ME, Yu YY, Zheng Z, Robbins PF, Theoret MR, Wunderlich JR, Hughes MS, Restifo NP, Rosenberg SA. High efficiency TCR gene transfer into primary human lymphocytes affords avid recognition of melanoma tumor antigen glycoprotein 100 and does not alter the recognition of autologous melanoma antigens. Journal of Immunology 2003;171(6) 3287-3295.

[52] Robbins PF, Morgan RA, Feldman SA, Yang JC, Sherry RM, Dudley ME, Wunderlich JR, Nahvi AV, Helman LJ, Mackall CL, Kammula US, Hughes MS, Restifo NP, Raf-

feld M, Lee CC, Levy CL, Li YF, El-Gamil M, Schwarz SL, Laurencot C, Rosenberg SA. Tumor regression in patients with metastatic synovial cell sarcoma and melanoma using genetically engineered lymphocytes reactive with NY-ESO-1. Journal of Clinical Oncology 2011;29(7) 917-924.

[53] Zhang G, Wang L, Cui H, Wang X, Zhang G, Ma J, Han H, He W, Wang W, Zhao Y, Liu C, Sun M, Gao B. Anti-melanoma activity of T cells redirected with a TCR-like chimeric antigen receptor. Sci Rep. 2014;4 3571.

[54] Hughes MS, Yu YY, Dudley ME, Zheng Z, Robbins PF, Li Y, Wunderlich J, Hawley RG, Moayeri M, Rosenberg SA, Morgan RA. Transfer of a TCR gene derived from a patient with a marked antitumor response conveys highly active T-cell effector functions. Human Gene Therapy 2005;16(4) 457-472.

[55] Willemsen R, Ronteltap C, Heuveling M, Debets R, Bolhuis R. Redirecting human CD4+T lymphocytes to the MHC class I-restricted melanoma antigen MAGE-A1 by TCR alphabeta gene transfer requires CD8alpha. Gene Therapy 2005; 12(2) 140-146.

[56] Morgan RA, Dudley ME, Wunderlich JR, Hughes MS, Yang JC, Sherry RM, Royal RE, Topalian SL, Kammula US, Restifo NP, Zheng Z, Nahvi A, de Vries CR, Rogers-Freezer LJ, Mavroukakis SA, Rosenberg SA. Cancer Regression in Patients After Transfer of Genetically Engineered Lymphocytes. Science. 2006;314(5796) 126-129.

[57] Morgan RA, Chinnasamy N, Abate-Daga D, Gros A, Robbins PF, Zheng Z, Dudley ME, Feldman SA, Yang JC, Sherry RM, Phan GQ, Hughes MS, Kammula US, Miller AD, Hessman CJ, Stewart AA, Restifo NP, Quezado MM, Alimchandani M, Rosenberg AZ, Nath A, Wang T, Bielekova B, Wuest SC, Akula N, McMahon FJ, Wilde S, Mosetter B, Schendel DJ, Laurencot CM, Rosenberg SA. Cancer regression and neurological toxicity following anti-MAGE-A3 TCR gene therapy. J Immunother 2013;36(2) 133-151.

[58] Coccoris M, Swart E, de Witte MA, van Heijst JW, Haanen JB, Schepers K, Schumacher TN. Long-term functionality of TCR-transduced T cells in vivo. Journal of Immunology 2008; 180(10) 6536-6543.

[59] Rosenberg SA, Yannelli JR, Yang JC, Topalian SL, Schwartzentruber DJ, Weber JS, Parkinson DR, Seipp CA, Einhorn JH, White DE. Treatment of patients with metastatic melanoma with autologous tumor-infiltrating lymphocytes and interleukin 2. Journal of the National Cancer Institute 1994;86(15) 1159–1166.

[60] Seliger B. Molecular mechanisms of MHC class I abnormalities and APM components in human tumors. Cancer Immunology Immunotherapy 2008;57(11) 1719-1726.

[61] Sigalotti L, Fratta E, Coral S, Tanzarella S, Danielli R, Colizzi F, Fonsatti E, Traversari C, Altomonte M, Maio M. Intratumor heterogeneity of cancer/testis antigens expression in human cutaneous melanoma is methylation-regulated and functionally reverted by 5-aza-2'-deoxycytidine. Cancer Research 2004;64(24) 9167-9171.

[62]   Vitale M, Pelusi G, Taroni B, Gobbi G, Micheloni C, Rezzani R, Donato F, Wang X, Ferrone S. HLA class I antigen down-regulation in primary ovary carcinoma lesions: association with disease stage. Clinical Cancer Research 2005;11(1) 67-72.

[63]   Coccoris M, Straetemans T, Govers C, Lamers C, Sleijfer S, Debets R. T cell receptor (TCR) gene therapy to treat melanoma: lessons from clinical and preclinical studies. Expert Opinion on Biological Therapy 2010;10(4) 547-562.

[64]   Bendle GM, Linnemann C, Hooijkaas AI, Bies L, de Witte MA, Jorritsma A, Kaiser AD, Pouw N, Debets R, Kieback E, Uckert W, Song JY, Haanen JB, Schumacher TN. Lethal graft-versus-host disease in mouse models of T cell receptor gene therapy. Nature Medicine 2010; 16(5) 565-570.

[65]   Cohen CJ, Zhao Y, Zheng Z, Rosenberg SA, Morgan RA. Enhanced antitumor activity of murine-human hybrid T-cell receptor (TCR) in human lymphocytes is associated with improved pairing and TCR/CD3 stability. Cancer Research 2006;66(17) 8878-8886.

[66]   Kuball J, Dossett ML, Wolfl M, Ho WY, Voss RH, Fowler C, Greenberg PD. Facilitating matched pairing and expression of TCR chains introduced into human T cells. Blood 2007;109(6) 2331-2338.

[67]   Eshhar Z, Waks T, Gross G, Schindler DG. Specific activation and targeting of cytotoxic lymphocytes through chimeric single chains consisting of antibody-binding domains and the gamma or zeta subunits of the immunoglobulin and T-cell receptors. Proceedings of the National Academy of Sciences of the United States of America 1993;90(2) 720-724.

[68]   Cheadle EJ, Sheard V, Hombach, AA, Chmielewski M, Riet T, Berrevoets C, Schooten E, Lamers C, Abken H, Debets R, Gilham DE. Chimeric antigen receptors for T-cell based therapy. Methods Mol Biol 2012;907 645-666.

[69]   Hombach A, Heuser C, Sircar R, Tillmann T, Diehl V, Kruis W, Pohl C, Abken H. T cell targeting of TAG72+tumor cells by a chimeric receptor with antibody-like specificity for a carbohydrate epitope. Gastroenterol 1997;113(4), 1163 – 1170.

[70]   Hombach A, Abken H. Costimulation tunes tumor-specific activation of redirected T cells in adoptive immunotherapy," Cancer Immunology Immunotherapy 2007;56(5)731-737.

[71]   ClinicalTrials.gov A service of the U.S. National Institutes of Health. Trial ID: NCT00586391 http://clinicaltrials.gov/ct2/results?term=NCT+00586391

[72]   ClinicalTrials.gov A service of the U.S. National Institutes of Health. Trial ID: NCT00709033 http://clinicaltrials.gov/ct2/results?term=NCT+00709033

[73]   Hombach AA, Abken H. Costimulation by chimeric antigen receptors revisited the T cell antitumor response benefits from combined CD28-OX40 signalling. International Journal of Cancer 2011;129(12) 2935-2944.

[74] Hombach AA, Chmielewski M, Rappl G, Abken H. Adoptive immunotherapy with redirected T cells produces CCR7-cells that are trapped in the periphery and benefit from combined CD28-OX40 costimulation. Hum Gene Ther 2013;24(3) 259-269.

[75] Bridgeman JS, Hawkins RE, Hombach AA, Abken H, Gilham DE.Building better chimeric antigen receptors for adoptive T cell therapy. Current Gene Therapy 2010; 10(2) 77-90.

[76] Gilham DE, Debets R, Pule M, Hawkins RE, Abken H. CAR-T cells and solid tumors: tuning T cells to challenge an inveterate foe. Trends in Molecular Medicine 2012;18(7) 377-384.

[77] Reinhold U, Liu L, Lüdtke-Handjery HC, Heuser C, Hombach A, Wang X, Tilgen W, Ferrone S, Abken H. Specific lysis of melanoma cells by receptor grafted T cells is enhanced by anti-idiotypic monoclonal antibodies directed to the scFv domain of the receptor. The Journal of Investigative Dermatology 1999;112(5) 744-750.

[78] Burns WR, Zhao Y, Frankel TL, Hinrichs CS, Zheng Z, Xu H, Feldman SA, Ferrone S, Rosenberg SA, Morgan RA. A high molecular weight melanoma-associated antigen-specific chimeric antigen receptor redirects lymphocytes to target human melanomas. Cancer Research 2010;70(8) 3027-3033.

[79] Schmidt P, Kopecky C, Hombach A, Zigrino P, Mauch C, Abken H. Eradication of melanomas by targeted elimination of a minor subset of tumor cells. Proceedings of the National Academy of Sciences of the United States of America 2011;108(6) 2474-2479.

[80] Yvon E, Del Vecchio M, Savoldo B, Hoyos V, Dutour A, Anichini A, Dotti G, Brenner MK. Immunotherapy of metastatic melanoma using genetically engineered GD2-specific T cells. Clinical Cancer Research 2009;15(18) 5852-5860.

[81] Lo AS, Ma Q, Liu DL, Junghans RP. Anti-GD3 chimeric sFv-CD28/T-cell receptor zeta designer T cells for treatment of metastatic melanoma and other neuroectodermal tumors. Clinical Cancer Research 2010;16(10) 2769-2780.

[82] Kalos M, Levine BL, Porter DL, Katz S, Grupp SA, Bagg A, June CH. T cells with chimeric antigen receptors have potent antitumor effects and can establish memory in patients with advanced leukemia. Science Translational Medicine 2011;3(95) 95ra73.

[83] Porter DL, Levine BL, Kalos M, Bagg A, June CH. Chimeric antigen receptor-modified T cells in chronic lymphoid leukemia. The New England Journal of Medicine 2011;365(8) 725-733.

[84] Lamers CH, Sleijfer S, Vulto AG, Kruit WH, Kliffen M, Debets R, Gratama JW, Stoter G, Oosterwijk E. Treatment of metastatic renal cell carcinoma with autologous T-lymphocytes genetically retargeted against carbonic anhydrase IX: first clinical experience. Journal of Clinical Oncology 2006; 24(3) 20-22.

[85] Brentjens R, Yeh R, Bernal Y, Riviere I, Sadelain M. Treatment of chronic lymphocytic leukemia with genetically targeted autologous T cells: case report of an unforeseen adverse event in a phase I clinical trial. Molecular Therapy 2010;18(4) 666-668.

[86] Morgan RA, Yang JC, Kitano M, Dudley ME, Laurencot CM, Rosenberg SA. Case report of a serious adverse event following the administration of T cells transduced with a chimeric antigen receptor recognizing ERBB2. Molecular Therapy 2010;8(4) 843-851.

[87] Hawkins RE, Gilham DE, Debets R, Eshhar Z, Taylor N, Abken H, Schumacher TN, ATTACK Consortium. Development of adoptive cell therapy for cancer: a clinical perspective. Human Gene Therapy 2010;21(6) 665-672.

[88] Büning H, Uckert W, Cichutek K, Hawkins RE, Abken H. Do CARs need a driver's license? Adoptive cell therapy with chimeric antigen receptor-redirected T cells has caused serious adverse events. Human Gene Therapy 2010;21(9) 1039-1042.

[89] Zhou BB, Zhang H, Damelin M, Geles KG, Grindley JC, Dirks PB. Tumour-initiating cells: challenges and opportunities for anticancer drug discovery. Nature Reviews Drug Discovery 2009;8(10) 806-823.

[90] Al-Hajj M, Wicha MS, Benito-Hernandez A, Morrison SJ, Clarke MF. Prospective identification of tumorigenic breast cancer cells. Proceedings of the National Academy of Sciences of the United States of America 2003;100(7) 3983-3988.

[91] Dalerba P, Dylla SJ, Park IK, Liu R, Wang X, Cho RW, Hoey T, Gurney A, Huang EH, Simeone DM, Shelton AA, Parmiani G, Castelli C, Clarke MF. Phenotypic characterization of human colorectal cancer stem cells. Proceedings of the National Academy of Sciences of the United States of America 2007;104(24) 10158-10163.

[92] Singh SK, Clarke ID, Terasaki M, Bonn VE, Hawkins C, Squire J, Dirks PB. Identification of a cancer stem cell in human brain tumors. Cancer Research 2003;63(18) 5821-5828.

[93] Ricci-Vitiani L, Lombardi DG, Pilozzi E, Biffoni M, Todaro M, Peschle C, De Maria R. Identification and expansion of human colon-cancer-initiating cells. Nature 2007;445(7123) 111-115.

[94] Li C, Heidt DG, Dalerba P, Burant CF, Zhang L, Adsay V, Wicha M, Clarke MF, Simeone DM. Identification of pancreatic cancer stem cells. Cancer Research 2007;67(3) 1030-1037.

[95] Schatton T, Murphy GF, Frank NY, Yamaura K, Waaga-Gasser AM, Gasser M, Zhan Q, Jordan S, Duncan LM, Weishaupt C, Fuhlbrigge RC, Kupper TS, Sayegh MH, Frank MH. Identification of cells initiating human melanomas. Nature. 2008;451(7176) 345-349.

[96] Zabierowski SE, Herlyn M. Melanoma stem cells: the dark seed of melanoma. Journal of Clinical Oncology 2008;26(17) 2890-2894.

[97] Fang D, Nguyen TK, Leishear K, Finko R, Kulp AN, Hotz S, Van Belle PA, Xu X, Elder DE, Herlyn M. A tumorigenic subpopulation with stem cell properties in melanomas. Cancer Research 2005;65(20) 9328-9337.

[98] Boiko AD, Razorenova OV, van de Rijn M, Swetter SM, Johnson DL, Ly DP, Butler PD, Yang GP, Joshua B, Kaplan MJ, Longaker MT, Weissman IL. Human melanoma-initiating cells express neural crest nerve growth factor receptor CD271. Nature 2010;466(7302) 133-137.

[99] Quintana E, Shackleton M, Sabel MS, Fullen DR, Johnson TM, Morrison SJ. Efficient tumour formation by single human melanoma cells. Nature 2008;456(7222) 593-598.

[100] Quintana E, Shackleton M, Foster HR, Fullen DR, Sabel MS, Johnson TM, Morrison SJ. Phenotypic Heterogeneity among Tumorigenic Melanoma Cells from Patients that Is Reversible and Not Hierarchically Organized. Cancer Cell 2010;18(5) 510-523.

[101] Shakhova O, Zingg D, Schaefer SM, Hari L, Civenni G, Blunschi J, Claudinot S, Okoniewski M, Beermann F, Mihic-Probst D, Moch H, Wegner M, Dummer R, Barrandon Y, Cinelli P, Sommer L. Sox10 promotes the formation and maintenance of giant congenital naevi and melanoma. Nat Cell Biol 2012;14(8) 882-890.

[102] Schlaak M, Schmidt P, Bangard C, Kurschat P, Mauch C, Abken H. Regression of metastatic melanoma in a patient by antibody targeting of cancer stem cells. Oncotarget 2012;3(1) 22-30.

[103] Pinc A, Somasundaram R, Wagner C, Hörmann M, Karanikas G, Jalili A, Bauer W, Brunner P, Grabmeier-Pfistershammer K, Gschaider M, Lai CY, Hsu MY, Herlyn M, Stingl G, Wagner SN. Targeting CD20 in melanoma patients at high risk of disease recurrence. Mol Ther 2012;20(5) 1056-1062.

[104] Chmielewski M, Rappl G, Hombach AA, Abken H. T cells redirected by a CD3ζ chimeric antigen receptor can establish self-antigen-specific tumour protection in the long term. Gene Ther. 2013;20(2) 177-186.

[105] Kershaw MH, Westwood JA, Parker LL, Wang G, Eshhar Z, Mavroukakis SA, White DE, Wunderlich JR, Canevari S, Rogers-Freezer L, Chen CC, Yang JC, Rosenberg SA, Hwu P. A phase I study on adoptive immunotherapy using gene-modified T cells for ovarian cancer. Clin Cancer Res 2006;12(20.1) 6106-6115.

[106] Brentjens RJ, Davila ML, Riviere I, Park J, Wang X, Cowell LG, Bartido S, Stefanski J, Taylor C, Olszewska M, Borquez-Ojeda O, Qu J, Wasielewska T, He Q, Bernal Y, Rijo IV, Hedvat C, Kobos R, Curran K, Steinherz P, Jurcic J, Rosenblat T, Maslak P, Frattini M, Sadelain M. CD19-targeted T cells rapidly induce molecular remissions in adults with chemotherapy-refractory acute lymphoblastic leukemia. Sci Transl Med. 2013;5(177) 177ra38.

[107] Kaneko S, Mastaglio S, Bondanza A, Ponzoni M, Sanvito F, Aldrighetti L, Radrizzani M, La Seta-Catamancio S, Provasi E, Mondino A, Nagasawa T, Fleischhauer K, Russo V, Traversari C, Ciceri F, Bordignon C, Bonini C. IL-7 and IL-15 allow the generation

of suicide gene-modified alloreactive self-renewing central memory human T lymphocytes. Blood 2009; 113(5) 1006-1015.

[108] Suhoski MM, Golovina TN, Aqui NA, Tai VC, Varela-Rohena A, Milone MC, Carroll RG, Riley JL, June CH. Engineering artificial antigen-presenting cells to express a diverse array of co-stimulatory molecules. Mol Ther 2007;15(5) 981-988.

[109] Vera JF, Brenner LJ, Gerdemann U, Ngo MC, Sili U, Liu H, Wilson J, Dotti G, Heslop HE, Leen AM, Rooney CM. Accelerated production of antigen-specific T cells for preclinical and clinical applications using gas-permeable rapid expansion cultureware (G-Rex). J Immunother 2010;33(3) 305-315.

[110] Meidenbauer N, Marienhagen J, Laumer M, Vogl S, Heymann J, Andreesen R, Mackensen A. Survival and tumor localization of adoptively transferred Melan-A-specific T cells in melanoma patients. Journal of Immunology 2003;170(4) 2161-2169.

[111] Griffith KD, Read EJ, Carrasquillo JA, Carter CS, Yang JC, Fisher B, Aebersold P, Packard BS, Yu MY, Rosenberg SA. In vivo distribution of adoptively transferred indium-111-labeled tumor infiltrating lymphocytes and peripheral blood lymphocytes in patients with metastatic melanoma. Journal of the National Cancer Institute 1989;81(22) 1709-1717.

[112] Fisher B, Packard BS, Read EJ, Carrasquillo JA, Carter CS, Topalian SL, Yang JC, Yolles P, Larson SM, Rosenberg SA. Tumor localization of adoptively transferred indium-111 labeled tumor infiltrating lymphocytes in patients with metastatic melanoma. Journal of Clinical Oncology 1989;7(2) 250-261.

[113] Peng W, Ye Y, Rabinovich BA, Liu C, Lou Y, Zhang M, Whittington M, Yang Y, Overwijk WW, Lizée G, Hwu P. Transduction of tumor-specific T cells with CXCR2 chemokine receptor improves migration to tumor and antitumor immune responses. Clinical Cancer Research 2010;16(22) 5458-5468.

[114] Li Y, Liu S, Hernandez J, Vence L, Hwu P, Radvanyi L.MART-1-specific melanoma tumor-infiltrating lymphocytes maintaining CD28 expression have improved survival and expansion capability following antigenic restimulation in vitro. Journal of Immunology 2010;184(1) 452-465.

[115] Hernandez-Chacon JA, Li Y, Wu RC, Bernatchez C, Wang Y, Weber JS, Hwu P, Radvanyi LG. Costimulation through the CD137/4-1BB pathway protects human melanoma tumor-infiltrating lymphocytes from activation-induced cell death and enhances antitumor effector function. Journal of Immunology 2011;34(3) 236-250.

[116] Offringa R. Antigen choice in adoptive T-cell therapy of cancer. Current Opinion in Immunology 2009;21(2) 190-199.

[117] Overwijk WW, Theoret MR, Finkelstein SE, Surman DR, de Jong LA, Vyth-Dreese FA, Dellemijn TA, Antony PA, Spiess PJ, Palmer DC, Heimann DM, Klebanoff CA, Yu Z, Hwang LN, Feigenbaum L, Kruisbeek AM, Rosenberg SA, Restifo NP. Tumor

regression and autoimmunity after reversal of a functionally tolerant state of self-re-active CD8+T cells. The Journal of Experimental Medicine 2003;198(4) 569-580.

[118] Spiotto MT, Rowley DA, and Schreiber H. "Bystander" elimination of antigen loss variants in established tumors. Nature Medicine 2004; 10(3) 294-298.

[119] Schüler T, Blankenstein T. Cutting edge: CD8+effector T cells reject tumors by direct antigen recognition but indirect action on host cells. Journal of Immunology 2003;170(9) 4427-4431.

[120] Stewart-Jones G, Wadle A, Hombach A, Shenderov E, Held G, Fischer E, Kleber S, Nuber N, Stenner-Liewen F, Bauer S, McMichael A, Knuth A, Abken H, Hombach AA, Cerundolo V, Jones EY, Renner C. Rational development of high-affinity T-cell receptor-like antibodies. Proceedings of the National Academy of Sciences of the United States of America 2009;106(14) 5784-5788.

[121] Willemsen RA, Debets R, Hart E, Hoogenboom HR, Bolhuis RL, Chames P. A phage display selected fab fragment with MHC class I-restricted specificity for MAGE-A1 allows for retargeting of primary human T lymphocytes. Gene Therapy 2001;8(21) 1601-1608.

[122] Chmielewski M, Hombach A, Heuser C, Adams GP, Abken H.T cell activation by an-tibody-like immunoreceptors: increase in affinity of the single-chain fragment do-main above threshold does not increase T cell activation against antigen-positive target cells but decreases selectivity. Journal of Immunology 2004; 173(12) 7647-7653.

[123] Chmielewski M, Hombach AA, Abken H. CD28 cosignalling does not affect the acti-vation threshold in a chimeric antigen receptor-redirected T-cell attack. Gene Thera-py 2011;18(1) 62-72.

[124] Pule MA, Savoldo B, Myers GD, Rossig C, Russell HV, Dotti G, Huls MH, Liu E, Gee AP, Mei Z, Yvon E, Weiss HL, Liu H, Rooney CM, Heslop HE, Brenner MK. Virus-specific T cells engineered to coexpress tumor-specific receptors: persistence and an-titumor activity in individuals with neuroblastoma Nature Medicine 2008;14(11) 1264-1270.

[125] Antony PA, Piccirillo CA, Akpinarli A, Finkelstein SE, Speiss PJ, Surman DR, Palmer DC, Chan CC, Klebanoff CA, Overwijk WW, Rosenberg SA, Restifo NP. CD8+T cell immunity against a tumor/self-antigen is augmented by CD4+T helper cells and hin-dered by naturally occurring T regulatory cells. Journal of Immunology 2005;174(5) 2591-2601.

[126] Kofler DM, Chmielewski M, Rappl G, Hombach A, Riet T, Schmidt A, Hombach AA, Wendtner CM, Abken H. CD28 costimulation Impairs the efficacy of a redirected t-cell antitumor attack in the presence of regulatory t cells which can be overcome by preventing Lck activation. Mol Ther 2011;19(4) 760-767.

[127] [127]Leach DR, Krummel MF, Allison JP. Enhancement of antitumor immunity by CTLA-4 blockade. Science 1996;271(5256) 1734-1736.

[128] [128]Pedicord VA, Montalvo W, Leiner IM, Allison JP. Single dose of anti-CTLA-4 enhances CD8+T-cell memory formation, function, and maintenance. Proc Natl Acad Sci USA 2011;108(1) 266-271.

[129] Abate-Daga D, Hanada K, Davis JL, Yang JC, Rosenberg SA, Morgan RA. Expression profiling of TCR-engineered T cells demonstrates overexpression of multiple inhibitory receptors in persisting lymphocytes. Blood 2013;122(8) 1399-1410.

[130] Moon EK, Wang LC, Dolfi DV, Wilson CB, Ranganathan R, Sun J, Kapoor V, Scholler J, Puré E, Milone MC, June CH, Riley JL, Wherry EJ, Albelda SM. Multifactorial T-cell Hypofunction That Is Reversible Can Limit the Efficacy of Chimeric Antigen Receptor-Transduced Human T cells in Solid Tumors. Clin Cancer Res 2014;20(16) 4262-4273.

[131] Mackensen A, Meidenbauer N, Vogl S, Laumer M, Berger J, Andreesen R. Phase I study of adoptive T-cell therapy using antigen-specific CD8+T cells for the treatment of patients with metastatic melanoma. Journal of Clinical Oncology 2006;24(31) 5060-5069.

[132] Lozupone F, Rivoltini L, Luciani F, Venditti M, Lugini L, Cova A, Squarcina P, Parmiani G, Belardelli F, Fais S. Adoptive transfer of an anti-MART-1(27-35)-specific CD8+T cell clone leads to immunoselection of human melanoma antigen-loss variants in SCID mice. European Journal of Immunology 2003;33(2) 556-566.

[133] Becker JC, Varki N, Gillies SD, Furukawa K, Reisfeld RA. An antibody-interleukin 2 fusion protein overcomes tumor heterogeneity by induction of a cellular immune response," Proceedings of the National Academy of Sciences of the United States of America 1996;93(15) 7826-7831.

[134] Chmielewski M, Kopecky C, Hombach AA, Abken H. IL-12 release by engineered T cells expressing chimeric antigen receptors can effectively Muster an antigen-independent macrophage response on tumor cells that have shut down tumor antigen expression. Cancer Research 2011;71(17) 5697-5706.

[135] Boni A, Cogdill AP, Dang P, Udayakumar D, Njauw CN, Sloss CM, Ferrone CR, Flaherty KT, Lawrence DP, Fisher DE, Tsao H, Wargo JA. Selective BRAFV600E inhibition enhances T-cell recognition of melanoma without affecting lymphocyte function. Cancer Research 2010;70(13) 5213-5219.

[136] Wilmott JS, Long GV, Howle JR, Haydu LE, Sharma RN, Thompson JF, Kefford RF, Hersey P, Scolyer RA. Selective BRAF inhibitors induce marked T-cell infiltration into human metastatic melanoma. Clinical Cancer Research 2012;18(5) 1386-1394.

[137] Pegram HJ, Jackson JT, Smyth MJ, Kershaw MH, Darcy PK. Adoptive transfer of gene-modified primary NK cells can specifically inhibit tumor progression in vivo. Journal of Immunology 2008;181(5) 3449-3455.

[138] Kruschinski A, Moosmann A, Poschke I, Norell H, Chmielewski M, Seliger B, Kiessling R, Blankenstein T, Abken H, Charo J. Engineering antigen-specific primary human NK cells against HER-2 positive carcinomas," Proceedings of the National Academy of Sciences of the United States of America 2008;105(45) 17481-17486.

[139] Boissel L, Betancur-Boissel M, Lu W, Krause DS, Van Etten RA, Wels WS, Klingemann H. Retargeting NK-92 cells by means of CD19-and CD20-specific chimeric antigen receptors compares favorably with antibody-dependent cellular cytotoxicity. Oncoimmunology 2013;2(10) e26527.

[140] Jiang H, Zhang W, Shang P, Zhang H, Fu W, Ye F, Zeng T, Huang H, Zhang X, Sun W, Man-Yuen Sze D, Yi Q, Hou J. Transfection of chimeric anti-CD138 gene enhances natural killer cell activation and killing of multiple myeloma cells. Mol Oncol 2014;8(2) 297-310.

[141] Boissel L, Betancur M, Wels WS, Tuncer H, Klingemann H. Transfection with mRNA for CD19 specific chimeric antigen receptor restores NK cell mediated killing of CLL cells. Leuk Res 2009; 33(9), 1255-1259.

[142] Klingemann HG. Cellular therapy of cancer with natural killer cells-where do we stand? Cytotherapy 2013;15(10) 1185-1194.

[143] Müller T, Uherek C, Maki G, Chow KU, Schimpf A, Klingemann HG, Tonn T, Wels WS. Expression of a CD20-specific chimeric antigen receptor enhances cytotoxic activity of NK cells and overcomes NK-resistance of lymphoma and leukemia cells. Cancer Immunol Immunother 2008;57(3) 411-423.

[144] Chu J, Deng Y, Benson DM, He S, Hughes T, Zhang J, Peng Y, Mao H, Yi L, Ghoshal K, He X, Devine SM, Zhang X, Caligiuri MA, Hofmeister CC, Yu J. CS1-specific chimeric antigen receptor (CAR)-engineered natural killer cells enhance In Vitro and In Vivo anti-tumor activity against human multiple myeloma. Leukemia 2014;28(4) 917-927.

[145] Uherek C, Tonn T, Uherek B, Becker S, Schnierle B, Klingemann HG, Wels W. Retargeting of natural killer-cell cytolytic activity to ErbB2-expressing cancer cells results in efficient and selective tumor cell destruction. Blood 2002;100(4) 1265-1273.

[146] Tavri S, Jha P, Meier R, Henning TD, Müller T, Hostetter D, Knopp C, Johansson M, Reinhart V, Boddington S, Sista A, Wels WS, Daldrup-Link HE. Optical imaging of cellular immunotherapy against prostate cancer. Mol Imaging2009;8(1) 15-26.

[147] Esser R, Müller T, Stefes D, Kloess S, Seidel D, Gillies SD, Aperlo-Iffland C, Huston JS, Uherek C, Schönfeld K, Tonn T, Huebener N, Lode HN, Koehl U, Wels WS. NK cells engineered to express a GD2-specific antigen receptor display built-in ADCC-

like activity against tumour cells of neuroectodermal origin. J Cell Mol Med 2012;16(3) 569-581.

[148] Imai C, Iwamoto S, Campana D. Genetic modification of primary natural killer cells overcomes inhibitory signals and induces specific killing of leukemic cells. Blood 2005;106(1) 376-383.

[149] Altvater B, Landmeier S, Pscherer S, Temme J, Schweer K, Kailayangiri S, Campana D, Juergens H, Pule M, Rossig C. 2B4 (CD244) signaling by recombinant antigen-specific chimeric receptors costimulates natural killer cell activation to leukemia and neuroblastoma cells. Clin Cancer Res2009;15(15) 4857-4866.

[150] Sahm C, Schönfeld K, Wels WS. Expression of IL-15 in NK cells results in rapid enrichment and selective cytotoxicity of gene-modified effectors that carry a tumor-specific antigen receptor. Cancer Immunol Immunother 2012;61(9) 1451-1461.

5

Current Insights Into Canine Cutaneous Melanocytic Tumours Diagnosis

Luis Resende, Joana Moreira, Justina Prada,
Felisbina Luisa Queiroga and Isabel Pires

1. Introduction

Skin melanoma is a devastating disease, frequently diagnosed in human and dogs, accounting for 0,8% - 2% of all skin tumors in latter species [1].

Melanocytic tumours are common neoplasms in dogs, accounting for 4 to 7% of neoplastic lesions in general, and up to 7% of all malignant tumours [2,3]. They generally arise on the oral cavity (Figure 1), lip, skin (Figure 2) and digit, amongst other locations (Figure 3) [4].

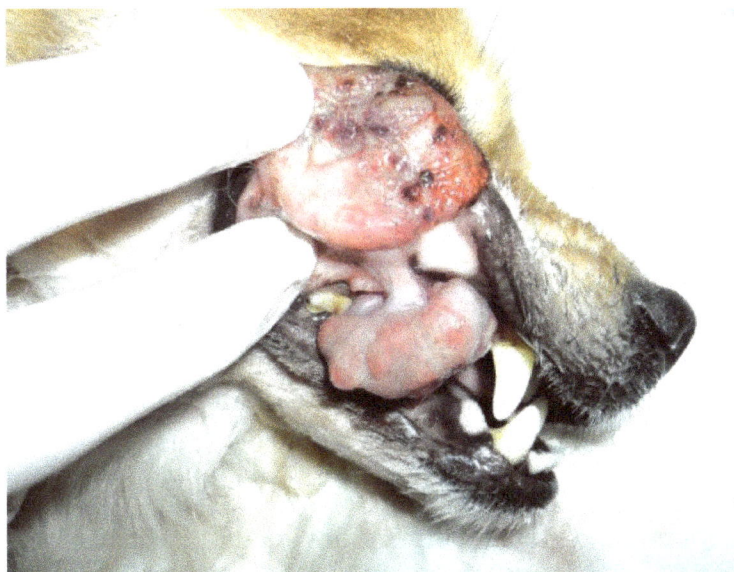

Figure 1. Canine oral melanoma (courtesy of Dr. Abel Fernandes).

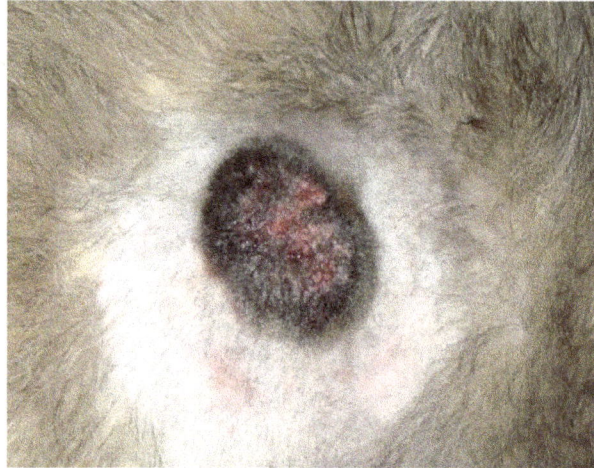

Figure 2. Canine cutaneous melanoma.

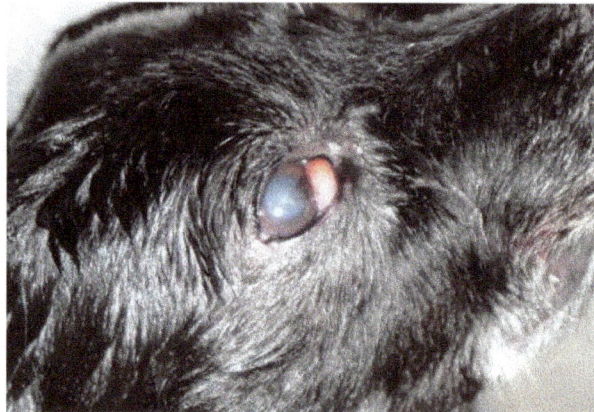

Figure 3. Canine ocular melanoma.

Biologic behaviour of these tumours is often related to its location. Over 85% of melanocytic lesions located on haired skin are described as of benign behaviour. The majority of oral and mucocutaneous junction melanomas, with the exception of the eyelid, and 50% of digital melanomas originated from the nail bed are reported as malignant [5,6].

Cutaneous canine melanocytic lesions are usually benign [7,8]. They are generally detected at a late stage, when excision is rarely curative and metastasis is often detectable in regional lymph nodes [7]. Malignant tumors are found most frequently on the head, ventral abdomen, and scrotum [7]; in the last one, they represent 3,1% of all cutaneous malignant melanomas and 4,7% of scrotal tumours [9]. Amelanotic lesions can occur as cutaneous neoplasms, but are more frequent in the oral cavity, and tend to be behaviorally malignant [10].

Metastasis are often found on regional lymph nodes and lungs, but organs as brain, heart and spleen are also commonly affected [11].

Veterinary nomenclature of canine melanocytic tumours has been subjected to many controversies and changes over time. Through this article, in accordance with the revised World

Health Organization classification system, and in order to simplify and avoid confusion, the authors describe benign lesions as melanocytoma, whereas malignant lesions are referred to as melanoma [12].

Etiology of this neoplasms is still uncertain, and several factors may be related, such as consanguinity, trauma, chemical exposure, hormones and genetic susceptibility [10]. Unlike humans, ionizing solar radiation exposure doesn't seem to be related to canine melanoma initiation [4].

Canine melanocytic tumour diagnosis often represents a challenge for the pathologist, since a high number of neoplastic lesions are quite similar in terms of its clinical and histologic appearance, including carcinoma, sarcoma, lymphoma and plasmocitoma, amongst others [10]. Indeed, cutaneous neoplasms with malignant behavior are more difficult to distinguish histologically from benign neoplasms than oral or lip neoplasms [13].

Diagnosis is usually based on fine-needle aspiration citology, but biopsy for histopathological examination is essential to determine its malignant potential [4,14]. The most reliable histologic criteria is the mitotic index, defined as the total number of mitotic figures observed per ten high-power light microscopic fields, which is known to be 90% accurate [5,6,15].

Immunochemistry has arised as an extremely useful tool, for both diagnostic and prognostic purposes. A positive diagnostic for melanocytic neoplasms is obtained with a positive labelling of S100 protein, vimentine, Neuron Specific Enolase (NSE) and a simoultaneous negative labelling with cytokeratine [16].

The treatment of choice for local cutaneous melanomas is surgical excision; tumours with benign histopathology criteria have an excellent prognostic after this surgery. However, for malignant tumors, the prognostic is guarded, since metastatic rates of 30-75% have been reported [5,6].

Alternative therapy methods described in the literature include systemic chemotherapy, radiotherapy [17], photodynamic therapy [18], local hyperthermia [19,20] and intralesional injection of cisplatin or carboplatin.

The poor responses to the conventional therapy are leading to a development of new immunotherapy procedures – including intralesional adenoviral vector-mediated transfer of CD40L, a tumor necrosis factor gene [21], therapy with a plasmid DNA encoding staphylococcal enterotoxin B [22], and systemic tratment with liposome-encapsulated muramyl tripeptide [23].

At last, the most promising therapy appears to be a xenogenetic human tyrosinase DNA vaccine, with minimal local reaction and no systemic toxicity signs, and a great clinical responde with significant increasing of the survival time [24].

In this paper, the authors aim to contribute to the understanding of melanocytic tumours in the dog, making a critical review of the literature and discussing the parameters currently considered valid for diagnosis use in canine melanocytic neoplams.

2. Signalment

Cutaneous melanocytic tumours are most common in older dogs (mean age of 9 years old) [25], with a higher mean age for dogs with malignant melanocytic tumours (12 years). However, age has not been related with the patient clinical outcome and survival time [26].

Although all breeds of dog (and crossbred animals) may be affected, some breeds are reported as predisposed, including Schnauzer, Doberman, Scottish Terrier, Irish Setter, Golden Retriever, Chow Chow, Cocker Spaniel, German Shepherd and Rottweiler [4,27]. Breed predisposition is thought to be related to an underlying genetic risk and/or increased pigmentation in the described above breeds [4].

One study [6] has also established a relationship between patient breed and tumour behavior, likely due to genetic susceptibility, as prior described. In the referred work, melanocytic lesions tended to be behaviorally benign in Doberman pinschers and miniature schnauzers, while miniature poodles were the mostly affected breed with malignant melanoma. However, it must be noted that oral neoplasms were also included in that study.

An early report described a higher frequency of these lesions in male dogs [28], but recent literature denies gender predisposition [6,27,29-31].

3. Pathogenesis

Melanin is a dark-brown pigment synthetized by melanocytes, dendritic cells found within the basal layer of the epidermis. These cells are dispersed from each other, located between basal keratinocytes, forming adherent and regulatory junctions mediated by epithelial cadherin (E-cadherin) molecules. After its synthesis, melanin is retained in melanosomas and transferred to the adjacent keratinocytes [32].

Conversion of normal melanocytes to clusters of neoplastic melanocytes is a process composed by a series of events: initiation, promotion, transformation and metastasis [4].

Little is known about initiation on most animal melanomas, but ionizing solar radiation exposure – the main initiator factor in Human melanomas [33] - doesn't seem to be related to canine melanomas [4]. A higher incidence of spontaneously mutated cells due to familiar clustering through inbreeding may be a critical initiation factor in domestic animals.

Malignant transformation of canine cutaneous melanocytomas is very uncommon. Regarding cutaneous melanomas, there are a few published case reports, including one by Valentine and team [34], which have described a single case of malignant transformation of a congenital melanocytic nevus is a Golden retriever. Conroy [35] described two cases of melanoma originated from junctional or dermal hamartomas and a single case of a primary melanomas originated from a subcutaneous melanocytoma have also been reported [36]. In summary, canine cutaneous melanomas are thought to arise *de novo* from epidermal and dermal melanocytes.

Promotion phase is related to mutated cells proliferation, with subsequent amplification of cell population and origin of additional mutations [4]. Melanoma promoters include chronic trauma, chemical exposure, drugs and hormones [10], and its action results in reactive hyperplasia of the epithelium, with disruption of regular keratinocyte-melanocyte interactions and proliferation of initiated cells.

The next step in carcinogenesis involves a series of transformation events. Recent developments in genetic and molecular study techniques have identified the role of a few tumour suppressors in melanoma cell lines, giving new insights on the importance of these molecules in canine melanoma development. A reduction or loss of *p16* expression was one of the most commonly found changes, in both benign and malignant tumours, suggesting that inactivation of this pathway is a critical step in the pathogenesis of melanoma [37]. Altered expression of *PTEN*, *TP53*, *Rb* and *p21* have also been related to its progression [38], as well as the presence of various oncogenes (as a result of proto-oncogenes mutation), such as *c-myc*, *c-erb-B-2*, *c-yes*, *c-kit* and *ras* [4].

After local proliferation phase, neoplastic cells may acquire a malignant behavior, and disseminate through hematic or lymphatic vessels to various other organs, originating secondary neoplasms known as metastasis. This complex process has it start with loss of adhesion and detachment of neoplastic cells from the primary mass, hematic and lymphatic vessels intravasion and attachment and proliferation within a secondary location [4].

Metastasis process is dependent of various adhesion molecules regulation by neoplastic cells. Several studies have shown an association between decreased and altered expression of E-cadherin, a calcium-dependent adhesion molecule responsible for melanocyte-keratinocyte interaction, and canine cutaneous melanoma progression [39,40]. CD44, a second transmembrane glycoprotein which facilitates metastasis, is required for several processes, including hyaluronate degradation, cell aggregation and migration, angiogenesis and hematopoiesis [4]. Down-regulation of regular CD44 plus up-regulation of CD44v5 has also been associated with melanoma metastasis, particularly with lymph node metastasis [41].

Autonomous growth is a key requirement for both primary and secondary neoplastic development. The most important autocrine growth factors in animal melanoma include basic fibroblast growth factor (*bFGF*), melanoma growth stimulatory activity or growth regulated proteins, platelet-derive growth factor-A, α-melanocyte stimulating hormone, and a series of interleukins (*IL-8*, *IL-10* and *IL-18*) [4].

4. Gross morphologic features

Macroscopically, canine malignant melanoma cannot be differentiated from melanocytoma [42]. Melanomas in dogs tend to be dermal in location, unlike Human melanomas – which are intraepidermal with some degree of dermal invasion. Prognostic schemes, such as Clark's level or Breslow thickness, built nased on depht of dermal invasion, are not applicable on canine lesions [43].

Canine melanocytomas share some aspects with Human benign melanocytic lesions, in terms of clinical evolution most common metastatic locations [42], and genetic alterations [44].

Cutaneous melanocytomas are usually symmetrical, circumscribed, but encapsulated [43], solitary, black, brown, or gray cutaneous alopecic nodules [43,45] with a variable size with range of 1-4 cm in diameter (Figure 4 and Figure 5) [43]. Epidermis is usually intact, and alopecia is frequent. Epidermal cells may be hyperpigmented, and the majority of dermal cells are replaced by the tumoral ones, which in larger masses might also extends into the subcutaneous tissue. The tumors may have a varieated appearance, with areas of pigmentation intermingled with no pigmented regions [42].

Canine cutaneous malignant melanomas can vary considerably in appearance, regardless of the location. Melanomas tend to be asymmetrical. The asymmetry may be most readily recognizable in the epidermal component of junctional tumors [43]. Melanomas size vary from some milimiteres to as large as 10 centimeters in diameter (mean range being 1 to 3 cm in diameter) [43], but this is not a reliable indicator of malignancy [13,42]. The color is variable, ranging from gray or brown to black, red, or even dark blue [7]. Cutaneous melanoma presentation includes smooth domes, sessile nodules, polypoid, plaquelike [7,43], or even lobulated masses [7]. The larger ones are often ulcerated [7,43]. The tumors may invade deeply into the subcutaneous tissue and along fascial planes [42].

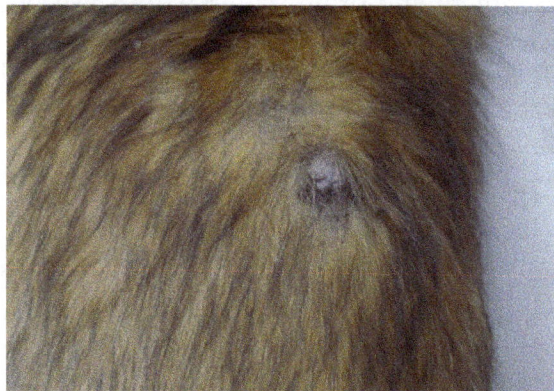

Figure 4. Canine cutaneous melanoma.

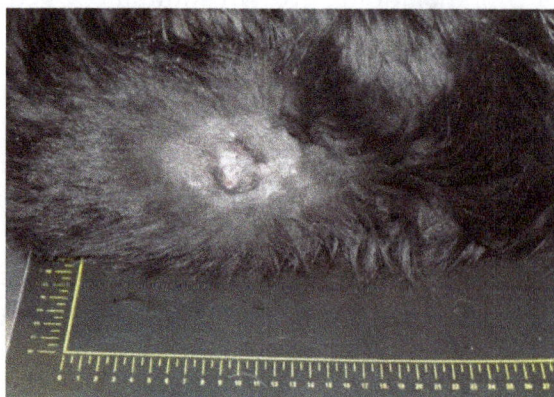

Figure 5. Canine cutaneous melanoma.

5. Cytological diagnosis

Microscopic examination of a cytological specimen obtained through fine needle aspiration has become a valuable technique to obtain a preliminary, and often definitive, diagnosis [46]. Being a quick, non-evasive and inexpensive procedure, it can also provide information on the stage, prognosis and metastasis evidence. Its main limitation reside on the fact that non-pigmented melanomas may strongly resemble other neoplastic lesions, and the amount of cytological sample might be very small and not fully representative of the lesion [4,46].

Several studies in Human cancer have described a strong accuracy in cytological examination in comparison with histopathological findings [47,48], but there are only few studies on the subject in Veterinary Medicine [49]. For instance, Ghisleni and others [50] evaluated a series of cutaneous and subcutaneous masses from dogs and cats through histopathology and cytology, describing an agreement between both techniques in 90.9% of the samples.

Melanocytic tumours are characterized by the presence of cells with abundant cytoplasmatic melanin granules. Neoplastic cells may appear with an epithelial (cohesive cells), mesenchymal (single oval or spindle-shaped cells) or round cell morphology. Nuclei may present a central or eccentric location, and is often solitary, though multinucleated forms are occasionally found. Nucleoli tends to be very prominent, with variable shapes such as round, oval or angular. These cells have a light basophilic cytoplasm, with a moderate to high nuclear-cytoplasmatic ratio. Varying degrees of pigmentation might be found within the same tumour smear [4,46], (Figure 6 and Figure 7).

Malignant criteria consist, most importantly, of marked anisokaryosis and nuclear pleomorphism, but also of the presence of large and atypical nucleoli [46]. Mitotic index, the most reliable criteria in histopathological evaluation, has no use in cytology. Regional lymph nodes are the most commonly evaluated site while monitoring for metastasis [4].

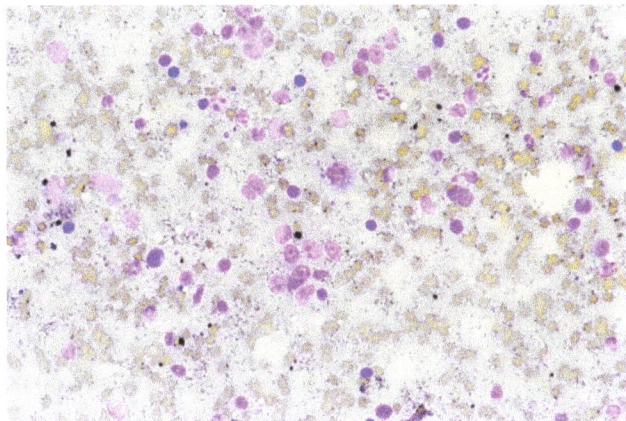

Figure 6. Canine cutaneous melanoma (Wright, 100x).

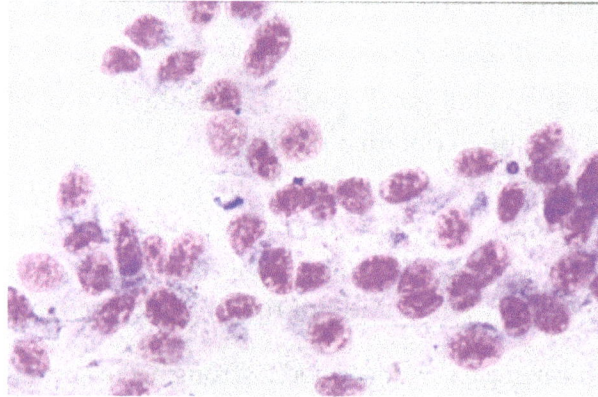

Figure 7. Canine cutaneous melanoma (Wright, 400x).

6. Histological diagnosis

Histological characteristics of canine melanocytic neoplasms were defined by World Health Organization, in *International Histological Classification of Tumours of Domestic Animals*, back in 1974 (Figure 8 and Figure 9) [13].

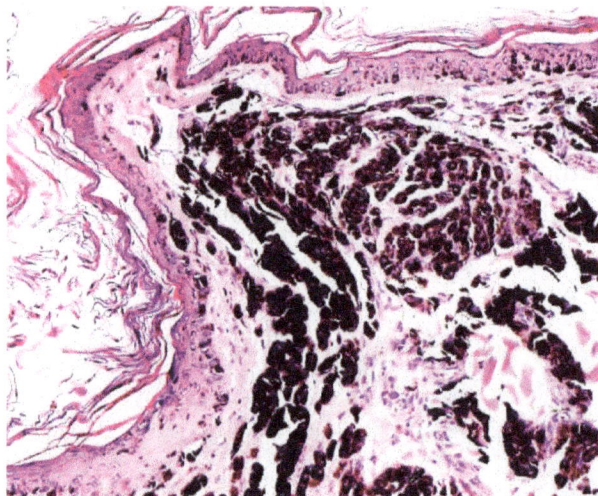

Figure 8. Canine cutaneous melanocytoma (H&E, 200x).

Histological appearance does not always correlate well with biological behavior [8]. More recent studies have provided a numerical "tumor score" taking into consideration mitotic index, nuclear atypia, inflammation, necrosis and volume which appears to have improved correlation between histology and behavior [8].

The term nevus, commonly used in describing pigmented melanocytic lesions of the epidermis and dermis in humans, is not used in veterinary dermatopathology [7].

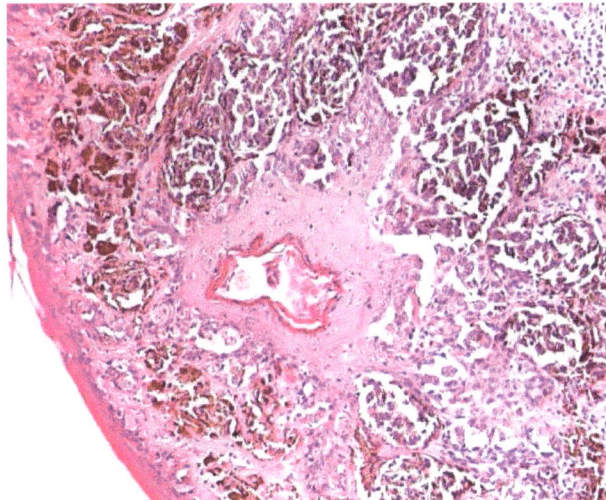

Figure 9. Canine cutaneous melanoma (H&E, 200x).

In this chapter we review several histological parameters on their ability to diagnose and predict prognosis (i.e., prediction of mortality) of canine melanocytic neoplasms. Malignancy celular features include a characteristic large nucleous, nuclear atypia, hyperchromasia, abnormal chromatin clumping and anomalous mitotic figures [51].

6.1. Predominant cell type

Melanocytic neoplasms are generally composed of one of the following cell types: epithelioid (Figure 10), spindle, mixed (Figure 11), dendritic [51,52], and round cells [43]. Other less commonly described cell types include signet ring and ballon cells [51]. All these cell types may occur either alone or in combination [43]. In melanomas, ganglion cell and multinucleated giant cell forms also may be observed [43]. The epithelioid cell type is the most common type in all locations, whereas a mixture of cell types is seen with less frequency [51].

The epithelioid cells are round, with discrete cell borders, abundant glassy cytoplasm, appearing arranged in sheets and larger nests [43]. Similar to their spindle-shaped counterparts melanomas may exhibit large ovoid nuclei and prominent nucleoli [7,43], marked anisokaryosis and variable chromatin patterns [43].

The spindle cell tumors are arranged in streams and interweaving bundles, resembling fibrosarcoma or neurofibrosarcoma presentation. In malignant lesions, the nuclei are large and fusiform with prominent nucleoli [7,43], and moderate to marked nuclear pleomorphism is seen [43]. Spindle cell predominant morphology was statistically associated with benignity in one study (in 71% melanocytomas in contrast to 29% melanomas) [43]. The mixed type consists of both cell morphologies and patterns [7].

Dendritic melanocytes have a highly angular shape, sometimes with long cytoplasmic processes, and are usually arranged in small nests [43] or organized in tightly swirling streams, often with a fingerprint pattern [7]. The dendritic or whorled forms occurs only in the skin [53].

Round cells tumors have round to polygonal cells arranged in sheets as dense packets of cells, the packets being separated by a scant stroma. The nuclei is large and round in melanomas [43].

The signet-ring cell tumors consist of compact neoplastic clusters, with round to ovoid cells presenting a faintly-eosinophilic cytoplasm and an intensely-stained periphery. A vesicular nuclei, crescent-shaped, and with a peripheral location, gives the cell a signet-ring appearance [52].

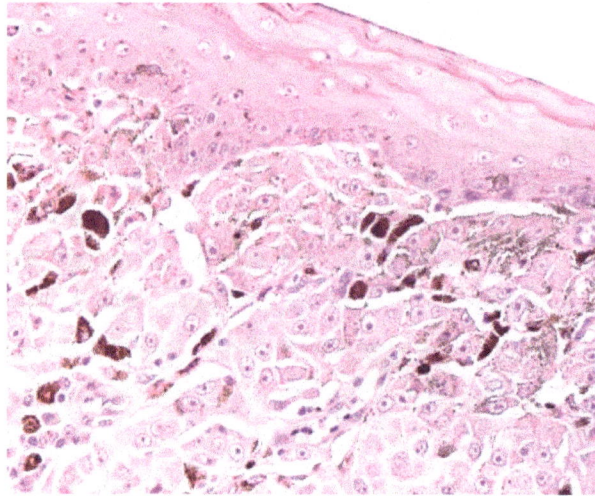

Figure 10. Epithelioid cell canine cutaneous melanoma (H&E, 400x).

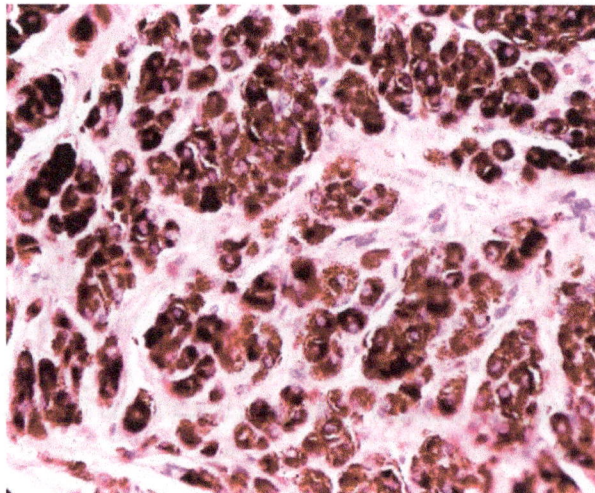

Figure 11. Mixed cell canine cutaneous melanoma (H&E, 400x).

Balloon cells are found organized in groups, separated by collagenous septa [52]. The cells are round to polyhedral and have clear or faintly eosinophilic cytoplasm [43,52]. In melanomas, the nuclei are round situated mainly at the periphery of the tumor cells [52]. Usually contains one central prominent nucleolus [7], which sometimes is difficult to detect. Heterochromatin, which is sparse, is dispersed throughout the nuclei [52].

Benign melanocytic cells present an enlarged vesicular nuclei with small nucleoli. Nuclear shape vary on according to the predominant tumour cell type. Mitotic figures are rare, and mitotic atypia is rarely observed. [43].

Although cell type appears to play some role in the prognosis of ocular melanocytic neoplasms, this feature lacked significance in prognosis of melanocytic tumors occurring in the mouth, feet, buccal mucosa and skin of dogs in several studies [8]. On the contrary, the epithelioid shape was associated with an unfavorable course, for 8/15 cases. The difference seems to be significant (p = 0,03) [12].

6.2. Nuclear atypia

One of the major criteria of malignancy in melanocytic neoplasms arising at any pigmented anatomic site is nuclear atypia. This feature is more valuable in epithelioid tumours than in spindle, whorled type or signet-ring cells, due to the insufficient nuclear detail associated with the later neoplasms [8,44,54]. However, not all studies are consensual [12].

Well-differentiated tumoral melanocytes have a small nucleus with one central nucleolus [8]. In contrary, undifferentiated tumours generally present cells with multiple, large, irregular and eccentrically nucleoli [8].

Several criteria are used to estimate nuclear atypia, including the percentage of nuclei involved [8]. Figures 12 and 13 (below) present moderate and severe nuclear atypia, respectively.

6.3. Mitotic index

In animal cutaneous and eye melanocytic neoplasms, mitotic index (MI) is the most reliable histological feature for distinguishing malignant from benign tumors [44,51], and also in predicting the clinical course of the disease [8]. In cutaneous melanoma, an MI of ≥3/10 hpf is significantly correlated with decreased survival [55].

The number of mitoses is usually lower in melanocytomas [<3 mitotic figures per 10 high power fields (hpf)] than melanomas [42,44,53].

In one study, the mitotic index was strongly correlated with the clinical outcome of tumors. For tumors with a favorable outcome, the mean value of the number of mitosis (on 10 randomly selected high power fields) was 1,98 (from 0 to 27). For tumors with a malignant behavior, it was 18,53 (from 0 to 75) [12].

The evaluation of the MI in conjunction with nuclear atypia classification (Figure 13) offers a more precise value the histological diagnosis [8].

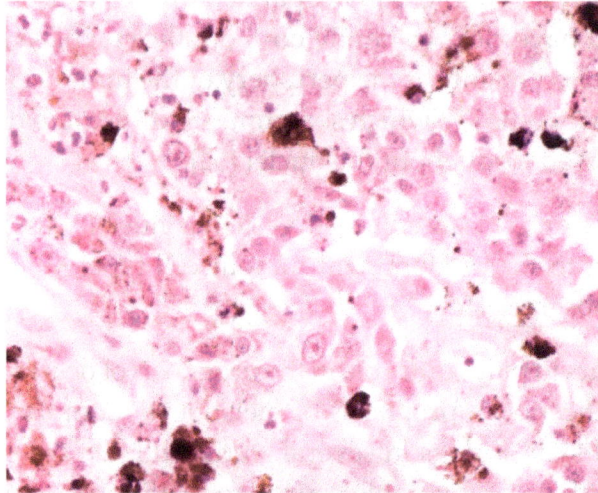

Figure 12. Canine cutaneous melanoma with moderate diferenciation (H&E, 400x).

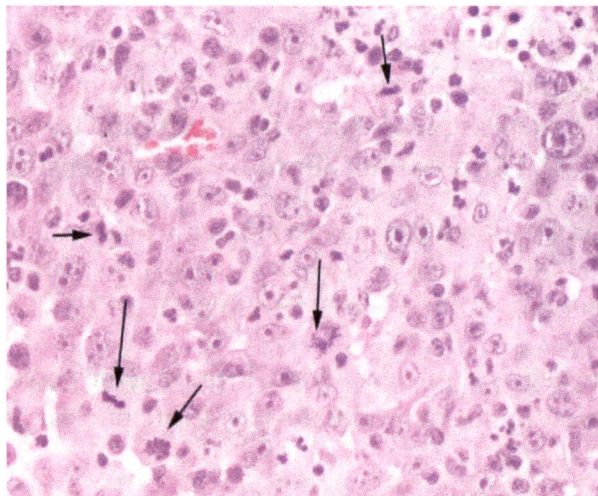

Figure 13. Canine cutaneous melanoma with evident nuclear atypia and numerous mitosis (arrow), (H&E, 400x).

6.4. Cellular pleomorphism

Cellular pleomorphism criteria include several features, such as cell size and shape, pigmentation degree and nuclear features (including prominence of nucleoli and chromatin pattern). The usefulness of these parameters as individual prognostic factors is doubtful; however, it increases when these are used together [8,27].

6.5. Degree of pigmentation

Degree of pigmentation is highly variable, even within a single smear (Figures 14, 15 and 16). Even on histological evaluation of amelanotic-classified tumours is common to detect a few very fine pigment granules in some cells. These are generally punctuate, spherical or elongated, as observed in pigmented keratinocytes. Cells with a very fine pigment may present a dusty gray appearance, instead of the typical granulation image [7]. In summary, it can be difficult to accurately diagnose an amelanotic melanocytic neoplasm and to define the degree of pigmentation [13].

Individual tumoral cells possess a different amount of melanin, which granules are generally small and uniform in size within the same cell. Splindle, round to polygonal, and balloon cells have sparsely-distributed melanin granules, while large epithelioid and dendritic cells are known to have a higher degree of pigmentation [43].

The majority of canine melanocytomas (except for ballon cell ones) have marked to moderate melanin pigmentation overall, especially in the superficial aspect of the tumors [43]. Similarly to cellular morphology, the degree of pigmentation of neoplastic cells was not an indicator of prognosis [12].

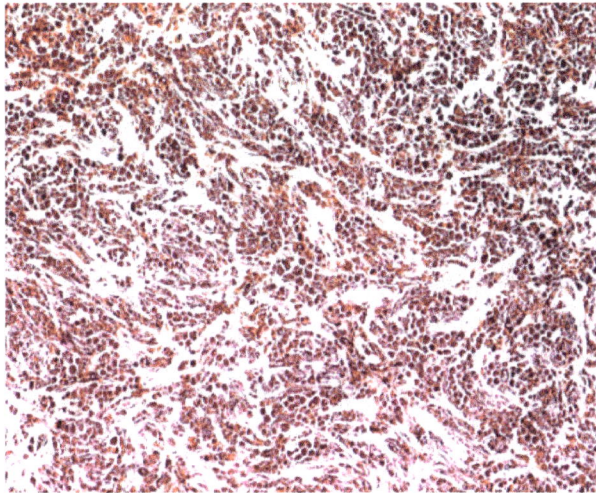

Figure 14. Canine cutaneous melanoma with marked pigmentation (H&E, 400x).

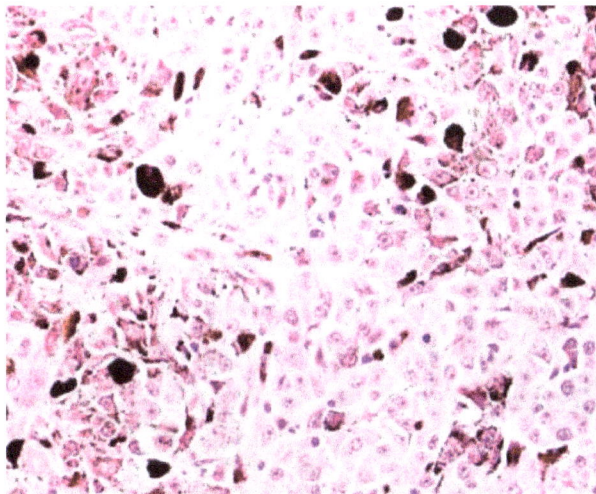

Figure 15. Canine cutaneous melanoma with moderate pigmentation (H&E, 400x).

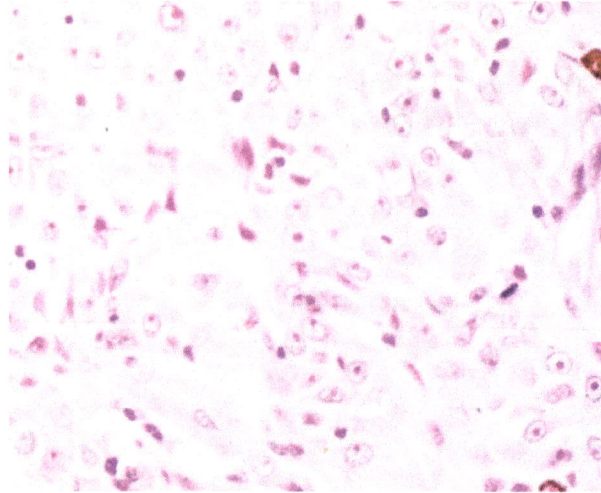

Figure 16. Amelanotic melanoma (H&E, 400x).

6.6. Junctional activity

Junctional activity refers to the proliferation of neoplastic melanocytes at the interface between the epidermis and dermis or epithelium and submucosa [53].

The presence or absence of junctional activity is not specific to melanoma and often occurs in melanocytomas [7], however, malignant melanomas arising in the skin often show marked junctional activity, (Figure 17 and Figure 18) [42].

Junctional activity was not statistically associated with survival for skin neoplasms in one study [8]. In contrast, another work considered junctional activity as an independent prognostic factor (p =0,0239) for cutaneous melanocytic neoplasms, and found that its occurrence was associated with a longer survival time (p = 0,0046) [55].

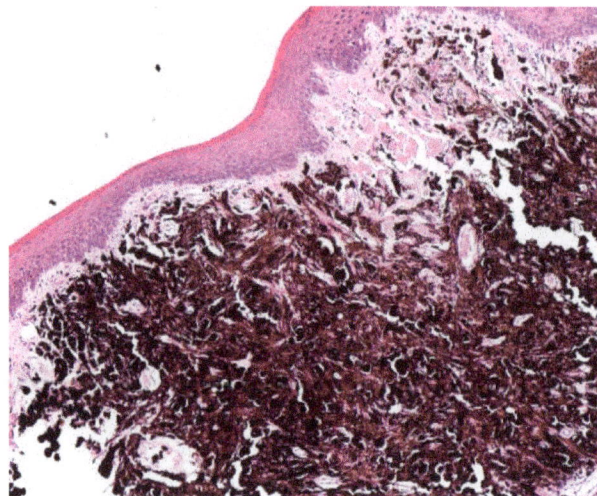

Figure 17. Canine cutaneous melanoma without junctional activity (H&E, 200x).

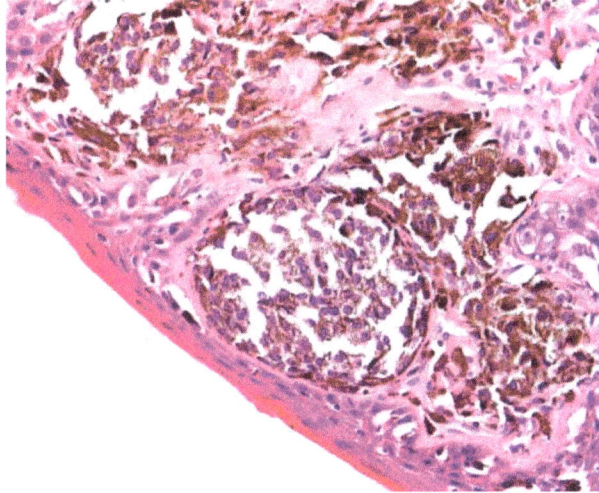

Figure 18. Canine cutaneous melanoma with junctional activity (H&E, 400x).

6.7. Intraepithelial neoplastic cells

The presence of intraepidermal tumoural cells can be graded as absent, slight (25% of neoplastic melanocytes in epidermis), moderate or prominent (more than 50% of tumour cells are present in the epidermis) [44]. However, this feature appears not to be of prognostic significance [8].

In a recent study was found that the samples of canine melanomas presented medium to prominent scatter of intraepidermal melanocytes, lower pigmentation, and higher nesting of intraepidermal melanocytes, in comparison with melanocytomas [44].

In most melanocytomas, the overlying epidermis is hyperpigmented, regardless of the presence or absence of intraepidermal clusters of neoplastic melanocytes [43].

6.8. Ulceration

Canine melanomas are most frequently ulcerated [44] and particularly larger masses [43] than melanocytomas.

According to Laprie and team [55], ulceration might be taken as a prognostic marker for this neoplasms. In the referred work, the presence of an ulcerated epidermis was associated with a shorter survival time (p = 0,0023) and shown to be an independent prognostic factor (p = 0,0065) [55]. However, two other studies found no correlation between ulceration and clinical evolution of lip, nail bed [27] or cutaneous melanocytic neoplasms [12,27].

6.9. Level of infiltration/invasion

Melanocytic tumours strictly limited to the dermis, with a shallow depth, are associated with a greater survival time (p < 0,0001), and deep level of infiltration has been shown to be a significant prognostic factor (p = 0,0012) [55]. One other study that evaluated the level of invasion (in cutaneous and subcutaneous tissues) concluded that tumors confined to the superficial dermis were associated with a benign course in 94% of cases. On the other hand, tumors reaching the deep dermis and the subcutis showed a malignant behavior; however, the sample number were too low to allow for a conclusion [12].

6.10. Necrosis

Necrosis is a common feature, particularly in larger masses [43]. The presence of necrosis was correlated with malignancy and with a short survival time in a study set of 389 melanocytic neoplasms containing both benign and malignant lesions from various locations (mouth, feet and lip, skin) [8]. In other report with a set of 38 malignant melanomas from various locations, no correlation was found with survival time [54]. In summary, necrosis is considered of limited prognostic value in animals [7].

6.11. Morphologic classification

Melanocytomas include dermal, compound, and balloon cell tumors, as well as multiple dysplastic melanocytoma syndrome in dogs [43].

Dermal melanocytoma are strictly intradermal in location and larger tumours may extend into the subcutis [43]. Melanocytomas are generally composed by spindle cells disposed in bundles, nests and whorles, with a moderate cellular concentration and a lack of stromal collagen [43,45]. Melanophages might be dispersed throughout the tumoral nodule or in aggregates [43]. Mitotic figures are ocasionally seen (inferior to 1 per 10 high power fields), and mitotic atypia is not observed [43].

Some dermal melanocytomas are composed of epithelioid or dendritic cells that are heavily pigmented [43]. Nuclear morphology may be obscured by the large amount of pigment [43]. Although nuclei may be large, there is minimal nuclear pleomorphism [43].

A compound melanocytoma has a wedge-shaped configuration, and its description refers to the fact of including both junctional and dermal components. A numerous and densely packed tumor cell population is present in the dermis, while a variable amount of tumor cells accumulate in clusters and nests within the epidermis, along the dermal–epidermal junction and in the outer follicular wall – this pattern is referred to as 'junctional activity' [43].g

Balloon cell melanocytoma have a dermal location, and are predominantly composed of large round cells [43,45], although some fusiform or polygonal melanocytes might be present [42], with an abundant, pale eosinophilic and finely granular cytoplasm [42,43,45]. These lesions often lack readily visible pigmentation; however, dust-like melanin granules may be detected in small numbers [42,43]. Nuclei are small, uniform, and ovoid [43,45] and mitotic figures are rarely observed [42,43].

Multiple dysplastic melanocytoma syndrome mostly resemble compound melanocytomas on low magnification. However, their incidence increases in larger lesions. Also, cytologic atypia and mitotic figures are present and some of the proliferating melanocytes have irregularly shaped and enlarged hyperchromatic nuclei [43].

Canine melanocytoma–acanthomas are mixed tumors that are composed of a benign melanocytic proliferation, resembling compound melanocytoma, and a benign epithelial proliferation [43,45]. The epithelial component usually appears follicular and resembles an isthmus-type tricholemmoma or infundibular keratinizing acanthoma [43]. The epithelial population forms a mass in the dermis composed of cords and nests with occasional small cystic structures containing keratin [45]. Melanocytic cells form nests in the epidermis and sometimes in the cords of epithelial cells within the dermal mass; melanocytic spindle cells can form whorls and bundles between the epithelial cords and nests [45]. A dermal melanocytoma– acanthoma has been immunophenotyped in a German Shepherd dog identifying the presence of keratinocytes and melanocytes [56].

Dermal melanomas have no junctional activity, but in some cases the tumour might extend deeply into the subcutaneous tissue. There might be a predominance of a certain cell type, but most tumors reveal a mixture of spindle cells, round to polygonal cells, and/or epithelioid cells. While spindle cells are poorly pigmented, more round and epithelioid cells tend to have a moderate to abundant amont of melanin granule [43]. Other important features in this kind of neoplastic lesions include a marked nuclear pleomorphism, nucleolar prominence, a moderate mitotic rate (3 or greater per 10 high power fields), atypical mitotic figures, asymmetry of the tumor nodule and a lymphoplasmacytic cell population [43].

Melanomas have an obvious 'junctional activity' pattern, with tumor cells distributed through the dermal–epidermal junction, as well as at higher levels of the epidermis, particularly in those of the nail bed and lip [43]. The intraepidermal element is mainly composed of epithelioid melanocytes, disposed individually or arranged in nests and clusters [43]. Tumours with numerous melanocytes distributed through all levels of the epidermis are referred to as lesions with a 'pagetoid' pattern [43]. Other melanomas present numerous individual neoplastic melanocytes present within the basal cell layer only, which is also referred to as an 'atypical lentiginous infiltrate' [43].

Spindle cell and desmoplastic melanomas, a subgroup of dermal melanomas, is composed predominantly of spindled melanocytes densely packed, or arranged loosely within abundant pale stroma [43]. Occasionally, there is a prominent fibroblastic component associated with the spindle shaped melanocytes, and collagen may become more abundant than the tumor cells [43]. The vast majority are amelanotic, thus a Fontana–Masson stain usually is necessary to detect the presence of melanin granules; cells are usually arranged in bundles or palisades, mimicking tumors of neural origin [43].

Balloon cell melanoma (clear cell melanoma), possess large cells with a clear eosinophilic cytoplasm [43]. The majority of balloon cell melanomas are amelanotic [43]. Some dust-like melanin granules may be present in a few tumor cells, and Fontana–Masson staining may be required for their demonstration [43,45]. These cells have a large vesicular nuclei with a prominent nucleoli [7,43]. Mitotic activity is generally low [43,45] and these dermal masses exhibit no junctional activity [45].

Signet-ring melanomas are composed of round to polygonal cells [45,52], with a pale eosinophilic cytoplasm and a darker periphery [52]. The nuclei are vesicular, crescent shaped and located at the periphery, giving the cells the appearance of signet-rings [52]. Nucleoli are prominent and occasional multinucleated cells may be present [45].

7. Histochemical diagnosis

The histological diagnosis of melanoma can be a challenge for the pathologist, especially in amelanotic tumours. On the other hand, in tumours heavily pigmented the observation of cellular features could be very difficult, requiring the use of bleaching, a histochemical method where melanin is extracted [7].

In cases where the diagnosis of a melanocytic tumor is not evident, histochemical methods specific for the cells producing melanin, such as DOPA (dihydroxyphenylalanine) reaction can be used [7,43].

8. Molecular diagnostic methods

A diagnosis of melanocytic tumors in dogs is not always easy to obtain only by conventional histological methods. Melanoma is often similar to other tumours types and has a highly variable histologic pattern which implies an accurate differential diagnosis. Furthermore, the distinction between benign and malignant tumors is not always easy [7]. Thus, it is essential the research of additional tools that can be used in melanocytic tumours diagnosis and to achieve a more accurate prognosis [57].

8.1. Classical diagnostic markers

Several markers are used to evaluate the presence of proteins normally found in melanocytes or in cells of neuroectoderm origin. The most common antibodies used are S-100 protein, *melanoma-associated antigen* (Melan-A)/MART-1, HMB-45, MEL-1, vimentin, *Neuron Specific Enolase* (NSE), microphthalmia transcription factor (MiTF), PNL2, tyrosinase, and tyrosinase-related proteins 1 and 2 (TRP-1 and TRP-2). Tumor cells are usually positive for vimentin, S100, neuron-specific enolase, and Melan-A, and negative for cytokeratin [7]. However, there is a heterogeneneity of antigen expression. The majority of melanomas are S100 positive, but other tumour types are also positive to this protein. NSE is also positive in smooth muscle and neuroendocrine tumours. Melan-A and HMB-45 expression is not a constant in every canine melanocytic tumours. Vimentin is expressed in other tumours as sarcomas [7,58-61]. HMB-45, tyrosinase, and tyrosine hydroxylase showed 100% specific but low sensitivities. One study refers that PNL2, TRP-1, and TRP-2 seems to be highly sensitive and specific for the diagnosis of canine amelanotic tumours, but it was only performed in oral melanomas [62].

In the absence of an ideal marker that excludes definitively other tumour types, confirms a diagnosis of canine melanoma and positively reacts with tumour cells in all melanomas, a diagnostic panel must be performed, including different antibodies [58-61].

8.2. Growth fraction

The proliferative activity has provided valuable information on cell growth kinetics and consequently tumour behavior in melanocytic tumours [63]. There are some markers that estimate tumor proliferation, by identifying steps associated with cell cycle [64].

MIB-1 is the monoclonal antibody which is reactive against Ki-67 nuclear antigen, a protein present in all active phases of the cell cycle (G1, S, G2 and M) while being absent in resting phase (G0) [65,66].

In canine melanocytic tumours, Ki-67 may be useful in distinction between benign and malignant tumors: melanocytomas seem to have a significant lower growth fraction than malignant melanomas [67]. Furthermore, KI-67 could be an important prognosis factor in canine cutaneous melanocytic tumours [64,68].

8.3. DNA ploidy

Changes in DNA content may reflect chromosomal alterations and represent tumour genetic instability [69-72]. Changes in the DNA ploidy constitute an early event in carcinogenesis [73,74] and detection of aneuploid cell population of pre-neoplastic lesions can be considered a factor risk of the emergence of malignant tumours [75]. Although usually benign tumors were diploid [76] and aneuploidy were malignant [77], diploidy is not synonymous of a benign behavior [78]. Moreover, not all malignant tumors are aneuploid [79,80].

There are few studies about the ploidy assessment in canine melanocytic tumors [81,82] and its usefulness is still discussed. DNA index and ploidy balance seem to provide an additional tool to evaluate melanocytic tumors, being useful in the distinction of benign and malignant melanocytic tumours, mainly in amelanotic lesions [82]. Flow cytometry apparently has a limited utility for predicting the biological behavior of pigmented canine melanomas. DNA content and nuclear morphometric variables have little value in predicting survival time [83].

8.4. c-kit expression

The c-Kit protein (CD117), a transmembrane receptor that belongs to RTK III family, is a growth factor for melanocyte migration and proliferation. A loss-of-function KIT mutation are usually related with human melanocytic tumors [84,85].

In canine cutaneous melanocytic tumours, c-kit immunolabeling (both extension and intensity) were generally higher in melanocytomas than in malignant melanomas. The lack of c-kit expression in canine cutaneous malignant melanomas might be used as a criteria of tumor aggressiveness, helping to achieve a proper diagnosis [86].

8.5. Matrix metalloproteinase 2 and 9 expression

MMPs are zinc- and calcium-dependent proteases that promove not only the disruption and remodeling of structural barriers [87-89] but also a response to signaling molecules, acting as ligand for cellular adhesion receptors [90-92].

MMP-2 is widely distributed and constitutively expressed by most cells [93,94]. This protease has major roles reducing cell adhesion, stimulating cell migration and differentiation, and acting as an anti-inflammatory factor [95]. MMP-9 expression is normally induced, while almost MMPs are constitutively secreted after their translation [93,96], and may act as anti- or pro-inflammatory factors [95].

MMPs play a pivotal role in cancer development and progression [92,94,96-98] contributing to tumour proliferation, invasion, intravasation into circulation, extravasation, migration to metastatic sites and angiogenesis [90,94,99-101], deregulate the balance between growth and antigrowth signals in the tumour microenvironment [97,102,103], orchestrate inflammation [94,102,104], and evade apoptosis [89,91,102].

In canine cutaneous melanocytic tumours, MMP-2 and MMP-9 may be taken as a complement to histology in tumour diagnosis, especially in borderline lesions. Both MMP-2 and MMP-9 were expressed in the majority of canine cutaneous melanocytic tumours. MMP-2 is most commonly expressed in melanocytomas than in melanomas [105]. MMP-9 was overexpressed in malignant melanomas, compared with its expression in melanocytomas [106].

Additionally, in canine malignant melanomas a switch may occur in the MMP expression profile during tumour progression; meaning that the aggressiveness, evaluated by nuclear grade, seems to be associated with a decrease of MMP-9 and an increase of MMP-2 expression [105].

8.6. Inflammatory cells associated to tumour

The tumour associated inflammatory infiltrate may be modulate and determine tumor behavior [107]. The most studied cells in CCMT are macrophages and T-lymphocyte, however, studies on the matter are scarce.

8.6.1. Tumour Associated Macrophages (TAMs)

Macrophages constitute the most abundant leukocytes in the tumor environment, recruited by a number of chemoattractants that are produced by the tumor cells and tumor-associated stroma [108,109]. TAMs play a critical role in tumour progression and invasion by inducing neovascularization, suppressing immunocompetent cells and supporting cancer stem cells [110-113].

One study published by our group found that canine cutaneous melanocytomas present a lower number of TAMs than malignant melanomas. TAMs could constitute an important marker of canine melanocytic aggressiveness, being implicated in the progression of melanocytic precursor lesions to malignant melanoma [114].

8.6.2. T-Lymphocytic Infiltrate (TLI)

In spite of the fact that the role of the T-lymphocytic infiltrate in cancer tumourigenesis remains controversial, several studies showed that the presence of TILs are related to tumoural behavior in different tumour types [115,116].

Preliminary studies of our group showed that there is a difference between TILs in benign and malignant melanocytic neoplasms, whereas all melanocytomas presented little or even absence of TILs and melanomas had a more intense TILs, (Figure 19), [117].

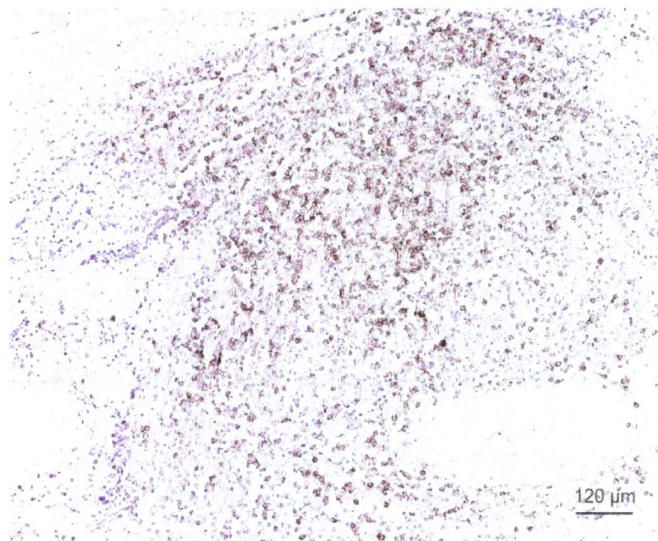

Figure 19. Abundant CD3+TILs in canine cutaneous melanoma (IHC, 100x), courtesy of Dr. Patricia Monteiro.

8.7. E-cadherin/β-catenin

Epithelial cadherin (E-cadherin) is a transmembranar glycoprotein which belongs to a family of cell to cell adhesion molecules dependent of the present of calcium molecules to bind cytoskeleton proteins through catenins. A decreased or altered expression of E-cadherin molecules often represents an increased invasiveness of tumour cells and ultimately malignancy in animal and human epithelial tumours [118,119].

In canine melanocytic tumours, the benign lesions present a membranous labelling (Figure 20) and the malignant ones an erroneous labelling, with a cytoplasmatic predominant immunostaining. Additionally, a loss of E-cadherin expression is noted in melanoma [120]. A loss of membrane E-cadherin/β-catenin complex is also detected in canine melanoma showing that a disruption of E-cadherin/β-catenin complexes and a increase of β-catenin may be associated with canine melanocytic tumours progression and aggressiveness [121].

8.8. Cox-1 and Cox-2 expression

Cyclooxygenase (COX), also known as the prostaglandin H-synthase, is an enzyme envolved on prostanoids biosynthesis. Cox-1 and Cox-2 are the two cyclooxigenase isoforms identified to date, similar in its structure but produced by different genes. The biological functions are also different: Cox-1, constitutively expressed in many tissues, plays an important role in the regulation of normal physiological, while Cox-2 is usually absent from normal cells but induced by growth factors, inflammatory reactions, tumour promoters and oncogenes [122-125].

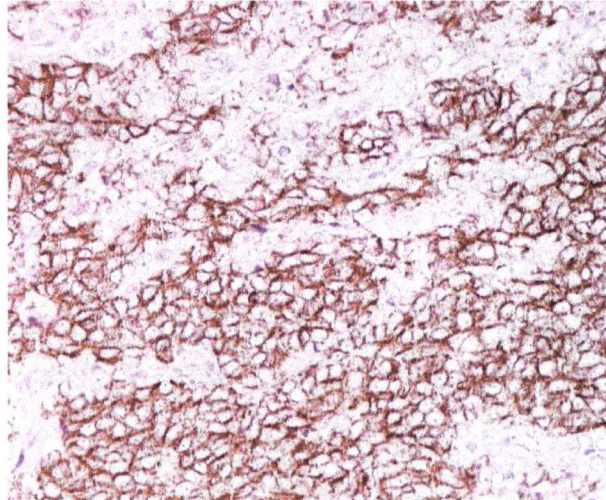

Figure 20. Strong membranar E-cadherin expression (IHC, 200x), courtesy of Dr. Mariana Santos.

Cox-1 and Cox-2 expression was recently described in canine melanocytic tumours [126-128]. Cox-1 is expressed in almost every tumours, both benign and malignant melanocytic skin lesions. Regarding Cox-2, melanocytomas did not present a positive immunolabelling, but in melanomas Cox-2 expression was present in more than 50% of the tumours [114,127]. The differences observed suggest that Cox-2 expression could be a useful tool in canine melanoma diagnosis, particularly in borderline lesions.

COX-2 expression was also observed in tumours with epithelium ulceration, necrosis, high mitotic index and nuclear grade and in less pigmented neoplasms, which could represent the higher aggressiveness of Cox-2 positive melanocytic tumours. In canine malignant melanomas, Cox-2 is associated with a higher cellular proliferation [114]. Besides the relation with tumour behavior [127], Cox-2 over-expression relates with a poor overall survival [129].

8.9. Angiogenesis

Vascular system is essential in oxygen and nutrients supply, elimination of metabolism products and promoting efficient access of leukocytes [130].

Angiogenesis is a complex process by which new blood vessels develop from pre-existing vasculature [131-133]. It is a fundamental requirement for organs development. Angiogenesis is also implicated in the pathogenesis of different pathological alterations, such as cancer and inflammation [134-136].

The tumor-associated neovascularization, by establishing continuity with the systemic circulation, allows tumor cells expressing their critical advantage in growth and facilitates metastization [137-139].

8.9.1. Vascular endothelial growth factor

Angiogenesis is a delicate process, tightly regulated by the balance of pro- and anti-angiogenic factors [140]. Among the angiogenic factors, VEGF is the more powerful and ubiquitous vascular endothelial growth factor, capable of inducing proliferation, migration, specialization and survival of endothelial cells [141,142]. Functions of VEGF family members related to neoplastic pathogenesis are linked not only to its angiogenic capacity [143], but also with the lymphangiogenesis [144,145], immunosuppression [146-148], stimulation and recruitment of endothelial and hematopoietic precursors of the bone marrow [149,150] and anti-apoptotic activity [150].

In canine melanomas, the only study published on VEGF expression is in oral melanomas. High blood concentrations of VEGF were correlated to a shorter survival time in dogs receiving definitive therapy and were associated with tumour stage [151].

This is a promising area, since VEGF may be a good indicator of preneoplastic change in melanocytic lesions [137,152]. VEGF plays a role in human melanoma progression [153,154] with a strong involvment in the switch from the radial to the vertical growth phase and the metastatic phase. So, anti-angiogenic agents might even interfere with or block melanoma progression [155].

Preliminary studies performed by Gomes J and Pires I (data unpublished) show that VEGF may be useful as a discriminating factor between malignant melanoma and benign, since it is more intensely expressed in melanomas (Figure 21) than in melanocytomas.

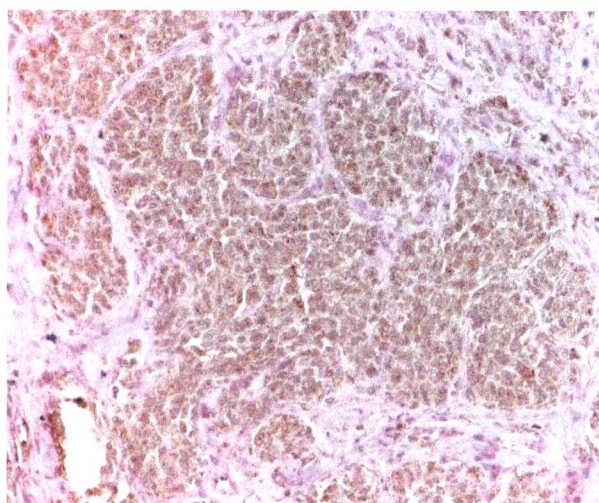

Figure 21. Canine cutaneous melanoma with a strong and diffuse VEGF expression (IHC, 200x), courtesy of Dr. Joana Gomes.

8.9.2. Microvessel Density (MVD)

Tumor angiogenesis can be estimated through a quantification of microvessel density (MVD). The most widely used method is the immunohistochemical methods, in which specific markers for endothelial cells are employed, as von Willebrand factor (Figure 22), CD34 and CD31 [156-158].

MVD seems to be important for diagnostic purposes in canine MT's. MVD is significantly higher in melanoma than in melanocytomas [159] and its expression has been associated with a high mitotic index, necrosis and ulceration (study performed by Gomes J and Pires I, data unpublished). However, its prognostic significance is still discussable [159,160].

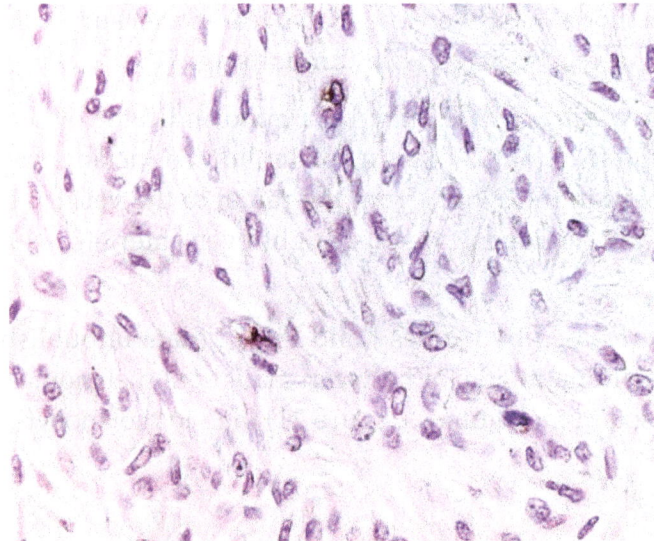

Figure 22. Tumoural neovessels positive to von Willebrand factor (IHC, 400x), courtesy of Dr. Joana Gomes.

9. Conclusions

The incidence of melanoma is increasing annually both in man and in dog. Given that dogs and humans share the same environment and similarities between human and canine melanoma it is urgent to discuss common mechanisms in melanoma development in both species.

Melanoma diagnosis in dogs can be challenging due to the variety of its histological appearances, especially when pathologists are facing amelanotic or metastatic lesions. Although the definitive diagnosis of a melanoma is often difficult by the lack of specific markers that can distinguish these lesions, immunohistochemistry plays a key role in the differential diagnosis with other neoplasms.

Additionally, the distinction between benign and malignant melanocytic tumours is not always easy, especially in borderline lesions, thus the importance of a strong knowledge of new markers of malignancy for the establishment of a definitive diagnosis and a correct therapy managment and prognosis establishment.

Author details

Luis Resende[1], Joana Moreira[2], Justina Prada[3], Felisbina Luisa Queiroga[4] and Isabel Pires[3*]

*Address all correspondence to: ipires@utad.pt

1 Veterinary Faculty, Lusófona University, Lisbon, Portugal

2 Department of Veterinary Sciences, University of Trás-os-Montes and Alto Douro, Portugal

3 Animal and Veterinary Research Centre (CECAV), Department of Veterinary Sciences, University of Trás-os-Montes and Alto Douro, Portugal

4 Center for Research and Technology of Agro-Environment and Biological Sciences (CIT-AB), Department of Veterinary Sciences, University of Trás-os-Montes and Alto Douro, Portugal

References

[1] Grandi F, Rocha RM, Miot HA, Cogliati B, Rocha NS. Immunoexpression of S100A4 in canine skin melanomas and correlation with histopathological parameters. Veterinary Quarterly 2014 1-7.

[2] Goldschmidt MH. Benign and malignant melanocytic neoplasms of domestic animals. The American Journal of Dermatopathology 1985;7 203-12.

[3] Cotchin E. Melanotic tumours of dogs. Journal of Comparative Pathology and Therapeutics 1955;65 115-IN14.

[4] Smith SH, Goldschmidt MH, McManus PM. A Comparative Review of Melanocytic Neoplasms. Veterinary Pathology 2002;39(6) 651-78.

[5] Aronsohn MG, Carpenter JL. Distal extremity melanocytic nevi and malignant melanomas in dogs. Journal of American Animal Hospital Association 1990;26 605-12.

[6] BoVeterinary Pathologylon B, Calderwood Mays MB, Hall BJ. Characteristics of canine melanomas and comparison of histology and DNA ploidy to their biologic effect. Veterinary Pathology 1990;27 96-102.

[7] Smith SH, Goldschmidt MH, McManus PM. A comparative review of melanocytic neoplasms. Veterinary Pathology 2002;39(6) 651-78.

[8] Spangler WL, Kass PH. The histologic and epidemiologic bases for prognostic considerations in canine melanocytic neoplasia. Veterinary Pathology 2006;43(2) 136-49.

[9]   Trappler MC, Popovitch CA, Goldschmidt MH, Goldschmidt KH, Risbon RE. Scrotal tumors in dogs: A retrospective study of 676 cases (1986–2010). Canadian Veterinary Journal 2014;55.

[10]   Ramos-Vara J, Beissenherz M, Miller M, Johnson G, Pace L, Fard A, Kottler S. Retrospective study of 338 canine oral melanomas with clinical, histologic, and immunohistochemical review of 129 cases. Veterinary Pathology 2000;37(6) 597-608.

[11]   Kim D, Royal A, Villamil J. Disseminated melanoma in a dog with involvement of leptomeninges and bone marrow. Veterinary Pathology 2009;46(1) 80-3.

[12]   Lacroux C, Raymon-Letron I, Bourges-Abella N, Lucas MN, Deviers A, Serra F, Degorce-Rubiales F, Delverdier M. Study of canine cutaneous melanocytic tumours: evaluation of histological and immunohistochemical prognostic criteria in 65 cases. Revue Médicine Vétérinaire 2012;163(8-9) 393-401.

[13]   Smedley RC, Spangler WL, Esplin DG, Kitchell BE, Bergman PJ, Ho HY, Bergin IL, Kiupel M. Prognostic markers for canine melanocytic neoplasms: a comparative review of the literature and goals for future investigation. Veterinary Pathology 2011;48(1) 54-72.

[14]   Morrison WB. Tumors of the Skin and Subcutis. In: Morrison WB. (ed.) Cancer in Dogs and Cats: Medical and Surgical Management. University of Minnesota: Williams & Wilkins; 1998. p 499-500.

[15]   Millanta F, Fratini F, Corazza M, Castagnaro M, Zappulli V, Poli A. Proliferation activity in oral and cutaneous canine melanocytic tumors: correlation with histological parameters, location, and clinical behaviour. Research in Veterinary Sciences 2002;73 45-51.

[16]   Sulaimon SS, Kitchell BE, Ehrhart EJ. Immunohistochemical Detection of Melanomaspecific Antigens in Spontaneous Canine Melanoma. Journal of Comparative Pathology 2002;127(2–3) 162-8.

[17]   Banks W, Morris E. Results of radiation treatment of naturally occurring animal tumors. Journal of the American Veterinary Medical Association 1975;166(11) 1063.

[18]   Frimberger AE, Moore AS, Cincotta L, Cotter SM, Foley JW. Photodynamic therapy of naturally occurring tumors in animals using a novel benzophenothiazine photosensitizer. Clinical Cancer Research 1998;4(9) 2207-18.

[19]   Gillette EL. Hyperthermia effects in animals with spontaneous tumors. National Cancer Institute monograph 1982;61 361-4.

[20]   Marmor JB, Pounds D, Hahn N, Hahn GM. Treating spontaneous tumors in dogs and cats by ultrasound-induced hyperthermia. International Journal of Radiation Oncology Biology Physics 1978;4(11–12) 967-73.

[21]   Westberg S, Sadeghi A, Svensson E, Segall T, Dimopoulou M, Korsgren O, Hemminki A, Loskog AS, Totterman TH, von Euler H. Treatment efficacy and immune stimu-

lation by AdCD40L gene therapy of spontaneous canine malignant melanoma. J Immunother 2013;36(6) 350-8.

[22] Dow SW, Elmslie RE, Willson AP, Roche L, Gorman C, Potter TA. In vivo tumor transfection with superantigen plus cytokine genes induces tumor regression and prolongs survival in dogs with malignant melanoma. Journal of Clinical Investigation 1998;101(11) 2406.

[23] MacEwen EG, Kurzman ID, Vail DM, Dubielzig RR, Everlith K, Madewell BR, Rodriguez CO, Phillips B, Zwahlen CH, Obradovich J. Adjuvant therapy for melanoma in dogs: results of randomized clinical trials using surgery, liposome-encapsulated muramyl tripeptide, and granulocyte macrophage colony-stimulating factor. Clinical Cancer Research 1999;5(12) 4249-58.

[24] Bergman PJ, McKnight J, Novosad A, Charney S, Farrelly J, Craft D, Wulderk M, Jeffers Y, Sadelain M, Hohenhaus AE, Segal N, Gregor P, Engelhorn M, Riviere I, Houghton AN, Wolchok JD. Long-Term Survival of Dogs with Advanced Malignant Melanoma after DNA Vaccination with Xenogeneic Human Tyrosinase: A Phase I Trial. Clinical Cancer Research 2003;9(4) 1284-90.

[25] Vail DM, Withrow SJ. Chapter 18 - Tumors of the Skin and Subcutaneous Tissues. In: Withrow SJ, Vail DM. editors. Withrow & MacEwen's Small Animal Clinical Oncology (Fourth Edition). Saint Louis: W.B. Saunders; 2007. p 375-401.

[26] Smedley R, Spangler W, Esplin D, Kitchell B, Bergman P, Ho H-Y, Bergin I, Kiupel M. Prognostic Markers for Canine Melanocytic Neoplasms A Comparative Review of the Literature and Goals for Future Investigation. Veterinary Pathology 2011;48(1) 54-72.

[27] Schultheiss PC. Histologic Features and Clinical Outcomes of Melanomas of Lip, Haired Skin, and Nail Bed Locations of Dogs. Journal of Veterinary Diagnostic Investigation 2006;18(4) 422-5.

[28] Orkin M, Schwartzman RM. A Comparative Study of Canine and Human Dermatology. The Journal of Investigative Dermatology 1959;32 451-66.

[29] de Camargo LP, Conceição LG, dos Santos Costa PR. Neoplasias melanocíticas cutâneas em cães: estudo retrospectivo de 68 casos (1996-2004). Brazilian Journal of Veterinary Research and Animal Science 2008;45(2) 138-52.

[30] Goldschmidt M, Hendrick M. Tumors of the skin and soft tissues. Tumors in Domestic Animals, Fourth Edition 2008 45-117.

[31] Spangler W, Kass P. The histologic and epidemiologic bases for prognostic considerations in canine melanocytic neoplasia. Veterinary Pathology 2006;43(2) 136-49.

[32] Junqueira L, Carneiro J. Pele e Anexos. Histologia Básica. Rio de Janeiro, RJ, Brazil 2004. p 359-70.

[33] Marks R. Epidemiology of melanoma. Clinical and Experimental Dermatology 2000;25(6) 459-63.

[34] Valentine B, McManus P, Knox A. Malignant transformation of a giant congenital pigmented nevus (hamartoma) in a dog. Veterinary Dermatology (United Kingdom) 1999.

[35] Conroy JD. Melanocytic Tumors of Domestic Animals: With Special Reference to Dogs. Archives of Dermatology 1967;96(4) 372-80.

[36] Mulligan R. Melanoblastic tumors in the dog. American Journal of Veterinary Research 1961;22 345-51.

[37] Koenig A, Bianco S, Fosmire S, Wojcieszyn J, Modiano J. Expression and significance of p53, rb, p21/waf-1, p16/ink-4a, and PTEN tumor suppressors in canine melanoma. Veterinary Pathology 2002;39(4) 458-72.

[38] Dobson JM. Breed-predispositions to cancer in pedigree dogs. International Scholarly Research Notices 2013;2013.

[39] Hsu M-Y, Meier FE, Nesbit M, Hsu J-Y, Van Belle P, Elder DE, Herlyn M. E-cadherin expression in melanoma cells restores keratinocyte-mediated growth control and down-regulates expression of invasion-related adhesion receptors. The American Journal of Pathology 2000;156(5) 1515-25.

[40] Meier F, Satyamoorthy K, Nesbit M, Hsu M-Y, Schittek B, Garbe C, Herlyn M. Molecular events in melanoma development and progression. Front Biosci 1998;3(D) 1005-10.

[41] Seiter S, Schadendorf D, Herrmann K, Schneider M, Rösel M, Arch R, Tilgen W, Zöller M. Expression of CD44 variant isoforms in malignant melanoma. Clinical Cancer Research 1996;2(3) 447-56.

[42] Goldschmidt MH, Hendrick MJ. Tumors of the Skin and Soft Tissues. In: M. DJ. (ed.) Tumors in Domestic Animals. Fourth Edition ed. Iowa State: Iowa State Press; 2002. p 78-83.

[43] Gross TL, Ihrke PJ, Walder EJ, Affolter VK. Melanocytic tumors. In: Gross TL, Ihrke PJ, Walder EJ, Affolter VK. editors. Skin Diseases of the Dog and Cat: Blackwell Science Ltd; 2005. p 813-36.

[44] Campagne C, Jule S, Alleaume C, Bernex F, Ezagal J, Chateau-Joubert S, Estrada M, Aubin-Houzelstein G, Panthier JJ, Egidy G. Canine melanoma diagnosis: RACK1 as a potential biological marker. Veterinary Pathology 2013;50(6) 1083-90.

[45] Ginn PE, Mensett JEKL, Rukich PM. The skin and appendages. In: Grant M. (ed.) Jubb, Kennedy & Palmer's Pathology of Domestic Animals. Ontario, Canada: Grant, M.; 2007. p 759-60.

[46] Friedrichs KR, Young KM. Diagnostic cytopathology in clinical oncology. Withrow and MacEwen's Small Animal Clinical Oncology 2013 111.

[47] Daskalopoulou D, Gourgiotou K, Thodou E, Vaida S, Markidou S. Rapid cytological diagnosis of primary skin tumours and tumour-like conditions. Acta Dermato-Venereologica 1997;77(4) 292-5.

[48] Dey P, Mallik M, Gupta S, Vasishta R. Role of fine needle aspiration cytology in the diagnosis of soft tissue tumours and tumour-like lesions. Cytopathology 2004;15(1) 32-7.

[49] Simeonov RS. The accuracy of fine-needle aspiration cytology in the diagnosis of canine skin and subcutaneous masses. Comparative Clinical Pathology 2012;21(2) 143-7.

[50] Ghisleni G, Roccabianca P, Ceruti R, Stefanello D, Bertazzolo W, Bonfanti U, Caniatti M. Correlation between fine-needle aspiration cytology and histopathology in the evaluation of cutaneous and subcutaneous masses from dogs and cats. Veterinary Clinical Pathology 2006;35(1) 24-30.

[51] Liu W, Bennet M, Helm T. Canine melanoma: a comparison with human pigmented epithelioid melanocytoma. International Journal of Dermatology 2011;50 1542-5.

[52] Cangul IT, van Garderen E, van der Linde-Sipman JS, van den Ingh TS, Schalken JA. Canine balloon and signet-ring cell melanomas: a histological and immunohistochemical characterization. Journal of Comparative Pathology 2001;125(2-3) 166-73.

[53] Goldschmidt MH, Dustan RW, Stannard AA, von Tscharner C, Walder EJ, Yager JA. Melanocytic tumors and tumor-like lesions. In: Goldschmidt MH, Dustan RW, Stannard AA, von Tscharner C, Walder EJ, Yager JA. editors. Washington DC: Armed Forces Institute of Pathology; 1998. p 38-48.

[54] Millanta F, Fratini F, Corazza M, Castagnaro M, Zappulli V, Poli A. Proliferation activity in oral and cutaneous canine melanocytic tumours: correlation with histological parameters, location, and clinical behaviour. Research in Veterinary Sciences 2002;73(1) 45-51.

[55] Laprie C, Abadie J, Amardeilh MF, Net JLLE, Lagadic M, Delverdier M. MIB-1 immunoreactivity correlates with biologic behaviour in canine cutaneous melanoma. Veterinary Dermatology 2001;12(3) 139-47.

[56] De los Monteros AE, de las Mulas JM, Fernández A, Orós J, Rodríguez F. Immunohistopathologic Characterization of a Dermal Melanocytoma-Acanthoma in a German Shepherd Dog. Veterinary Pathology 2000;37(3) 268-71.

[57] USDA licenses DNA vaccine for treatment of melanoma in dogs. Journal of American Veterinary Medical Association 2010;236(5) 495.

[58]   Koenig A, Wojcieszyn J, Weeks BR, Modiano JF. Expression of S100a, vimentin, NSE, and melan A/MART-1 in seven canine melanoma cells lines and twenty-nine retrospective cases of canine melanoma. Veterinary Pathology 2001;38(4) 427-35.

[59]   Sulaimon S, Kitchell B, Ehrhart E. Immunohistochemical detection of melanoma-specific antigens in spontaneous canine melanoma. Journal of Comparative Pathology 2002;127(2-3) 162-8.

[60]   Ramos-Vara JA, Beissenherz ME, Miller MA, Johnson GC, Pace LW, Fard A, Kottler SJ. Retrospective study of 338 canine oral melanomas with clinical, histologic, and immunohistochemical review of 129 cases. Veterinary Pathology 2000;37(6) 597-608.

[61]   Sandusky GE, Jr., Carlton WW, Wightman KA. Immunohistochemical staining for S100 protein in the diagnosis of canine amelanotic melanoma. Veterinary Pathology 1985;22(6) 577-81.

[62]   Smedley RC, Lamoureux J, Sledge DG, Kiupel M. Immunohistochemical diagnosis of canine oral amelanotic melanocytic neoplasms. Veterinary Pathology 2011;48(1) 32-40.

[63]   Rieger E, Hofmann-Wellenhof R, Soyer HP, Kofler R, Cerroni L, Smolle J, Kerl H. Comparison of proliferative activity as assessed by proliferating cell nuclear antigen (PCNA) and Ki-67 monoclonal antibodies in melanocytic skin lesions. A quantitative immunohistochemical study. Journal of Cutaneous Pathology 1993;20(3) 229-36.

[64]   Millanta F, Fratini F, Corazza M, Castagnaro M, Zappulli V, Poli A. Proliferation activity in oral and cutaneous canine melanocytic tumours: correlation with histological parameters, location, and clinical behaviour. Research in Veterinary Sciences 2002;73(1) 45-51.

[65]   Gerdes J, Schwab U, Lemke H, Stein H. Production of a mouse monoclonal antibody reactive with a human nuclear antigen associated with cell proliferation. International Journal of Cancer 1983;31(1) 13-20.

[66]   Gerdes J, Li L, Schlueter C, Duchrow M, Wohlenberg C, Gerlach C, Stahmer I, Kloth S, Brandt E, Flad HD. Immunobiochemical and molecular biologic characterization of the cell proliferation-associated nuclear antigen that is defined by monoclonal antibody Ki-67. American Journal of Pathology 1991;138(4) 867-73.

[67]   Laprie C, Abadie J, Amardeilh MF, Net JL, Lagadic M, Delverdier M. MIB-1 immunoreactivity correlates with biologic behaviour in canine cutaneous melanoma. Veterinary Dermatology 2001;12(3) 139-47.

[68]   Roels S, Tilmant K, Ducatelle R. PCNA and Ki67 proliferation markers as criteria for prediction of clinical behaviour of melanocytic tumours in cats and dogs. Journal of Comparative Pathology 1999;121(1) 13-24.

[69]   Grollino MG, Cavallo D, Di Silverio F, Rocchi M, De Vita R. Interphase cytogenetics and flow cytometry analyses of renal tumours. Anticancer Research 1993;13(6A) 2239-44.

[70]   Yamal JM, Cox D, Hittelman WN, Boiko I, Malpica A, Guillaud M, MacAulay C, Follen M, Vlastos AT. Quantitative histopathology and chromosome 9 polysomy in a clinical trial of 4-HPR. Gynecology Oncology 2004;94(2) 296-306.

[71]   Kronenwett U, Castro J, Roblick UJ, Fujioka K, Ostring C, Faridmoghaddam F, Laytragoon-Lewin N, Tribukait B, Auer G. Expression of cyclins A, E and topoisomerase II alpha correlates with centrosome amplification and genomic instability and influences the reliability of cytometric S-phase determination. BMC Cell Biology 2003;4 8.

[72]   Sidoni A, Cavaliere A, D'Amico GA, Brachelente G, Bucciarelli E. Biopathological significance of single cell DNA aneuploidy measured by static cytometry in breast cancer. Breast 2001;10(4) 325-9.

[73]   Li R, Sonik A, Stindl R, Rasnick D, Duesberg P. Aneuploidy vs. gene mutation hypothesis of cancer: recent study claims mutation but is found to support aneuploidy. Proceedings of the National Academy of Sciences USA 2000;97(7) 3236-41.

[74]   Postier RG, Lerner MR, Lightfoot SA, Vannarath R, Lane MM, Hanas JS, Brackett DJ. DNA ploidy and markovian analysis of neoplastic progression in experimental pancreatic cancer. Journal of Histochemistry Cytochemistry 2003;51(3) 303-9.

[75]   Elkowitz D, Daum F, Markowitz J, Proccaccino J, Boas E, Cuomo J, Kahn E. Risk factors for carcinoma of the pelvic ileal pouch/anal canal in ulcerative colitis. Annals of Clinical & Laboratory Science 2004;34(2) 143-9.

[76]   Cohen C. Image cytometric analysis in pathology. Human Pathology 1996;27(5) 482-93.

[77]   Nordemar S, Hogmo A, Lindholm J, Tani E, Sjostrom B, Auer G, Munck-Wikland E. The clinical value of image cytometry DNA analysis in distinguishing branchial cleft cysts from cystic metastases of head and neck cancer. Laryngoscope 2002;112(11) 1983-7.

[78]   Harada K, Nishizaki T, Ozaki S, Kubota H, Okamura T, Ito H, Sasaki K. Cytogenetic alterations in pituitary adenomas detected by comparative genomic hybridization. Cancer Genetics and Cytogenetics 1999;112(1) 38-41.

[79]   Frazier KS, Hines ME, 2nd, Hurvitz AI, Robinson PG, Herron AJ. Analysis of DNA aneuploidy and c-myc oncoprotein content of canine plasma cell tumors using flow cytometry. Veterinary Pathology 1993;30(6) 505-11.

[80]   Lewis JE, Olsen KD, Sebo TJ. Carcinoma ex pleomorphic adenoma: pathologic analysis of 73 cases. Human Pathology 2001;32(6) 596-604.

[81] Johnson TS, Raju MR, Giltinan RK, Gillette EL. Ploidy and DNA distribution analysis of spontaneous dog tumors by flow cytometry. Cancer Research 1981;41(8) 3005-9.

[82] Bolon B, Calderwood Mays MB, Hall BJ. Characteristics of canine melanomas and comparison of histology and DNA ploidy to their biologic behavior. Veterinary Pathology 1990;27(2) 96-102.

[83] Roels SL, Van Daele AJ, Van Marck EA, Ducatelle RV. DNA ploidy and nuclear morphometric variables for the evaluation of melanocytic tumors in dogs and cats. American Journal of Veterinary Research 2000;61(9) 1074-9.

[84] Pilloni L, Bianco P, Difelice E, Cabras S, Castellanos ME, Atzori L, Ferreli C, Mulas P, Nemolato S, Faa G. The usefulness of c-Kit in the immunohistochemical assessment of melanocytic lesions. European Journal of Histochemistry 2011;55(2) e20.

[85] Yarden Y, Kuang WJ, Yang-Feng T, Coussens L, Munemitsu S, Dull TJ, Chen E, Schlessinger J, Francke U, Ullrich A. Human proto-oncogene c-kit: a new cell surface receptor tyrosine kinase for an unidentified ligand. EMBO Journal 1987;6(11) 3341-51.

[86] Gomes J, Queiroga FL, Prada J, Pires I. Study of c-kit immunoexpression in canine cutaneous melanocytic tumors. Melanoma Research 2012;22(3) 195-201.

[87] Foda HD, Zucker S. Matrix metalloproteinases in cancer invasion, metastasis and angiogenesis. Drug Discovery Today 2001;6(9) 478-82.

[88] Stamenkovic I. Extracellular matrix remodelling: the role of matrix metalloproteinases. Journal of Pathology 2003;200(4) 448-64.

[89] Szabo KA, Ablin RJ, Singh G. Matrix metalloproteinases and the immune response. Clinical and Applied Immunology Reviews 2004;4(5) 295-319.

[90] López-Otín C, Palavalli LH, Samuels Y. Protective roles of matrix metalloproteinases: From mouse models to human cancer. Cell Cycle 2009;8(22) 3657-62.

[91] Cauwe B, Van den Steen PE, Opdenakker G. The biochemical, biological, and pathological kaleidoscope of cell surface substrates processed by matrix metalloproteinases. Critical Reviews in Biochemistry and Molecular Biology 2007;42 113-85.

[92] Sternlicht MD, Werb Z. How matrix metalloproteinases regulate cell behavior. Cell and Developmental Biology 2001;17 463-516.

[93] Bergman RL. Matrix Metalloproteinases 2 and 9 in Normal Canine Cerebrospinal Fluid.Master thesis. Faculty of the Virginia Polytechnic Institute and State University 2001.

[94] Björklund M, Koivunen E. Gelatinase-mediated migration and invasion of cancer cells. Biochimica et Biophysica Acta (BBA) - Reviews on Cancer 2005;1755(1) 37-69.

[95] Visse R, Nagase H. Matrix Metalloproteinases and Tissue Inhibitors of Metalloproteinases. Circulation Research 2003;92(8) 827-39.

[96] Tonti Ga, Mannello F, Cacci E, Biagioni S. Neural stem cells at the crossroads: MMPs may tell the way. The International Journal of Developmental Biology 2009;53(1) 1-17.

[97] Handsley MM, Edwards DR. Metalloproteinases and their inhibitors in tumor angiogenesis. International Journal of Cancer 2005;115(6) 849-60.

[98] Galliera E, Tacchini L, Romanelli MM. Matrix metalloproteinases as biomarkers of disease: updates and new insights. Clin Chem Lab Med 2014.

[99] Chaudhary A, Singh M, Bharti A, Asotra K, Sundaram S, Mehrotra R. Genetic polymorphisms of matrix metalloproteinases and their inhibitors in potentially malignant and malignant lesions of the head and neck. Journal of Biomedical Science 2010;17(10).

[100] Joyce JA, Pollard JW. Microenvironmental regulation of metastasis. Nature Reviews Cancer 2009;9(4) 239-52.

[101] Mannello F, Medda V. Nuclear localization of Matrix metalloproteinases. Progress in Histochemistry and Cytochemistry 2012;47(1) 27-58.

[102] Kessenbrock K, Plaks V, Werb Z. Matrix Metalloproteinases: Regulators of the Tumor Microenvironment. Cell 2010;141(1) 52-67.

[103] Stamenkovic I. Matrix metalloproteinases in tumor invasion and metastasis. Seminars in Cancer Biology 2000;10(6) 415-33.

[104] Deryugina E, Quigley J. Matrix metalloproteinases and tumor metastasis. Cancer and Metastasis Reviews 2006;25(1) 9-34.

[105] Pires I, Gomes J, Prada J, Pereira D, Queiroga FL. MMP-2 and MMP-9 Expression in Canine Cutaneous Melanocytic Tumours: Evidence of a Relationship with Tumoural Malignancy2013. In: Lester D. (ed.) Recent Advances in the Biology, Therapy and Management of Melanoma. Rijeka: InTech; 2013.

[106] Docampo MJ, Cabrera J, Rabanal RM, Bassols A. Expression of matrix metalloproteinase-2 and -9 and membrane-type 1 matrix metalloproteinase in melanocytic tumors of dogs and canine melanoma cell lines. Am J Vet Res 2011;72(8) 1087-96.

[107] Le Bitoux MA, Stamenkovic I. Tumor-host interactions: the role of inflammation. Histochemical Cell Biology 2008;130(6) 1079-90.

[108] Guo C, Buranych A, Sarkar D, Fisher PB, Wang XY. The role of tumor-associated macrophages in tumor vascularization. Vascular Cell 2014;6(1) 2.

[109] Owen JL, Mohamadzadeh M. Macrophages and chemokines as mediators of angiogenesis. Frontiers Physiology 2013;4 159.

[110] Vinogradov S, Warren G, Wei X. Macrophages associated with tumors as potential targets and therapeutic intermediates. Nanomedicine (Lond) 2014;9(5) 695-707.

[111] Chanmee T, Ontong P, Konno K, Itano N. Tumor-associated macrophages as major players in the tumor microenvironment. Cancers (Basel) 2014;6(3) 1670-90.

[112] Brocker EB, Zwadlo G, Suter L, Brune M, Sorg C. Infiltration of primary and metastatic melanomas with macrophages of the 25F9-positive phenotype. Cancer Immunology & Immunotherapy 1987;25(2) 81-6.

[113] Bianchini F, Massi D, Marconi C, Franchi A, Baroni G, Santucci M, Mannini A, Mugnai G, Calorini L. Expression of cyclo-oxygenase-2 in macrophages associated with cutaneous melanoma at different stages of progression. Prostaglandins & Other Lipid Mediators 2007;83(4) 320-8.

[114] Pires I, Prada J, Coelho L, Garcia A, Queiroga FL. Tumour-Associated Macrophages (TAMs) and Cox-2 Expression in Canine Melanocytic Lesions. In: Murph M. (ed.) Melanoma in the Clinic - Diagnosis, Management and Complications of Malignancy. Rijeka: InTech; 2011.

[115] Carvalho MI, Pires I, Prada J, Queiroga FL. T-lymphocytic infiltrate in canine mammary tumours: clinic and prognostic implications. In Vivo 2011;25(6) 963-9.

[116] Kim JH, Yu CH, Yhee JY, Im KS, Sur JH. Lymphocyte infiltration, expression of interleukin (IL) -1, IL-6 and expression of mutated breast cancer susceptibility gene-1 correlate with malignancy of canine mammary tumours. J Comp Pathol 2010;142(2-3) 177-86.

[117] Monteiro P. Factores de prognóstico em melanomas em caninos. UTAD Vila Real; 2013.

[118] Makrilia N, Kollias A, Manolopoulos L, Syrigos K. Cell adhesion molecules: role and clinical significance in cancer. Cancer Investigation 2009;27(10) 1023-37.

[119] Patel SD, Chen CP, Bahna F, Honig B, Shapiro L. Cadherin-mediated cell-cell adhesion: sticking together as a family. Current Opinion Structural Biology 2003;13(6) 690-8.

[120] Santos M. Estudo da Immunoexpressão da caderina E em Tumores Melanocíticos do Cão. UTAD Vila Real; 2012.

[121] Han JI, Kim Y, Kim DY, Na KJ. Alteration in E-cadherin/beta-catenin expression in canine melanotic tumors. Veterinary Pathology 2013;50(2) 274-80.

[122] O'Banion MK, Winn VD, Young DA. cDNA cloning and functional activity of a glucocorticoid-regulated inflammatory cyclooxygenase. Proceedings of the National Academy of Sciences USA 1992;89(11) 4888-92.

[123] Williams CS, DuBois RN. Prostaglandin endoperoxide synthase: why two isoforms? Am J Physiol 1996;270(3 Pt 1) G393-400.

[124] Hla T, Bishop-Bailey D, Liu CH, Schaefers HJ, Trifan OC. Cyclooxygenase-1 and -2 isoenzymes. International Journal Biochemical Cell Biology 1999;31(5) 551-7.

[125] Dubois RN, Abramson SB, Crofford L, Gupta RA, Simon LS, Van De Putte LB, Lipsky PE. Cyclooxygenase in biology and disease. FASEB Journal 1998;12(12) 1063-73.

[126] Paglia D, Dubielzig RR, Kado-Fong HK, Maggs DJ. Expression of cyclooxygenase-2 in canine uveal melanocytic neoplasms. American Journal of Veterinary Research 2009;70(10) 1284-90.

[127] Pires I, Garcia A, Prada J, Queiroga FL. COX-1 and COX-2 expression in canine cutaneous, oral and ocular melanocytic tumours. Journal of Comparative Patholology 2010;143(2-3) 142-9.

[128] Mohammed SI, Khan KN, Sellers RS, Hayek MG, DeNicola DB, Wu L, Bonney PL, Knapp DW. Expression of cyclooxygenase-1 and 2 in naturally-occurring canine cancer. Prostaglandins Leukocyt Essential Fatty Acids 2004;70(5) 479-83.

[129] Martinez CM, Penafiel-Verdu C, Vilafranca M, Ramirez G, Mendez-Gallego M, Buendia AJ, Sanchez J. Cyclooxygenase-2 expression is related with localization, proliferation, and overall survival in canine melanocytic neoplasms. Veterinary Pathology 2011;48(6) 1204-11.

[130] Thomas KA. Vascular endothelial growth factor, a potent and selective angiogenic agent. Journal Biology Chemestry 1996;271(2) 603-6.

[131] Robinson CJ, Stringer SE. The splice variants of vascular endothelial growth factor (VEGF) and their receptors. Journal Cell Science 2001;114(Pt 5) 853-65.

[132] Folkman J, D'Amore PA. Blood vessel formation: what is its molecular basis? Cell 1996;87(7) 1153-5.

[133] Risau W. Mechanisms of angiogenesis. Nature 1997;386(6626) 671-4.

[134] Ferrara N, Keyt B. Vascular endothelial growth factor: basic biology and clinical implications. EXS 1997;79 209-32.

[135] Ferrara N, Davis-Smyth T. The biology of vascular endothelial growth factor. Endocrine Reviews 1997;18(1) 4-25.

[136] Marneros AG. Tumor angiogenesis in melanoma. Hematology Oncology Clinics of North America 2009;23(3) 431-46.

[137] Einspahr JG, Thomas TL, Saboda K, Nickolof BJ, Warneke J, Curiel-Lewandrowski C, Ranger-Moore J, Duckett L, Bangert J, Fruehauf JP, Alberts DS. Expression of vascular endothelial growth factor in early cutaneous melanocytic lesion progression. Cancer 2007;110(11) 2519-27.

[138] Papetti M, Herman IM. Mechanisms of normal and tumor-derived angiogenesis. American Journa Physiology Cell Physiology 2002;282(5) C947-70.

[139] Mittal K, Ebos J, Rini B. Angiogenesis and the tumor microenvironment: vascular endothelial growth factor and beyond. Seminars Oncology 2014;41(2) 235-51.

[140] Benazzi C, Al-Dissi A, Chau CH, Figg WD, Sarli G, de Oliveira JT, Gartner F. Angiogenesis in spontaneous tumors and implications for comparative tumor biology. Scientific World Journal 2014;2014 919570.

[141] Ruhrberg C. Growing and shaping the vascular tree: multiple roles for VEGF. Bioessays 2003;25(11) 1052-60.

[142] Hoeben A, Landuyt B, Highley MS, Wildiers H, Van Oosterom AT, De Bruijn EA. Vascular endothelial growth factor and angiogenesis. Pharmacological Reviews 2004;56(4) 549-80.

[143] Goel HL, Mercurio AM. VEGF targets the tumour cell. Nature Reviews Cancer 2013;13(12) 871-82.

[144] Baldwin ME, Stacker SA, Achen MG. Molecular control of lymphangiogenesis. Bioessays 2002;24(11) 1030-40.

[145] Nagy JA, Vasile E, Feng D, Sundberg C, Brown LF, Detmar MJ, Lawitts JA, Benjamin L, Tan X, Manseau EJ, Dvorak AM, Dvorak HF. Vascular permeability factor/vascular endothelial growth factor induces lymphangiogenesis as well as angiogenesis. Journal Experimental Medicine 2002;196(11) 1497-506.

[146] Gabrilovich D, Ishida T, Oyama T, Ran S, Kravtsov V, Nadaf S, Carbone DP. Vascular endothelial growth factor inhibits the development of dendritic cells and dramatically affects the differentiation of multiple hematopoietic lineages in vivo. Blood 1998;92(11) 4150-66.

[147] Ohm JE, Gabrilovich DI, Sempowski GD, Kisseleva E, Parman KS, Nadaf S, Carbone DP. VEGF inhibits T-cell development and may contribute to tumor-induced immune suppression. Blood 2003;101(12) 4878-86.

[148] Ohm JE, Carbone DP. VEGF as a mediator of tumor-associated immunodeficiency. Immunology Research 2001;23(2-3) 263-72.

[149] Hattori K, Dias S, Heissig B, Hackett NR, Lyden D, Tateno M, Hicklin DJ, Zhu Z, Witte L, Crystal RG, Moore MA, Rafii S. Vascular endothelial growth factor and angiopoietin-1 stimulate postnatal hematopoiesis by recruitment of vasculogenic and hematopoietic stem cells. Journal Experimental Medice 2001;193(9) 1005-14.

[150] Xie K, Wei D, Shi Q, Huang S. Constitutive and inducible expression and regulation of vascular endothelial growth factor. Cytokine Growth Factor Rev 2004;15(5) 297-324.

[151] Taylor KH, Smith AN, Higginbotham M, Schwartz DD, Carpenter DM, Whitley EM. Expression of vascular endothelial growth factor in canine oral malignant melanoma. Veterinary Comparative Oncology 2007;5(4) 208-18.

[152] Simonetti O, Lucarini G, Brancorsini D, Nita P, Bernardini ML, Biagini G, Offidani A. Immunohistochemical expression of vascular endothelial growth factor, matrix met-

alloproteinase 2, and matrix metalloproteinase 9 in cutaneous melanocytic lesions. Cancer 2002;95(9) 1963-70.

[153] Bayer-Garner IB, Hough AJ, Jr., Smoller BR. Vascular endothelial growth factor expression in malignant melanoma: prognostic versus diagnostic usefulness. Modern Pathology 1999;12(8) 770-4.

[154] Brychtova S, Bezdekova M, Brychta T, Tichy M. The role of vascular endothelial growth factors and their receptors in malignant melanomas. Neoplasma 2008;55(4) 273-9.

[155] Vacca A, Ria R, Ribatti D, Bruno M, Dammacco F. Angiogenesis and tumor progression in melanoma. Recenti Prog Med 2000;91(11) 581-7.

[156] Wang Y, Yao X, Ge J, Hu F, Zhao Y. Can Vascular Endothelial Growth Factor and Microvessel Density Be Used as Prognostic Biomarkers for Colorectal Cancer? A Systematic Review and Meta-Analysis. ScientificWorldJournal 2014;2014 102736.

[157] Nico B, Benagiano V, Mangieri D, Maruotti N, Vacca A, Ribatti D. Evaluation of microvascular density in tumors: pro and contra. Histology Histopathology 2008;23(5) 601-7.

[158] Fanelli M, Locopo N, Gattuso D, Gasparini G. Assessment of tumor vascularization: immunohistochemical and non-invasive methods. International Journal Biological Markers 1999;14(4) 218-31.

[159] Cuitino MC, Massone AR, Idiart JR. Lack of prognostic significance of angiogenesis in canine melanocytic tumours. Journal of Comparative Pathology 2012;147(2-3) 147-52.

[160] Mukaratirwa S, Chikafa L, Dliwayo R, Moyo N. Mast cells and angiogenesis in canine melanomas: malignancy and clinicopathological factors. Veterinary Dermatology 2006;17(2) 141-6.

6

New Insights in Cutaneous Melanoma Immune-Therapy— Tackling Immune-Suppression and Specific Anti-Tumoral Response

Monica Neagu and Carolina Constantin

1. Introduction

In this chapter the maturity of immune-therapy in cancer, with emphasis on melanoma will be discussed.

The heterogeneity of melanoma tumour regarding primary and metastatic variants will be argued. Therefore the mutational heterogeneity of this type of tumor triggers complex immune-therapy approach. Notions such as *Immune-therapy* will be tackled, meaning targeting immune elements like immune suppression and using immune drugs like monoclonal antibodies against targets that can or not be immune elements. The chapter will end with the importance of designing complex immune-therapies like abolishing the immune-suppression and enhancing the specific anti-tumoral effect.

Physiologically, the immune system can recognize cells that display an aberrant proliferation like neoplasia. The immune system is equipped with cells that can destroy cancer cells them during their early development. Years ago, when the theory of immunoediting was initiated [1], immunosurveillance was defined as a complex pathway that supervises and controls the elimination of transformed self cells/tissue. When the immune system cannot properly control these aberrantly proliferating cells, and the equilibrium is deregulated, tumour cells escape and form a clinically significant tumoral tissue [2].

In cancer immune-therapy, several approaches that aim to start and sustain the immune response and eventually elicit an immunological memory were lately tackled. The therapy armentarium that started the "bumpy road" from bench to bedside comprises cancer vaccines, adoptive T cell therapy, anti-tumor antibodies, immune checkpoint blockade and/or various immune combinations. Some of the conclusions of the last Congress of SITC (*Society for*

Immunotherapy of Cancer) is that combining these above mentioned immune approaches with other immunomodulators (e.g. cytokines, cyclic dinucleotides) and/or indoleamine 2,3-dioxygenase (IDO) inhibitors can increase the efficacy of immunotherapy [3] and hopefully replace in the future routine approaches such as chemotherapy/radiotherapy.

Early diagnosed stages of melanoma are resolved mainly by surgery and large margin excision, but for advanced stages, systemic therapies, whether chemotherapy, immune-therapy or combined ones have had very low efficacy. Advanced melanoma remains a continuous clinical provocation for the physicians who use therapeutical approaches with low response rates, un-manageable toxicities, and reduced efficacy.

One of the main *molecular hurdles* in cutaneous melanoma is the heterogeneity of tumors. A tumoral tissue has cells with different characteristics in terms of proliferation, invasive-ness and pheno/genotype. In melanoma, aggressiveness has a distinct cellular genotype and in the tumor dynamic development, cells go through several phenotype switching [4]. Specific genetic expression studies have identified more than 100 genes over-expressed in cells with a higher proliferative capacity or in cells that were committed to invade tissues [5].

Recently, a study was published on single melanoma cells and the report shows that there are 114 genes expression that could distinguish the proliferative and invasive phenotype of cells. Among these genes, regulatory networks were found along with genes that encode for pluripotency factor (e.g. POUF51); all these genes were found associated with cell's tumori-genic potential. Authors report that among the regulatory network genes, MITF (microphthal-mia-associated transcription factor) is one of the key players in the heterogeneous character of tumour cells populations. Moreover, the heterogeneity of cells depends on the 2D or 3D status of the cell cultures, thus TPBG (trophoblast glycoprotein) is expressed in a melanoma cell line, 501Mel, only in 3D cultures [4]. In the same way, in 1205Lu melanospheres, PI3K/AKT (phosphatidylinositol 3' –kinase/protein kinase B) signaling pathway is enhanced [4], while DAPK1 (death-associated protein kinase 1) expression is decreased in 501Mel experimental tumors, finding that is in line with the hypermethylated gene promoter associated to melano-ma [6]. This study emphasizes that when transformed melanocytes start to organize in growing tumors, the heterogeneity of the cellular populations' increases, the tumoral tissue having MITF-low/negative cells [4, 7]. In experimental tumour spheres, cells that grow on the exterior layers have an active proliferation, while in the interior of the tumour, due to hypoxic conditions, cells are arrested in the G1 phase [8]. The overall mechanism is that 3D growth enhances tumour-initiating properties [9].

Cell's heterogeneity is important from the immunological point of view. Tumour heteroge-neous tissues have different expression of tumor antigens, thus any type of therapy that addresses only one tumour epitope is proned to have low efficacy. This is the rationale to investigate tumor antigens and evaluate the patient's immune responses prior to any immune-therapy [10].

Extensive studies performed by large groups of researchers and extended networks like *Melanoma Research Networks* established in Europe, Canada, and New Zeeland have provided seminal scientific information regarding melanoma's immune biology. All these insights have led to an actual scientific leap by the development of the first immune-therapies that proved efficacy in advanced melanoma treatment. Therefore drugs that aim intracellular pathways such as mitogen-activated protein kinase (MAPK) pathway, or antibodies that aim CTLA4 (cytotoxic T lymphocyte-associated protein 4), or PD1/PD1-L (programmed cell death 1/ programmed cell death 1 ligand) have recently followed the bench to bedside path [11]. Building upon the early success of these therapies, trials involving new classes of drugs and combinations of these drugs are underway [12].

Starting from 2011, metastatic melanoma beneficiated from four new approved drugs, all these drugs proving in clinical trials the improvement of patient's survival. From this four drugs, one is a B-Raf enzyme inhibitor (vemurafenib), one is an inhibitor of the associated enzyme B-Raf (dabrafenib), and one is a MEK inhibitor (trametinib); the only one that is an actual immune-therapy, is an anti-CTLA-4 (ipilimumab) antibody [13]. Therefore searching new efficacious immune-therapies in this disease is still an open subject of intense research.

This chapter summarizes the main achievements gathered in the last 3 years regarding immune-therapy as the ultimate approach for melanoma treatment.

2. Reducing specific immune-suppression

Until recently, the approved therapy armentarium in advanced melanoma was comprising only dacarbazine (DTIC), hydroxyurea, while the only approved immune agent was high-dose interleukin-2 (IL-2) [14]. These drugs cannot provide satisfactory overall survival (OS) rates in advanced stages. After searching various combination of immune-therapies, from vaccination [15] to drugs that inhibit immune-signaling pathways [16], in 2011 FDA approved, ipilimumab and vemurafenib, agents that significantly increased OS and long-term improvement in advanced melanoma [17].

In this case, monoclonal antibodies (mAbs) as immune-therapy agents have the intrinsic role to establish an antineoplastic action through stimulation of a specific immune response. This action can be performed by inducing *de novo* primary response and/or by eliciting an already existing antitumor action, but repressed in these patients.

The most advanced, in terms of positive research results, were the immune-related drugs that abrogated the immune –suppression such as CTLA4 or PD-1. Other mAbs were designed to aim toward stimulation of co-stimulatory receptors, molecules that are expressed by antigen presenting cells (APC); the aimed molecules were CD40 or OX40 (member 4 tumor necrosis factor receptor superfamily) or GITR (TNFRSF18), expressed on activated T lymphocytes.

Tremelimumab, also an anti CTLA4 mAb, is being evaluated in solid tumors. Nivolumab, an anti PD-1 mAb is also in the evaluation phase. This year (2014) clinical trials assessing OX40- and GITR-activating mAbs were initiated as well [18].

2.1. Anti-CTLA-4 antibodies

Activated T lymphocytes express transiently CTLA-4 transmembrane protein, while on T regulatory lymphocytes (Tregs) this protein is expressed constitutively. Two possible mechanisms are known accounting for CTLA-4 immune-suppressive effect. One of the mechanisms is the competitive binding to B7-1 and B7-2 in the detriment of the normal binding to CD28, delivering thus an immune-suppressive signal [19]. Actually CTLA-4 competes with the binding of CD28 to B7, thus hindering a normal activation. The other possible mechanism is that cells expressing CTLA-4, endocytose the appropriate ligands of other cells, as such, CD28 cannot trigger activation [20].

Overall in cancer research, drugs that aim B7 family can enhance the therapeutic panel and thorough studies are further needed for elucidating these regulatory pathways [21].

The particular action of monoclonal anti-CTLA-4 antibody is to link to CTLA-4, blocking the inhibitory immune-suppressive signal, T cell can perform thus its activation pathways, proliferate while infiltrating the tumors, and in the end, set off tumour apoptosis. Designed to bind to CTLA-4, ipilimumab was approved by FDA in 2011 for advanced melanoma [22] and in the same year the European Commission issued a marketing authorization for ipilimumab [23].This type of immune-drug aims to downregulate the inhibitory activity of T-lymphocytes leading to the normal activation of T cells by allowing the binding of CD28 to B7, this costimulatory process participates to the main coupling of MHC (major histocompatibility complex) that presents the tumour antigen to TCR (T cell receptor). Re-establishing these physiological molecular interactions, T-cells can mount an efficient antitumor immune response (Figure 1) [24]. CTLA-4 expressed on T cells is omnipresent and is not dependent upon the tumour's particularities, thus the drug's action should not be dependent on tumor's characteristics.

EMA recommendation after analyzing the post-phase III results extended clinical trials [25,17] is a dose of intravenously 3 mg/kg ipilimumab over a 90 min period, this procedure needs to be repeated every 3 weeks; overall four doses should be administered [23]. If the patients are treated in combination with DTIC it is recommended that a dose of 10 mg/kg should be used [25,17].

The actual clinical results of using this immune-therapy showed that patients with advanced melanoma increased their median OS to 10 months when compared to the 6 months OS in gp100 melanoma vaccine. When comparing OS in patients treated with ipilimumab in combination with DTIC, OS was 11 months, while DTIC monotherapy just 9 months.

As stated above ipilimumab's action is not dependent on specific and individual tumor cell mutations, hence it can be efficient in different patients and stages [26, 27]. The beneficial clinical results regarding OS were registered as independent of various parameters such as age, gender, stage and/or previous therapy regimens.

Investigating the patients survival curves it has been shown that there are groups surviving more than 4 years [28], and that their clinical response was durable during the follow-up [29]. Durability is an important differentiating criterion when recommending first-line therapy with immunomodulators in comparison to the duration obtained in kinase inhibitors treatment.

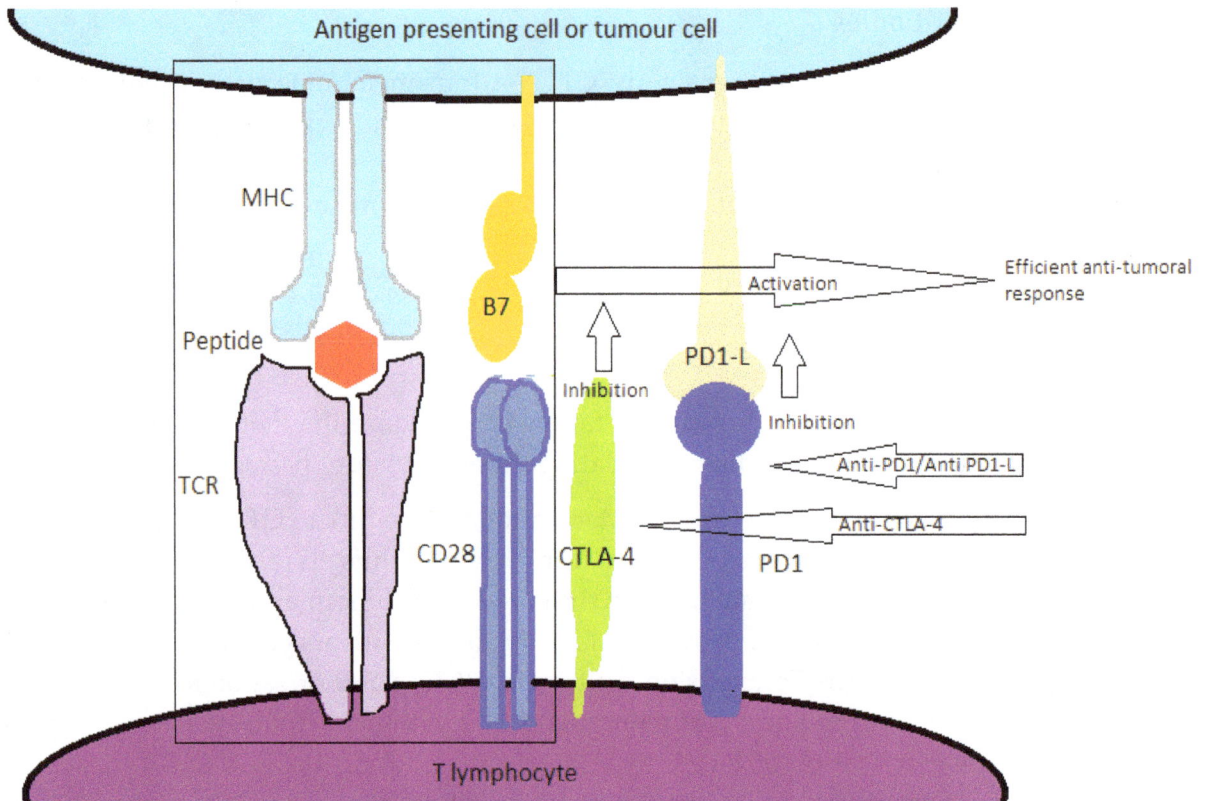

Figure 1. Main immune-suppression molecular mechanisms that can be overridden by therapeutical monoclonal antibodies targeting CTLA-4 and PD1.

As we are focusing on an immune therapy and as *immune memory* is a characteristic of this process, it was a logic approach to see what the effects are when ipilimumab gets another round of therapy. The National Comprehensive Cancer Network (NCCN) recommendation show that ipilimumab re-treatment can be done when the first round induced intolerable toxicity and/or for patients relapsing after the first therapy or proving at least 3 months stable disease [30]. Adverse reaction during re-treatment are similar to those for the first approach (see below) and no actual predisposition was noted regarding first encountered toxicity with the re-treatment one. Authors report that retreatment with ipilimumab is a feasible therapy and, currently a phase II trial (http://trialsunited.com/studies/NCT01709162) focuses on the immune response parameters in ipilimumab re-treatment [31].

Non-cutaneous melanomas were also therapeutic targets for ipilimumab therapy. Thus, in an Australian study published in 2014 over 100 patients were followed after ipilimumab therapy. Median OS for mucosal and uveal melanoma patients was half of that registered in cutaneous melanoma patients. This report underlines the severities of adverse effects, even death-related to therapy cases, thus administration and follow-up by an experienced clinical team is extremely necessary in this type of clinical trials [32].

Stage IV patients presenting brain metastasis were another therapy target group as blood-brain barrier is permeable to activated T lymphocytes, cells capable of inducing a local immune response [33]. In a large study comprising over 800 patients with brain metastasis treated with ipilimumab, up to 25% survived at least 1 year, as the un-treated median OS is only 5 months [34].

Adverse reactions in ipilimumab therapy are associated with hyper-immune reactions, but these can be solved by the physician using additional classic therapies. Over 10% of patients experienced gastrointestinal deregulations (e.g. diarrhea, nausea, vomiting, decreased appetite and abdominal pain), rash, pruritus, fatigue. Side-effects are manageable by the physician and, seldom, the severity can lead to treatment discontinuation (www.ema.europa.eu). These immune-related adverse effects (irAEs) are mild to moderate toxicity and are experienced by around 60% of the patients, while around 15% developed grade 3 or 4 toxicity [25]. Endocrine system – related adverse effects were also reported in this therapy; in patients group receiving ipilimumab, 8% have experienced hypophysitis and 6% hypothyroidism/thyroiditis. Combined therapy, ipilimumab and nivolumab, induce in 22% of the patients thyroiditis or hypothyroidism and in 9% hypophysitis. Authors report hormone replacement as adjuvant therapy and immediate initiation of this therapy reverses symptoms [35]. If the ipilimumab therapy is combined with vemurafenib, important hepatotoxicity was reported, thus caution should be taken when combining immune-therapy with this B-Raf enzyme inhibitor [36].

2.2. Anti-PD-1 or PD-1L antibodies

2.2.1. Nivolumab

In July 2014, the first human monoclonal antibody against programmed death receptor-1 was announced as approved in Japan-*Nivolumab* [37]. As shown above in Figure 1, it targets a negative regulatory molecule that sustains immunosuppression. After accomplishing phase I and II clinical trials, around 25% of stage III and IV patients had a good clinical response when 2 mg/kg intravenous nivolumab was administered every 3 weeks. The clinical outcome was very optimistic in this study, patients did not progress in their disease for a median of 172 days, and at the time of publication (July 2014) median OS was still not achieved.

Nivolumab displayed a good tolerability profile; grade 3 or 4 adverse effects were reported in les than 18 % of patients, mainly an increased γ-glutamyl transferase [38].

Another group studying T lymphocyte interaction with tumour cell, interaction mediated by PD-1 receptor linking to PD-L 1, has shown that in phase I/II studies this antibody can lead to tumor regression and can enhance OS in various cancers including skin melanoma. Studying antibodies that target PD-1 or PD-1L (e.g. nivolumab, MK-3475, pidilizumab, MPDL3280A, BMS-936559, MEDI4736, MSB0010718C) the authors show that the positive clinical response goes to a maximum of 50% response rate when antibodies against PD-1 combined with anti-CTLA-4 were used. The clinical responses start early upon treatment and continue after the treatment is finished [39].

Another study published in 2014 searched to evaluate the survival of patients upon discontinuation of the therapy. After enrolling over 100 patients with advanced melanoma, the authors concluded that the median OS was 16.8 months [40].

Melanoma patients along with other cancer diagnosed patients were treated with anti-PD-1 (nivolumab). This early-phase clinical trial published in 2014 aimed to elucidate the link between PD-1, PD-L1, and PD-L2 expression, immune cell infiltration and the clinical efficacy of this therapy. The degree of PD-L1 expression depicted on tumor cells was associated with its receptor PD-1 expressed by lymphocytes. The other ligand of PD-1, PD-L2 corroborated with PD-L1 expression. The expression of PD-L1 on the tumors was correlated with the clinical efficacy of the anti-PD-1 therapy, and the found best correlation when compared to other studied factors, such as PD-1 expression and/or TIL (tumor infiltrating lymphocytes). The study concludes that, when achieving maximum efficacy with novilumab, tumor PD-L1 expression is the base of anti-PD-1 therapeutical blockade [41].

In 2013, results from phase I clinical trials, of nivolumab and MK-3475 (anti-PD-1 and anti-PD-L1 antibodies) were released. For MK-3475 an objective response of 38 % with only 13 % of the patients reporting grade 3/4 toxicities was shown [42]. These results were probably the ground for further approval (see below).

Phase III clinical trails are on-going and, it seems that PD-1-PD-L1 triggers a sequence of intracellular signaling that brings important clinical benefits [43].

Adverse effects in this type of therapy are of low grade, the physician can impose a good patient management [39] and long-term safety is acceptable [40].

2.2.2. Pembrolizumab

In September 2014, FDA granted accelerated approval to pembrolizumab (formerly known as MK-3475), an antibody targeting PD-1, to be used following ipilimumab therapy. A recently published report showed the efficacy and safety results of this antibody at two doses (2 mg/kg and 10 mg/kg) given every 21 days. The enrolled patients that received the therapy were refractory to ipilimumab therapy. Similar safety profiles were reported whether patients were treated with 2 mg/kg or 10 mg/kg and authors show that no drug-related deaths were registered [44]. Another published study had similar results with the difference that the response rate between patients with or without prior ipilimumab treatment were not statistically different. Positive clinical outcome was registered with the overall median progression-free survival exceeding 7 months. Patients with advanced melanoma, prior refractory to ipilimumab, proved in this study a high rate of tumor regression [45].

Drug-related adverse effects were fatigue in one third of the patients and around 20% of them experienced pruritus and rash. Grade 3 fatigue was the single drug-related grade 3 to 4 adverse effect in 3% of the patients [44].

The positive results in a difficult to manage patients, like the ones refractory to ipilimumab, probably accelerated this drug authorization with two months ahead of its planned approval and the clinical study is still on going [46].

After ipilimumab approval, finding another antibody that could be used as immune-therapy for blocking an immune checkpoint like PD-1 and PD-1L gained an intense research frenzy in the last years.Therapeutical approaches that use immunomodulatory drugs have completely different mode of action in comparison to the well-known chemotherapeutical procedures. From this point of view investigating the intimate mechanisms that underlie their effect is of outmost importance because it can reveal new signaling molecules, future to be drug targets. Moreover biomarkers that can clinically predict the patient response could optimize the approach and personalize the immune-therapy [47].

2.3. Biomarkers for clinical benefit prediction

In the last couple of years there is a less abundant literature focusing on predictive and/or prognostic biomarkers in the immune-therapy of cutaneous melanoma. Biomarkers that were published lately range from classic serum LDH, to membrane molecules and circulating cells without any *clear-cut biomarker* that could predict the immune-therapy efficacy.

In the last year researchers were focusing on biomarkers that can predict immune-therapy with ipilimumab outcome. Thus some studies show that ipilimumab therapy was correlated with an increase in peripheral blood absolute lymphocyte count when patients had a good clinical outcome in terms of OS. More specifically OS was 11.9 months for patients that had more than 1,000 lymphocyte count / μL peripheral blood in comparison to OS of 1.4 months in patients with lower counts [48, 49]. These results were confirmed this year when increased absolute lymphocyte count was associated with increased progression free survival (PFS) but not with OS. Any other parameters including classic serum LDH did not relate to OS or PFS [32].

Another cell biomarker, forkhead box P3 (FoxP3) expressed by T-regs, was correlated with positive clinical outcome in advanced melanoma patients [50].

Correlations were investigated regarding circulatory myeloid-derived suppressor cells (MDSC) in treated patients. Authors report that circulatory MDSC with Lin(-) CD14(+) HLA-DR(-) phenotype are increased in patients compared to normal. After surgically removing the tumour and subjecting patients' to ipilimumab treatment, this immune parameter did not change. Then again, an interesting finding was that patients could be stratified in the ipilimumab-responders and non-responders based on the lower and respectively higher concentration of circulatory MDSC, thus pinpointing these cells as possible predictive markers of response to ipilimumab. This candidate immune-marker did not correlate with baseline serum LDH, but showed higher values in severe metastasis compared to localized metastasis to skin and/or to lymph nodes [51].

As to the possible efficacy biomarkers for nivolumab therapy, in a phase I clinical trial, stage III or IV patients were followed after this therapy by several biomarkers evaluation. This recent study reports that high circulatory T lymphocytes with NY-ESO-1 and MART-1-specific CD8(+) phenotype are associated with disease progression. After therapy, increased circulatory Tregs and decreased antigen-specific T cells are the two immune biomarkers that were found associated with disease progression. The expression of PD-L1 on the tumor did not correlate with the clinical response [52].

2.4. Animal models studying immune-therapy mechanisms

There are few studies focusing on animal models that bring new data regarding the intimate cellular mechanisms in immune-therapy. Having in mind the fact that these recent immune-therapies are limited to certain groups of patients, the published animal models searched for the resistance mechanisms that could hinder this therapy.

In 2013, the role of IDO upon an experimental anti CTLA-4 blockade was shown. Authors used IDO knockout mice and showed that, upon treatment with anti-CTLA-4 antibody, B16 melanoma was growing more slowly and that, the animals' overall survival increased compared to normal mice expressing IDO. The mechanisms were similar when the animal model was treated with anti PD-1/ anti-PD-L1 and GITR. The authors show in this animal model that CTLA-4 and IDO inhibitors converge and that the inhibitory role of IDO can be the background mechanisms accounting for the resistance to anti-CTLA-4 therapy. Moreover, the process is T lymphocyte dependent and, if this resistance is overridden, effector T cells are found increased in tumour infiltration, the effector-to-regulatory T cell ratio increases as well [53]. The molecular mechanisms of IDO expression are intimately related to the immune response. Several years ago it was reported that IDO expression is controlled by T activated lymphocytes through their secreted cytokines. IL-13 can repress the induction of IDO mediated by IFN-gamma [54]. Regarding possible emerging therapies, authors report that fludarabine that hinders the up-regulation of IDO in a T lymphocytes dependent manner, can be tested as a pre-treatment drug for melanoma patients. These patients can receive afterwards immuno-therapies that would have been less efficient when IDO was over-expressed [55].

Using animal models, new emerging therapies can be discovered, overriding the resistance to immune-therapies in certain patients groups.

3. Dendritic cells pulsed with specific antigens as inductors of specific immune-response

Treatment paradigms aim to include naturally occurring dendritic cells subsets in a single vaccine. The studies that are in the pre-clinical phases show synergistic effects between various antigen-presenting cells. We will present different types of methodologies to pulse dendritic cells, starting with mere cultivation of dendritic cells in total tumour lysates and ending with newer technologies such as electroporation mRNA-pulsed dendritic cells. Recently, the first clinical trials released their results and showed increased survival rates and broader anti-cancer immune responses. These new clinical findings will be presented.

In just a short period of time, the cancer immunotherapy field has gained new combatants through sipuleucel-T FDA approval, first DC immunovaccine for metastatic prostate cancer patients, followed closely by ipilimumab, an antibody specific to CTLA-4 as major target in metastatic melanoma [56]. Due to its clear tumor immunogenicity, melanoma treatment could be handled from an immunotherapeutic viewpoint. However, an important issue in melanoma immunovaccine success is the highly heterogeneous composition of antigens expressed within tumor site along with different genetic patterns of melanoma patients [57]. Deciphering this complex (intra)tumor heterogeneity of melanoma is directly linked to the possibility for clearly identifying, targeting and manageing drug-resistant cell subpopulations from the tumour site [58]. The genetic profile of melanoma patient is one of the foremost rationales for an autologous whole cell vaccine acting more efficiently in treating the micrometastasis than would an allogeneic designed one.

Revisiting the melanoma vaccines, it was pointed out that a preponderant cytokine-driven therapy activates a robust antitumoral T-cell mediated response representing a class of individualized auto-vaccination formula, surmounting thus the melanoma intratumoral heterogeneity [57]. Assembling a cancer vaccine aims to activate a specific anti-tumor immune response and/or to better access the tumor-associated antigens. In cutaneous melanoma, the pattern of tumor specific and tumor associated antigens is both large and heterogeneous, making melanoma immunogenicity exploitable in therapeutic approaches. Therefore, the plenty of discovered or yet hidden melanoma tumor antigens could open the way for vaccination of patients groups with the same vaccine type [59]. Being explored with synthetic peptides, whole tumor cells, cellular lysates or autologous immunovaccine, dendritic cells (DCs) take advantages in treatment or even in prevention approaches of cancer [60].

Dendritic cell in melanoma immunotherapy undergo a sequential number of actions. Thus, loading DCs with a tumor antigen and a specific adjuvant will induce the maturation state which involves antigens processing by proteasomal degradation and presenting the resulted peptides to T cells *via* MHC complex to stimulate further CD4+ cells, CD8+ cells as well as phagocytes and NK cells or, in certain activation conditions, induce Tregs that hamper antitumor responses [61].

3.1. Dendritic cells subsets

In malignant skin, the principal subsets of DC responsible for Ag-specific T cell immune response comprise *epidermal* (Langerhans cells) and *dermal* cell populations. The primary tumor site and the sentinel lymph nodes endure the immune-suppression generated by melanoma, this immune site being the field where T cells should start the fight against melanoma while being armed by activated DC to engender anti-melanoma immunity [62]. As in case of tumor associated macrophages, under the influence of tumor milieu DC are versatile players which could become *tumor-associated DC* enhancing Immune-suppression by sustaining T cell regulatory activity [63] (Table 1). Upon electrochemotherapy of tumor cells, for example, a relatively new approach to deliver better an antitumor drug, melanoma inflammatory infiltrate contains beside dermal DC, *plasmacytoid* DC cells for capturing tumor antigens to further elicit, along with dermal and Langerhans cells, a T cell antitumor response [64].

DCs subsets	Uptake receptors evaluated for immunotherapy of DC		
	Antigen uptake receptors	Unique receptors	TLR receptors
LC/dermal DC	FcR; DEC205; CD40; DCIR	Langerin	TLR-3
pDC	FcR; DEC205; CD40; DCIR	CD303; CD123; BDCA-2	TLR-7; TLR-9 specific to pDC
MoDC	FcR; DEC205; CD11c; CD40; DCIRDC-SIGN; MR		TLR-4; 8; 3; 7.

Table 1. DCs subsets and receptors for immunovaccine (LC – Langerhans cell; pDC - plasmacytoid-derived DC; MoDC – monocyte-derived DC; DEC205 – C-type lectin receptor on DC; BDCA-2 – blood dendritic cell antigen, specific to pDC subset; DCIR - dendritic cell immunoreceptor; DC-SIGN - dendritic cell specific ICAM-3 grabbing non-integrin; MR – mannose receptor; TLR – toll-like receptor)

3.2. Exploring dendritic cells in melanoma immunovaccine

As skin is an abundant cellular immune network and hence an accessible portal for thera-peutical approaches, DC cells remain an attractive target in melanoma therapy both as *ex-vivo*-generated or *in-vivo*-DC-targeting immunovaccine blueprint [65]. Peripheral blood and Langerhans cells are the main sources for DCs immunotherapy. Langerhans cells and mono-cyte-derived DCs elicit immune responses in comparable levels although the cytokine stimulation conditions are different. The initial therapeutical attempts with DCs vaccination was based on *ex-vivo* generated monocyte-derived DC pulsed with tumor lysates, peptide or tumor antigens which led to a tumor regression rate of 3-7%, having also a lower toxicity compared with standard therapeutical procedures [66]. In melanoma, DC derived from CD34+ progenitors prove better results compared with monocyte-DC vaccine in spite of the known heterogeneity of tumor antigens [10].

3.2.1. Loading DC with tumor associated-antigens

Loading effector immune cells with antigenic peptides or a whole tumor-associated antigen (TAA) was initially designed as an immune vaccination system with T lymphocytes *via* MHC molecules recognition. Due to possible issues related to molecule stability and/or delivery route, resulting in an ineffective antigen presentation, these approaches could fail in clinic due to a low response rate in patients. Using DC as tool for intracellular delivery of such tumor antigenic peptides, the process of antigen presentation to T cells could be improved [67]. Moreover, the Th1/Th2 balance could be regulated by such modified DC. Therefore, DCs loaded with MART-126-35 melanoma peptide were used in combination with anti-CTLA4 monoclonal antibody (tremelimumab) in advanced melanoma patients. Upon therapy, high levels of pro-inflammatory Th1 invariant natural killer T cells (iNKT) CD8(+) was associated with positive clinical responses, indicating that antitumor T cell activity could be immuno-modulated *via* iNKT cells by peptide-pulsed DCs [68]. In another recent study, high-risk stage III melanoma patients with lymph node resection were vaccinated with DC loaded with MHC I melanoma peptides respective to the patient's haplotype. The peptide pulsed DCs were well tolerated and elicited immune specific responses to melanoma antigens or/and IFN-γ-producing CD8+ cell response to melanoma peptides in 15 of 22 patients. The three-year overall survival rate was 68.2% vs. 25.7% in the control patients group [69].

Monocyte-derived DCs could be loaded in different conditions with a mixture of peptides, tumor lysates or even with a single tumor peptide such as from Mage-3A1. For 8 of 11 patients enrolled in the study it was registered an increase of Mage-3A1-specific (CD8+) T cells, with regression of a few metastases for 6 advanced melanoma patients; a lack of Mage 3A1 expression was observed in some non-regressed areas of melanoma [70]. Even immature DCs could be exploited in vaccination, thus DCs generated from CD34+ progenitor cells were cytokines-stimulated and pulsed *in vitro* with a pool of melanoma derived peptides [71].

Engineered DCs loaded with peptides or antigens could be delivered by lymphatic nodes or intradermally; the last type being the optimum method for generating T cell antitumor immunity [72].

3.2.2. DC electroporation with mRNA

Cellular electroporation is a transfection method to efficiently introduce mRNA encoding for a certain biomolecule in order to express at high level that specific antigen. A main advantage of mRNA transfection is the prolongation of the exposure and an accurate antigens processing. This approach was translated for DCs as a promising opportunity to facilitate access to tumor antigens and thus priming the T cell specific antitumor melanoma response, being applicable even in advanced stages of melanoma [73].

In the last few years, mRNA was proposed as an innovative vehicle for antigen delivery appropriate for cancer vaccination purposes. DCs were evaluated as the most suitable immune cells for mRNA transfection due to their professional quality in processing and presenting antigens for inducing specific immune responses by T cells. mRNA as an antigen delivery tool could generate a whole antigenic protein with all epitopes ready to be viewed by MHC molecules; last but not least, the interest mRNA molecule could be produced in large quantities with high purity.

The successful use of *ex vivo* mRNA-modified DCs for melanoma immunotherapy rely on DCs cellular subtype involved, the proper cellular activation and path of delivery [74]. The DCs *subtype* electroporated with mRNA in cancer vaccination purposes accounts for vaccination efficiency. pDCs cells loaded with melanoma antigenic peptides and further activated at CD40L elicit T cytotoxic anti-melanoma responses [75]. The cellular *activation* method of DC counts for CTL full activity and subsequently inhibition of Tregs. Engagement of TLR in DC activation proves to be a good approach in immunovaccine. Moreover, transfection with mRNA and activation of DC cells is the fundament of the TriMix mRNA set encoding for CD40L, CD70 and active form of TLR4. Thus in one clinical study with TriMix-DCs intradermally administrated, the efficacy of procedure was registered by means of the skin infiltrating CD8+ lymphocytes monitored by IL-12p70 as a marker of successful inoculation of the DC product [76]. The *delivery way* of modified DCs was compared in several clinical studies. The best way to target the lymph nodes in melanoma site by modified mRNA DCs is intradermic inoculation associated with an increased number of T cells although intranodally delivery reveal a higher number of DC. One recent study refers to DC electroporated with mRNA for gp100/tyrosinase antigens and injected in regional lymph nodes of melanoma patients prior to local surgery. The mRNA for electroporated melanoma antigen was immunohistochemically detected in T cells populations from both the primary and the adjacent lymph node concomitantly with a CD8+ T lymphocyte responses registered in 7 of 11 patients subjected to immunovaccination [77]. Some promising results in terms of safety, feasibility and immunogenic properties were obtained in patients with advanced cutaneous melanoma in a pilot study were DC were co-electroporated with mRNA encoding for CD40L, TLR4 and CD70 as a autologous TriMix-DC formula combined with IFN-α-2b sequential administration [76].

The foremost parameter to be monitored for immunovaccine efficacy is the induction or the enhancement of melanoma anti-tumor immune response. Several technologies like ELISPOT technique allows quantifying the precise number of active immune cells by counting antigen-specific cells that secrete a particular anti-tumor cytokine e.g. IFN-γ [59]. Since 2006, clinical studies with tumor mRNA transfected DCs administrated usually intradermic in patients with metastatic melanoma, detect an immunological T cell response with promising results at least for disease stabilization. In addition, advanced melanoma patients were treated intradermic with DCs simultaneously co-electroporated for 4 tumor antigens – Mage A3, Mage C2, Tyrosinase and gp100/DC-LAMP followed by TriMix mRNA single or in combination with additional therapy like IFNa-2b. In both clinical set-ups, the CD4/CD8 T cell responses were enhanced [74].

Recently, a small study on seven melanoma patients involved DCs from peripheral blood mononuclear cells pulsed with gp100 peptides and matured further *in vitro* with a cocktail of CD40L and INF-γ. It was noted a direct correlation between the clinical responses and levels of IL-12 produced by modified DCs. The highest levels of IL-12 were registered in one patient with complete remission. DCs from non-responding patients were unable to produce IL-12 without additional stimulation with TLR agonist, observation that induced a modification of the *in vitro* maturation protocol and thus contributed to the improvement of the clinical outcome [78].

4. Translating up-dated knowledge to clinics — Therapeutical future scenery

There is a recent trend that advises as first therapy a BRAF inhibitor in *advanced* stages, because, time-wise, these patients cannot build an effective immune response while in patients with less advanced stages, immune-therapy will lead to a better outcome whether the patient presents or not a BRAF mutation [79].

In the clinical management of melanoma it is certain that immune-therapy is one of the pillars. Among this new therapeutical approaches, MEK inhibitors can overcome the resistance induced by BRAF inhibitors [79, 80]. has shown in phase 3 clinical studies, an improved [81].

Combination of these antibodies with the new anti-CTLA4 drug induces an astonishing 80% or more tumor regression in patients (http://www.clinicaltrials.gov/show/ NCT01783938; http://trialsunited.com/studies/NCT01024231/) [82]. Newer therapeutical combination of ipilimumab with oncolytic immunotherapy with GM-CSF-expressing engineered herpes simplex virus, have shown in phase 3 clinical studies an improved OS in advanced melanoma [83].

On-going studies seek to establish the clinical boundaries of NK adoptive transfer in melanoma. Last year a study was published searching to rationalize the clinical trial framework [84] as the prior published results of a pilot trial showed no tumor regression in spite of the increased concentration of circulating autologous NK cells persistence [85].

Immunotherapy is the only therapeutical "light" that can increase OS in advanced melanomas. Eliciting an efficient immune response takes a certain amount of time in order to have an efficient anti-tumoral response, but as *immunological memory* is installed, the effect of immune-therapy persists in the absence of further immune-treatment.

We strongly believe, taking into account our experience in melanoma patients follow-up [86, 87] that immune-therapy is a major therapy weapon, increasing survival in advanced melanomas. The only draw-back is that, in order to develop its full efficacy, immune-therapy takes time, and this time interval can be up to 2–4 months. Thus, an early diagnostic in the metastatic stage would make a huge difference for a positive clinical outcome [88].

Besides imaging-based follow-up, immune parameters should complete the panel of investigation. New data regarding circulatory MDSC can enhance this panel and prospective clinical trials should soon validate them. Resistance to immune-therapy, like IDO expression opens new therapeutical avenues aiming at immune checkpoints and combining specific antibodies with IDO inhibitors.

5. Conclusion

The immune system is still not fully explored in this type of skin cancer [89, 90], thus new insights in tumour microenvironment and the involvement of innate immunity cells could enhance the panel of new therapeutical targets.

Balancing antitumor efficacy and reconstitution of a proper functioning immune system are processes aimed by immune-therapy in cutaneous melanoma. Owing to cutaneous melanoma immunogenic outline, this disease treatment could be addressed from an immunotherapeutic viewpoint. As we are facing the great success of having the first immune-therapy approved drug in melanoma, there is an open research combat of targeting personalized/individual antigens or undifferentiating antigens-stem-like to tackle the aggressive character of this disease.

Acknowledgements

The study was financed by the following Research Projects: PN-II-PT-PCCA-2013-4-1407, PN-II-ID-PCE-2011-3-0918 and PN.09.33-01.01/2009.

Author details

Monica Neagu* and Carolina Constantin

*Address all correspondence to: neagu.monica@gmail.com

Immunobiology Laboratory, Victor Babes National Institute of Pathology, Bucharest, Romania

References

[1] Dunn GP, Bruce AT, Ikeda H, et al. Cancer Immunoediting: From Immunosurveillance To Tumor Escape. Nature Immunology 2002; 3 991–998

[2] Dunn GP, Old LJ, Schreiber RD. The Immunobiology Of Cancer Immunosurveillance And Immunoediting. Immunity 2004; 21 137–148

[3] Raval RR, Sharabi AB, Walker AJ, Drake CG, Padmanee Sharma P. Tumor Immunology And Cancer Immunotherapy: Summary Of The 2013 SITC Primer. Journal for Immunotherapy of Cancer 2014; 2 14

[4] Ennen M, Keime C, Kobi D, Mengus G, Lipsker D, Thibault-Carpentier C, Davidson I. Single-Cell Gene Expression Signatures Reveal Melanoma Cell Heterogeneity. Oncogene 2014; doi: 10.1038/onc.2014.262. [Epub ahead of print]

[5] Widmer DS, Cheng PF, Eichhoff OM, Belloni BC, Zipser MC, Schlegel NC et al. Systematic Classification Of Melanoma Cells By Phenotype-Specific Gene Expression Mapping. Pigment Cell Melanoma Research 2012; 25 343–353

[6] Liu S, Ren S, Howell P, Fodstad O, Riker AI. Identification Of Novel Epigenetically Modified Genes In Human Melanoma Via Promoter Methylation Gene Profiling. Pigment Cell Melanoma Research 2008; 21 545–558

[7] Thurber AE, Douglas G, Sturm EC, Zabierowski SE, Smit DJ, Ramakrishnan SN et al. Inverse Expression States Of The BRN2 And MITF Transcription Factors In Melanoma Spheres And Tumour Xenografts Regulate The NOTCH Pathway. Oncogene 2011; 30 3036–3048

[8] Haass NK, Beaumont KA, Hill DS, Anfosso A, Mrass P, Munoz MA, Kinjyo I, Weninger W. Real-Time Cell Cycle Imaging During Melanoma Growth, Invasion, And Drug Response. Pigment Cell Melanoma Research 2014; 27(5) 764-776

[9] Perego M, Tortoreto M, Tragni G, Mariani L, Deho P, Carbone A et al. Heterogeneous Phenotype of Human Melanoma Cells with In Vitro and In Vivo Features of Tumor-Initiating Cells. The Journal of Investigative Dermatology 2010; 130 1877–1886

[10] Md. Selim Ahmed, Yong-Soo Bae. Dendritic Cell-Based Therapeutic Cancer Vaccines: Past, Present And Future. Clinical and Experimental Vaccine Research 2014;3 113-116

[11] Khattak M, Fisher R, Turajlic S, Larkin J. Targeted Therapy And Immunotherapy In Advanced Melanoma: An Evolving Paradigm. Therapeutic Advances in Medical Oncology 2013; 5 105–118

[12] Menzies AM, Long GV. New Combinations And Immunotherapies For Melanoma: Latest Evidence And Clinical Utility. Therapeutic Advances in Medical Oncology 2013; 5(5) 278–285

[13] Saraceni MM, Khushalani NI, Jarkowski A 3rd. Immunotherapy in Melanoma: Recent Advances and Promising New Therapies. Journal of Pharmacy Practice. 2014 Mar 27. Epub ahead of print]

[14] Garbe C, Eigentler TK, Keilholz U, Hauschild A, Kirkwood JM. Systematic Review Of Medical Treatment In Melanoma: Current Status And Future Prospects. Oncologist 2011;16(1) 5-24

[15] Slingluff CL JrPetroni GR, Olson W, Czarkowski A, Grosh WW, et al. Helper T-Cell Responses and Clinical Activity of a Melanoma Vaccine with Multiple Peptides from MAGE and Melanocytic Differentiation Antigens. Journal of Clinical Oncology 2008; 26, 4973-4980

[16] Bernardo-Faura M, Massen S, Falk CS, Brady NR, Eils R. Data-Derived Modeling Characterizes Plasticity of MAPK Signaling in Melanoma. PLOS Computational Biology 2014; 10(9) e1003795. doi:10.1371/journal.pcbi.1003795

[17] Robert C, Thomas L, Bondarenko I, et al. Ipilimumab Plus Dacarbazine for Previously Untreated Metastatic Melanoma. The New England Journal of Medicine 2011;364(26) 2517-2526

[18] Aranda F, Vacchelli E, Eggermont A, Galon J, Fridman WH, Zitvogel L, Kroemer G, Galluzzi L. Trial Watch: Immunostimulatory Monoclonal Antibodies in Cancer Therapy. Oncoimmunology 2014; 3(1) e27297

[19] Salama AK, Hodi FS. Cytotoxic T-Lymphocyte-Associated Antigen-4. Clinical Cancer Research 2011; 17 4622–4628

[20] Qureshi OS et al. Trans-Endocytosis Of CD80 And CD86: A Molecular Basis for the Cell-Extrinsic Function of CTLA-4. Science 2011; 332 600–603

[21] Ceeraz S, EC, Noelle RJ. B7 family checkpoint regulators in immune regulation and disease. Trends in Immunology 2013; 34 (11) 556-563

[22] Yervoy (ipilimumab) prescribing Information. Bristol-Myers Squibb Co. Revised December 2013. Available at: http://packageinserts.bms.com/pi/pi_yervoy.pdf. (accessed August 2014).

[23] Hanaizi Z, van Zwieten-Boot B, Calvo G, Sancho Lopez A, van Dartel M, Camarero J, Abadie E, Pignatti F. The European Medicines Agency Review of Ipilimumab (Yervoy) for the Treatment of Advanced (Unresectable Or Metastatic) Melanoma In Adults who Have Received Prior Therapy: Summary of the scientific assessment of the Committee for Medicinal Products for Human Use, European Journal of Cancer 2012; 48(2) 237–242

[24] Tarhini A, Lo E, Minor DR. Releasing the brake on the immune system: ipilimumab in melanoma and other tumors. Cancer Biotherapy and Radiopharmaceuticals 2010; 25(6) 601-613

[25] Hodi FS, O'Day SJ, McDermott DF, et al. Improved survival with ipilimumab in patients with metastatic melanoma. The New England Journal of Medicine 2010; 363(8) 711-723

[26] Wolchok JD, Weber JS, Maio M, et al. Four-Year Survival Rates for Patients with Metastatic Melanoma who Received Ipilimumab in Phase II Clinical Trials. Annals of Oncology 2013; 24(8) 2174-2180

[27] Eggermont AM. Can Immuno-Oncology Offer a Truly Pan-Tumour Approach to Therapy? Annals of Oncology 2012; 23(Suppl 8) viii53-57

[28] Olszanski AJ. Current and Future Roles of Targeted Therapy and Immunotherapy in Advanced Melanoma. Journal of Managed Care Pharmacy JMCP 2014; 20(4) 346-356

[29] Prieto PA, Yang JC, Sherry RM, et al. CTLA-4 Blockade with Ipilimumab: Long-Term Follow-Up of 177 Patients with Metastatic Melanoma. Clinical Cancer Research 2012;18(7) 2039-2047

[30] National Comprehensive Cancer Network website. NCCN Clinical Practice Guidelines in Oncology. Melanoma v2.2014. (Available at: http://www.nccn.org/professionals/physician_gls/pdf/melanoma.pdf)

[31] Robert C, Schadendorf D, Messina M, Hodi FS, O'Day S, for the MDX010-20 investigators. Efficacy and Safety of Retreatment with Ipilimumab in Patients with Pretreated Advanced Melanoma who Progressed After Initially Achieving Disease Control. Clinical Cancer Research 2013;19(8) 2232-2239

[32] Alexander M, Mellor JD, McArthur G, Kee D. Ipilimumab in Pretreated Patients with Unresectable Or Metastatic Cutaneous, Uveal And Mucosal Melanoma. Medical Journal of Australia 2014; 201(1) 49-53

[33] [Becher B, Bechmann I, Greter M. Antigen Presentation In Autoimmunity And CNS Inflammation: How T Lymphocytes Recognize The Brain. Journal of molecular medicine (Berlin, Germany) 2006; 84(7) 532-543

[34] Eigentler TK, Figl A, Krex D, et al. on behalf of the Dermatologic Cooperative Oncology Group and the National Interdisciplinary Working Group on Melanoma. Number Of Metastases, Serum Lactate Dehydrogenase Level, And Type Of Treatment Are Prognostic Factors In Patients With Brain Metastases Of Malignant Melanoma. Cancer 2011;117(8) 1697-1703

[35] Ryder M, Callahan M, Postow MA, Wolchok J, Fagin JA. Endocrine-Related Adverse Events Following Ipilimumab In Patients With Advanced Melanoma: A Comprehensive Retrospective Review From A Single Institution. Endocrine-related cancer 2014; 21(2) 371-381

[36] Ribas A, Hodi FS, Callahan M, Konto C, Wolchok J. Hepatotoxicity With Combination Of Vemurafenib And Ipilimumab. The New England Journal of Medicine 2013; 368(14) 1365-1366

[37] Nivolumab Receives Manufacturing and Marketing Approval in Japan for the Treatment of Unresectable Melanoma http://www.esmo.org/Oncology-News/Nivolumab-Receives-Manufacturing-and-Marketing-Approval-in-Japan-for-the-Treatment-of-Unresectable-Melanoma

[38] Deeks ED. Nivolumab: A Review Of Its Use In Patients With Malignant Melanoma. Drugs 2014;74(11) 1233-1239

[39] Lu J, Lee-Gabel L, Nadeau MC, Ferencz TM, Soefje SA. Clinical Evaluation Of Compounds Targeting PD-1/PD-L1 Pathway For Cancer Immunotherapy. Journal of oncology pharmacy practice: official publication of the International Society of Oncology Pharmacy Practitioners 2014; pii: 1078155214538087 [Epub ahead of print]

[40] Topalian SL, Sznol M, McDermott DF, et al. Survival, Durable Tumor Remission, and Long-Term Safety In Patients With Advanced Melanoma Receiving Nivolumab. Journal of Clinical Oncology 2014; 32(10) 1020-1030. doi: 10.1200/JCO.2013.53.0105.

[41] Taube JM, Klein A, Brahmer JR, Xu H, Pan X, Kim JH, Chen L, Pardoll DM, Topalian SL, Anders RA. Association of PD-1, PD-1 Ligands, and Other Features of the Tumor Immune Microenvironment with Response to Anti-PD-1 Therapy. Clinical Cancer Research 2014 Apr 8. [Epub ahead of print]

[42] Hamid O, Sosman JA, Lawrence DP, Sullivan RJ, Ibrahim N, Kluger HM, et al. Clinical activity, safety, and biomarkers of MPDL3280A, an engineered PD-L1 antibody in patients with locally advanced or metastatic melanoma (mM). 2013 ASCO Annual Meeting (May 31-June 4, 2013, Chicago, IL. 31(15suppl) 9010

[43] Mamalis A, Garcha M, Jagdeo J. Targeting the PD-1 pathway: a promising future for the treatment of melanoma. Archives of dermatological research 2014; 306(6) 511-519

[44] Robert C, Ribas A, Wolchok JD, Hodi FS, Hamid O, Kefford R, et al. Anti-programmed-death-receptor-1 treatment with pembrolizumab in ipilimumab-refractory advanced melanoma: a randomised dose-comparison cohort of a phase 1 trial. Lancet. 2014; 384(9948):1109-17

[45] Hamid O, Robert C, Daud A, Hodi FS, Hwu WJ, Kefford R, et al.Safety and tumor responses with lambrolizumab (anti-PD-1) in melanoma. N Engl J Med. 2013;369(2): 134-44.

[46] ClinicalTrials.gov identifier: NCT01295827

[47] Naidoo J, Page DB, Wolchok JD. Immune checkpoint blockade. Hematology/Oncology Clinics of North America 2014; 28(3) 585-600

[48] Ku GY, Yuan J, Page DB, et al. Single-Institution Experience With Ipilimumab In Advanced Melanoma Patients In The Compassionate Use Setting: Lymphocyte Count After 2 Doses Correlates With Survival. Cancer 2010;116(7) 1767–1775

[49] Berman DM, Wolchok J, Weber J, et al. Association Of Peripheral Blood Absolute Lymphocyte Count (ALC) And Clinical Activity In Patients (Pts) With Advanced

Melanoma Treated With Ipilimumab. Journal of Clinical Oncology 2009; 27(Suppl 15) Abstr 3020

[50] Hamid O, Chasalow SD, Tsuchihashi Z, et al. Association Of Baseline And On-Study Tumor Biopsy Markers With Clinical Activity In Patients (Pts) With Advanced Melanoma Treated With Ipilimumab. Journal of Clinical Oncology 2009; 27(Suppl 15) Abstr 9008

[51] Meyer C, Cagnon L, Costa-Nunes CM, Baumgaertner P, Montandon N, Leyvraz L, Michielin O, Romano E, Speiser DE. Frequencies Of Circulating MDSC Correlate With Clinical Outcome Of Melanoma Patients Treated With Ipilimumab. Cancer Immunology, Immunotherapy 2014; 63(3) 247-257

[52] Weber JS, Kudchadkar RR, Yu B, Gallenstein D, Horak CE, Inzunza HD, et al. Safety, efficacy, and biomarkers of nivolumab with vaccine in ipilimumab-refractory or -naive melanoma. Journal of Clinical Oncology 2013; 31(34) 4311-438

[53] Holmgaard RB, Zamarin D, Munn DH, Wolchok JD, Allison JP. Indoleamine 2,3-Dioxygenase Is A Critical Resistance Mechanism In Antitumor T Cell Immunotherapy Targeting CTLA-4. The Journal of Experimental Medicine 2013; 210(7) 1389-1402

[54] Godin-Ethier J, Pelletier S, Hanafi LA, Gannon PO, Forget MA, et al. Human activated T lymphocytes modulate IDO expression in tumors through Th1/Th2 balance. The Journal of Immunology 2009; 183 7752–7760

[55] Hanafi L-A, Gauchat D, Godin-Ethier J, et al. Fludarabine Downregulates Indoleamine 2,3-Dioxygenase in Tumors via a Proteasome-Mediated Degradation Mechanism, PLOS ONE 2014; 9(6) e99211

[56] Iversen TZ, Andersen MH, Svane IM. The Targeting of IDO-Mediated Immune Escape in Cancer. Basic & Clinical Pharmacology & Toxicology 2014; doi: 10.1111/bcpt. 12320.

[57] Elias EG, Sharma BK. Melanoma Vaccines, Revisited a Review, Update. G Ital Dermatol Venereol. 2014 Jul 31. [Epub ahead of print]

[58] Seftor EA, Seftor RE, Weldon DS, Kirsammer GT, Margaryan NV, Gilgur A, Hendrix MJ. Melanoma Tumor Cell Heterogeneity: A Molecular Approach to Study Subpopulations Expressing the Embryonic Morphogen Nodal. Semininars in Oncology 2014;41(2) 259-266. doi: 10.1053/j.seminoncol.2014.02.001.

[59] Butterfield LH, Buffo MJ. Immunologic Monitoring of Cancer Vaccine Trials Using the ELISPOT assay. Methods in Molecular Biology 2014;1102 71-82. doi: 10.1007/978-1-62703-727-3_5

[60] Ahmed MS, Bae YS. Dendritic cell-based therapeutic cancer vaccines: past, present and future. Clin Exp Vaccine Res. 2014 Jul;3(2):113-6. doi: 10.7774/cevr.2014.3.2.113.

[61] Shtivelman E, Davies MQ, Hwu P, Yang J, Lotem M, Oren M, Flaherty KT, Fisher DE. Pathways And Therapeutic Targets In Melanoma. Oncotarget 2014; 5(7) 1701-1752

[62] Oosterhoff D, Sluijter BJ, Hangalapura BN, de Gruijl TD. The Dermis as A Portal For Dendritic Cell-Targeted Immunotherapy Of Cutaneous Melanoma. Current Topics in Microbiology and Immunology 2012; 351 181-220.

[63] Benencia F, Muccioli M, Alnaeeli M. Perspectives On Reprograming Cancer-Associated Dendritic Cells For Anti-Tumor Therapies. Frontiers in Oncology 2014; 4 72. doi: 10.3389/fonc.2014.00072. eCollection 2014.

[64] Gerlini G, Di Gennaro P, Borgognoni L. Enhancing Anti-Melanoma Immunity By Electrochemotherapy and In Vivo Dendritic-Cell Activation. Oncoimmunology 2012;1(9) 1655-1657

[65] Palucka K, Banchereau J. Cancer Immunotherapy via Dendritic Cells. Nature Reviews Cancer 2012;12 265-277

[66] Butterfield LH. Dendritic Cells In Cancer Immunotherapy Clinical Trials: Are We Making Progress? Frontiers in Immunology 2013;4 454.

[67] Li H, Ma W. Intracellular Delivery Of Tumor Antigenic Peptides In Biodegradable-Polymer Adjuvant For Enhancing Cancer Immunotherapy. Current Medicinal Chemistry. 2014; 21(21) 2357-2366

[68] Ibarrondo FJ, Yang OO, Chodon T, Avramis E, Lee Y, Sazegar H, et al. Natural Killer T Cells In Advanced Melanoma Patients Treated With Tremelimumab. PLoS One 2013; 8(10) e76829. doi: 10.1371/journal.pone.0076829. eCollection 2013

[69] Markowicz S, Nowecki ZI, Rutkowski P, Lipkowski AW, Biernacka M, Jakubowska-Mucka A, et al. Adjuvant vaccination with melanoma antigen-pulsed dendritic cells in stage III melanoma patients. Medical Oncology 2012; 29(4) 2966-2977

[70] Thurner B, Haendle I, Roder C, Dieckmann D, Keikavoussi P, Jonuleit H, et al. Vaccination With Mage-3A1 Peptide-Pulsed Mature, Monocyte-Derived Dendritic Cells Expands Specific Cytotoxic T Cells And Induces Regression Of Some Metastases In Advanced Stage IV Melanoma. The Journal of experimental medicine. 1999; 190(11) 1669-1678

[71] Mackensen A, Herbst B, Chen JL, Kohler G, Noppen C, Herr W, et al. Phase I Study In Melanoma Patients Of A Vaccine With Peptide-Pulsed Dendritic Cells Generated In Vitro From CD34(+) Hematopoietic Progenitor Cells. International journal of cancer Journal international du cancer 2000; 86(3) 385-392

[72] Lesterhuis WJ, de Vries IJ, Schreibelt G, Lambeck AJ, Aarntzen EH, Jacobs JF, Scharenborg NM, van de Rakt MW, de Boer AJ, Croockewit S, van Rossum MM, Mus R, Oyen WJ, Boerman OC, Lucas S, Adema GJ, et al. Route Of Administration Modulates The Induction Of Dendritic Cell Vaccine-Induced Antigen-Specific T Cells In

Advanced Melanoma Patients. Clinical cancer research: an official journal of the American Association for Cancer Research 2011; 17(17) 5725-5735

[73] Aarntzen EH, Schreibelt G, Bol K, Lesterhuis WJ, Croockewit AJ, de Wilt JH, van Rossum MM, Blokx WA, Jacobs JF, Duiveman-de Boer T, Schuurhuis DH, Mus R, Thielemans K, de Vries IJ, Figdor CG, Punt CJ, et al. Vaccination With Mrna-Electro-porated Dendritic Cells Induces Robust Tumor Antigen-Specific CD4+ And CD8+ T Cells Responses In Stage III And IV Melanoma Patients. Clinical cancer research: an official journal of the American Association for Cancer Research 2012; 18(19) 5460-5470

[74] Van Lint S, Heirman C, Thielemans K, Breckpot K. mRNA: From A Chemical Blue-print for Protein Production to an Off-The-Shelf Therapeutic. Human vaccines & im-munotherapeutics 2013; 9(2) 265-274

[75] Salio M, Cella M, Vermi W, Facchetti F, Palmowski MJ, Smith CL, et al. Plasmacytoid Dendritic Cells Prime IFN-Gamma-Secreting Melanoma-Specific CD8 Lymphocytes And Are Found In Primary Melanoma Lesions. European Journal of Immunology 2003; 33 1052–1062

[76] Wilgenhof S, Van Nuffel AM, Corthals J, Heirman C, Tuyaerts S, Benteyn D, et al. Therapeutic vaccination with an autologous mRNA electroporated dendritic cell vac-cine in patients with advanced melanoma. Journal of Immunotherapy 2011; 34 448-456

[77] Schuurhuis DH, Verdijk P, Schreibelt G, Aarntzen EH, Scharenborg N, de Boer A, van de Rakt MW, Kerkhoff M, Gerritsen MJ, Eijckeler F, Bonenkamp JJ, Blokx W, van Krieken JH, Boerman OC, Oyen WJ, Punt CJ, Figdor CG, Adema GJ, de Vries IJ. In Situ Expression of Tumor Antigens by Messenger RNA-Electroporated Dendritic Cells in Lymph Nodes of Melanoma Patients. Cancer Research 2009; 69(7) 2927-2934

[78] Carreno BM, Becker-Hapak M, Huang A, Chan M, Alyasiry A, Lie WR, Aft RL, Cor-nelius LA, Trinkaus KM and Linette GP. IL-12p70-Producing Patient DC Vaccine Elicits Tc1-Polarized Immunity. The Journal of Clinical Investigation 2013; 123(8)3383-3394

[79] Flaherty KT, Robert C, Hersey P, et al., for the METRIC Study Group. Improved Sur-vival With MEK Inhibition In BRAF-Mutated Melanoma. The New England Journal of Medicine 2012; 367(2) 107-114

[80] Falchook GS, Lewis KD, Infante JR, et al. Activity of the Oral MEK Inhibitor Trameti-nib in Patients with Advanced Melanoma: A Phase 1 Dose Escalation Trial. The Lan-cet Oncology 2012; 13(8) 782-789

[81] Brahmer JR, Tykodi SS, Chow LQ, et al. Safety And Activity Of Anti-PD-L1 Antibody In Patients With Advanced Cancer. The New England Journal of Medicine 2012; 366(26) 2455-2465

[82] Wolchok JD, Kluger H, Callahan MK, et al. Nivolumab Plus Ipilimumab In Advanced Melanoma. The New England Journal of Medicine 2013; 369(2) 122-133

[83] Kaufman HL, Ruby CE, Hughes T, Slingluff CL Jr. Current Status of Granulocyte-Macrophage Colony-Stimulating Factor in the Immunotherapy of Melanoma. Journal for ImmunoTherapy of Cancer 2014; 13(2) 11

[84] Besser MJ1, Shoham T, Harari-Steinberg O, Zabari N, Ortenberg R, Yakirevitch A, Nagler A, Loewenthal R, Schachter J, Markel G. Development of allogeneic NK cell adoptive transfer therapy in metastatic melanoma patients: in vitro preclinical optimization studies. PLoS One 2013; 8(3) e57922

[85] Parkhurst MR, Riley JP, Dudley ME, Rosenberg SA. Adoptive Transfer Of Autologous Natural Killer Cells Leads To High Levels Of Circulating Natural Killer Cells But Does Not Mediate Tumor Regression. Clinical Cancer Research 2011; 17(9) 6287–6297

[86] Neagu M, Constantin C, Manda G et al. Biomarkers Of Metastatic Melanoma. Biomarkers In Medicine 2009; 3(1) 71-89

[87] Neagu M, Constantin C, Zurac S. Immune Parameters In Prognosis And Therapy Monitoring Of Cutaneous Melanoma Patients - Experience, Role And Limitations. BioMed Research International, special issue Molecular Biomarkers: Tools of Medicine (MBTM) 2013; 2013 Article ID 107940

[88] Gore M. Introduction Optimal approach for melanoma. European Journal of Cancer Supplements 2013; 11(2), 80

[89] Neagu M. The Immune System-A Hidden Treasure for Biomarker Discovery in Cutaneous Melanoma In: Makowski G.S. (ed.) Advances In Clinical Chemistry. Book Series: Advances in Clinical Chemistry; 2012. p89-140

[90] Neagu M, Constantin C, Tanase C. Immune-Related Biomarkers For Diagnosis/Prognosis And Therapy Monitoring Of Cutaneous Melanoma. Expert Review Of Molecular Diagnostics 2011; 10(7) 897-919

7

Acral Melanoma — A Distinct Molecular and Clinical Subtype

R. Barra-Martínez, N.E. Herrera-González,

F. Fernández –Ramírez and L.A. Torres

1. Introduction

Skin cancer represents one-third of all cancers that are diagnosed every year worldwide. From all types of skin cancer, cutaneous melanoma is the least frequent among this group of malignant tumors, it is however, the most highly invasive and metastatic tumor. It has also shown an important growth of around 150% in its appearance since 1971, having an estimation of 76,250 new cases diagnosed in the USA in 2012. In 1971 there was only 1 case in 600 white people. In the period of 1992 to 2004, its annual growth was of 3.1%. This led to an estimated incidence of 1 in every 90 white people by 2000. By 2010 it was 1 in every 50, for people above 50 years old in the USA. Its epidemiological importance lies in its high mortality rate, since it is the cause of 90% of deaths for skin cancer and it is potentially the most dangerous form of skin tumor [1]. The outlook for patients with advanced melanoma is often fatal due to a lack of effective treatments.

In Mexico, melanoma incidence is around 1.7 per 100 000 people, and the Histopathologic Record of Malignancies in 2001 reported that it is the second most frequent. Women are the gender most affected by Melanoma (1.6/1). The median age of presentation in this country is 54 years and in 77% of the cases there is no relation to sun exposure. On the other hand, it is important to point out that there is a lack of formal registration of neoplasias in health institutions of our nation [1, 2, 3].

There are four clinicopathological subtypes that Melanoma presents, which usually are correlated to ethnic differences and to exposition to UV radiation: Superficial spreading melanoma (SSM), Lentigo maligna melanoma (LMM), Nodular melanoma (NM) and Acral lentiginous melanoma (ALM) [1, 4]. SSM and LMM, are the most common among Caucasians and their presence has been directly related to sun exposure. Nodular melanoma is less frequent (10%) than SSM (70%), but both melanomas share pigmentary characteristics in patients. It is probable, however, that these two types of melanoma have a direct relation with sun exposure. However, this risk factor has not been proven in NM, given that this type can be found in any place on the body, not just in skin areas frequently exposed to sun light.

The most frequent subtypes of Melanoma in our population are, NM and ALM [4, 5] (Figure 1). Studies supporting the hypothesis that ALM may be a biological and genetically different subtype, will be mentioned in the following sections. Its distinct development pattern suggests that it may possess molecular and cellular uniqueness.

This may be because of different genetic alterations that control the transformation of melanocytes to acral melanoma, leading to the need for a specific-therapeutic target towards this subtype of melanoma with a high rate among Mexicans and Latin-Americans.

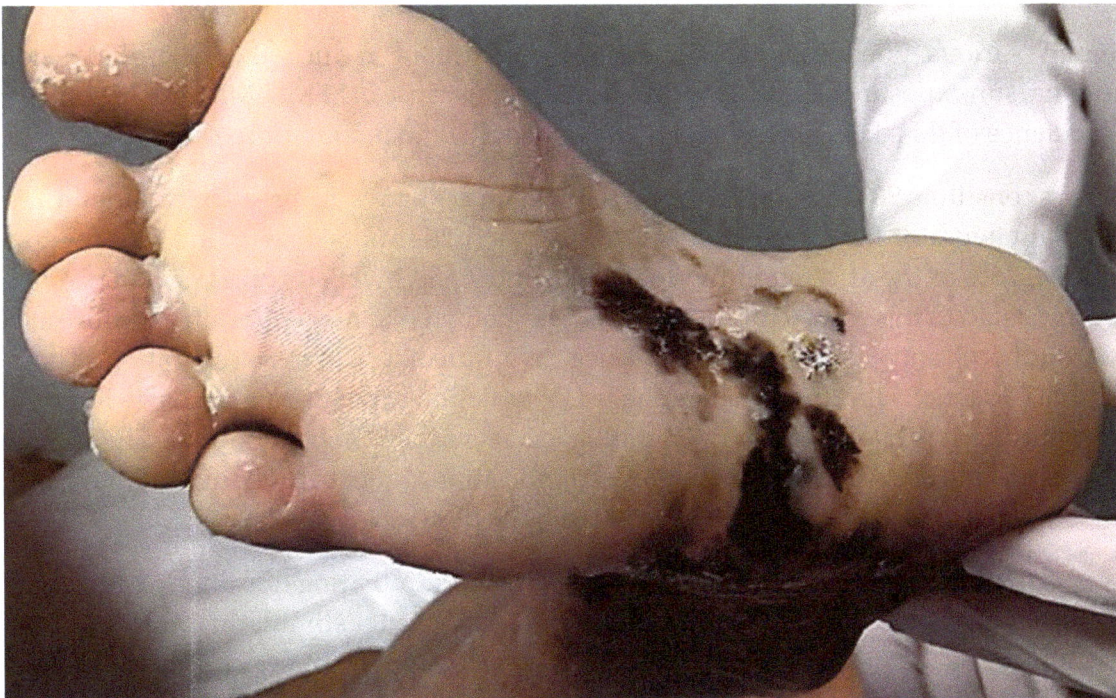

Figure 1. An indolent ALM subtype on the foot of a 58-year-old male patient, with 8 months of evolution. Nodular melanoma (NM) and Acral Lentiginous Melanoma (ALM) are the most frequent subtypes of Melanoma in our population. The lower extremities (mainly on the feet) are the most common anatomic locations reported for ALM.

2. Risk factors

Several studies have identified certain variables associated with an increased risk of developing melanoma: European ancestry, phenotype, UV radiation exposure, personal or family history of malignant melanoma, and molecular alterations are some of the most relevant [6]. Genetic alterations, will receive particularly emphasis later in this review. It is important to mention, that the risk factors traditionally associated with melanoma are related principally to Caucasians, where most clinical and basic studies are carried out. However, there are not enough studies supporting the predisposition of such factors for the subtypes of melanoma occuring in Mexican or Latin-American population.

Yamaguchi et al, reported that the risk factors traditionally described such as UV exposure, have a small influence in the pathogenesis of dark skin population. It has been postulated that UV radiation plays a smaller role in the pathogenesis of melanoma in the darker-skinned population. This is due to the fact that with an increase in melanin content, the larger melanosomes (in darker skin), absorb and scatter more energy than the smaller ones in lighter skin [7].

3. Sun exposure

Although various phenotypic characteristics enhance or reduce the risk of developing melanoma, sun exposure has been reported as the main cause of SSM, LMM and NM subtypes. The incidence of this disease is much higher in people who tend to burn rather than tan. (8)

UVA rays constitute 90% of solar radiation. However, UVB rays are greater risks for those who traditionally work or have recreational and daily activities outside. Among those with SSM and LMM, 75% of the affected individuals are sunburned by UVB rays. However, ALM has not been related to this risk factor. In addition, it is known that excessive sun exposure at early ages (childhood and adolescence) has a negative outcome in DNA reparation. The most important exogenous factor for melanoma is UV radiation exposure, particularly intermittent exposition, and it is known as the only etiological agent that can be modified. The increase in sun exposure and the damage to higher levels of the atmosphere because of contamination has resulted in an increase of the amount of radiation [9,10,11].

Sun exposure increases the expression of α-melanocyte stimulating hormone (α-MSH) and of the peptides of pro-opiomelanocortin in the skin. Melanocyte- stimulating hormone belongs to a group called the melanocortins. α-MSH is the most important melanocortin for pigmentation and shows a high affinity for melanocyte stimulating hormone receptor (MSHR). Once α-MSH binds to MSHR, cellular cAMP is activated, as well as other signal transduction pathways. The final result is the production of eumelanin.

Eumelanin, the primary pigment that colors the skin, hair and eyes in humans, also protects the body from UV and other hazardous radiations that can damage skin cells. When eumelanin has been crystalized, it forms both a geometric and a chemical disorder at the same time. It turns out that both kinds of disorders, may play a complementary role in producing eumelanin's broadband absorption. The tiny crystals of eumelanin have a chemically ordered state with intrinsic randomness: the orientations of the stacked molecules are arbitrary and the sizes of the crystals are different. That combination of order and disorder contributes to eumelanin's broadband absorption (12). Recently, it was reported that eumelanin is a naturally existing nanocomposite that has very critical macroscopic properties as a result of its nanostructure properties. All eumelanin molecules share very similar chemistry, although there are more than 100 variations. It has been proposed that the small variations from one molecule to another may contribute to the disorder that broadens the ability to absorb UV light (13).

Additionally, different alleles for melanocortin 1 receptor (MC1R) gene have been identified. The subtypes related to loss of function reduce the production of cAMP after stimulation of α-MSH, and thus increase the expression of pheomelanin. This is observed in individuals of light skin, increasing the risk of developing melanoma by the formation of free radicals after UV ray exposure.

Recently, a study was performed in 789 patients with diagnosis of melanoma. In order to characterize these patients according to their levels of sun exposure, three groups were established in the study: intermittent, chronic, and absence of exposure [14]. The vast majority of patients were in the first group. These melanomas were present in skin locations exposed to sun radiation in an intermittent manner. SSM and NM belong to this group. Multiple common and atypical nevi may constitute a marker of risk of these melanomas. The second group was formed by patients with melanomas in skin areas with chronic sun exposure, showing all the damage and premise typical of this location. LMM belongs to this group. Finally, the third group corresponds to melanomas present in skin areas with no sun exposure, usually diagnosed in late stages. This group includes ALM and mucosa melanoma, which usually are thicker at diagnosis and have worse prognosis [15, 16, 17]

4. Acral lentiginous melanoma

Acral lentiginous melanoma (ALM) distinguishes itself from the other subtypes for many characteristics, mainly histological and clinical-prognostic. A huge controversy regarding the cause of its worse prognosis, has been going on since its description.

ALM usually occurs on palmoplantar or subungual areas (Fig 2), lacking hair. Similar to NM, it is very aggressive when its proliferative vertical phase develops. It is more commonly found in individuals with dark skin (35-60%), oriental population and Afro-Caribbean. Considering its localization, it is thought to be UV-protected by the thickened stratum corneum and the nail matrix. ALM is rare in Caucasian populations (1-5%), but has a higher incidence among our population and Latin-Americans with dark skin(8, 9, 18). However, for individuals with lighter skin in our population, SSM is the most frequent.

According to the data of The National Cancer Institute Surveillance, Epidemiology and End Results, ALM is the least frequent histological subtype in the USA, with a 2-3% frequency. However, it shows a higher percentage among afroamerican people and Asians.

Reed described for the first time ALM as pigmented lesions of the extremities, mainly of the plantar and palmar regions, that were characterized by a phase of lentiginous (radial) growth, which evolved in months or years to the invasive vertical phase.(19)

Arrington was the first to notice that this type of melanoma was more prevalent among the African American population and that their prognosis was less favorable due to being diagnosed at an advanced stage. Yet, it was not documented by the SEER as a different histological subtype until 1986 [20]. Usually, ALM is not associated with nevi, family history or gene susceptibility known to melanoma. In its great majority, ALM are diagnosed as thick melanomas which in most cases are usually presented in their late phase, with a worse prognosis and a lower survival rate than the most common subtypes of melanoma associated with chronic sun exposure [20].

Pereda et al, reported the Clinical presentation of ALM in patients from Spain. In seventeen of them, ALM was found on a foot and in six on a hand. Four ALMs of the hand were subungueal. Most of the foot ALMs were located on the sole (twelve cases) [22].

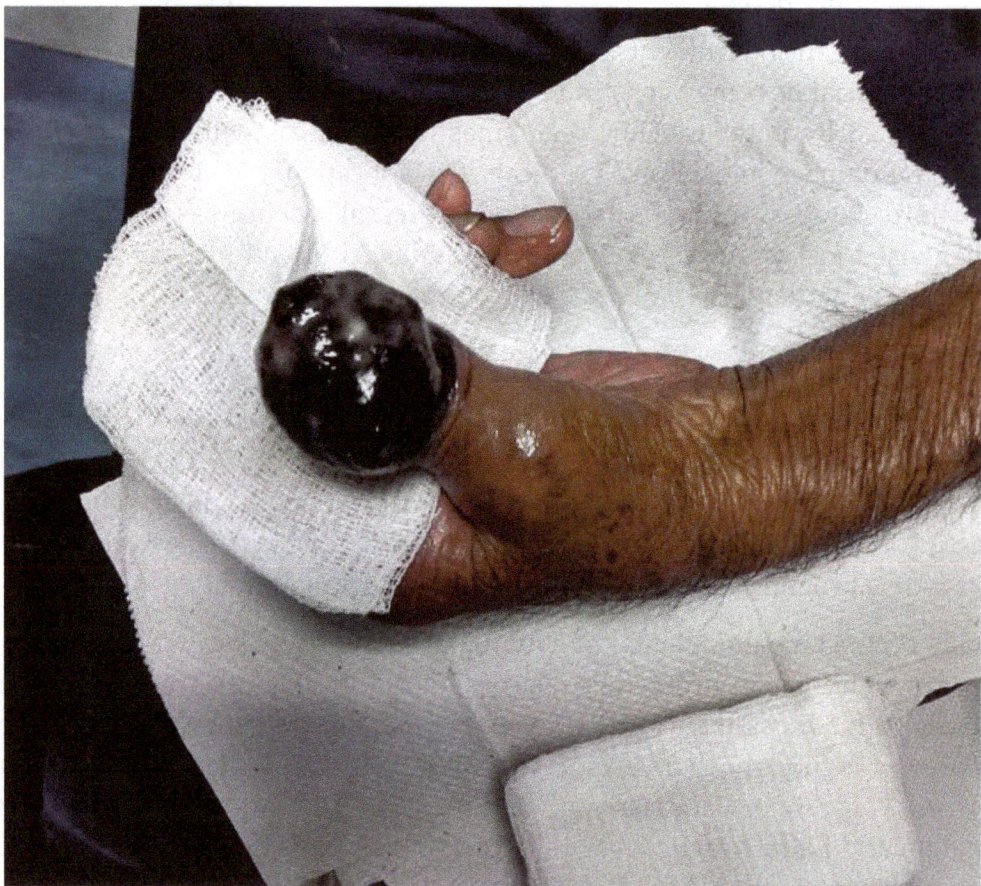

Figure 2. A subungueal tumor of a 71-year-old male patient with an advanced ALM (thick Breslow), on the thumb of the left hand. ALM is the most prevalent subtype in Mexicans and LatinAmericans. It is usually found on hands and feet: palms and soles, wrists and heels, and under the nails. ALM and NM are usually diagnosed in later stages, unlike SSM and LMM. The most affected sites are by far the feet and nails. Initially, they may be misdiagnosed as a mole, an ulcer, an abscess, a wart, a nail bed dystrophy or as the result of a trauma.

The most frequent location of ALM is in the feet (Figure 1), mainly the plantar region and the first finger, as in subungual areas in the majority of non caucasians racial groups. This has led to the conclusion that trauma may be an important factor of ALM, and not sun exposure [22]. Even when the superficial region of the palms and plantar region are similar, in the plantar region there is a continuous exposure to pressure, friction, maceration and irritation. Nevertheless, there are counterarguments towards this theory, including that the hands are more exposed to UV radiation and acute trauma. In addition, it has not been possible to prove changes in the incidence of plantar melanoma when some African tribes began urbanization and the use of shoes.

Another important factor in the predominance of plantar ALM, is the fact that there is a 50% greater amount of melanocytes there than in the palms [23, 24]. The research of Ghadially proposed that trauma during less than 12 months, did not increase the risk of melanoma in the Xiphophorus fish model [25]. Troyanova [26] described mechanical trauma on previous pigmented skin lesions as a risk factor for the formation of melanoma and remarks that trauma has to be carefully checked. Recently, an amelanotic subungueal melanoma arising after trauma was reported by Rangwala [27]. Melanomas formed on burns scars and tattoos have also been frequently publishedin recent years.Of 687 Chinese melanoma patients, 15.2% showed a strong association between trauma in the extremities and melanoma [28].

Clinical experience coming from medical attention given to patients of melanoma treated in two of the major oncological centers of our nation, shows that AM occurs in no photo exposed areas [5], mainly in lower extremities (more than 80% of the cases) and in subungual regions (Figure 3). This information has been reported by the Mixed Tumor Unit from the Oncologic Service (General Hospital of Mexico) and the Dermatologic Center "Ladislao de La Pascua", Mexico City [18]

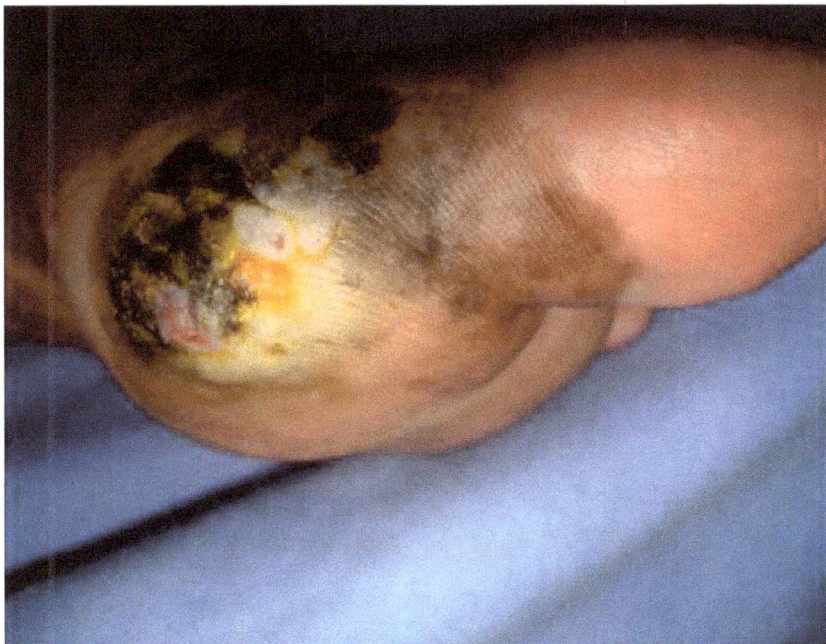

Figure 3. ALM on the foot of a 61-year-old male patient, with indolent growth. The Oncology Unit of the General Hospital of Mexico reports that more than 50% of ALMs are presented on the lower extremities (mainly on the soles and subungueal areas. Being the toe by far, the most affected).

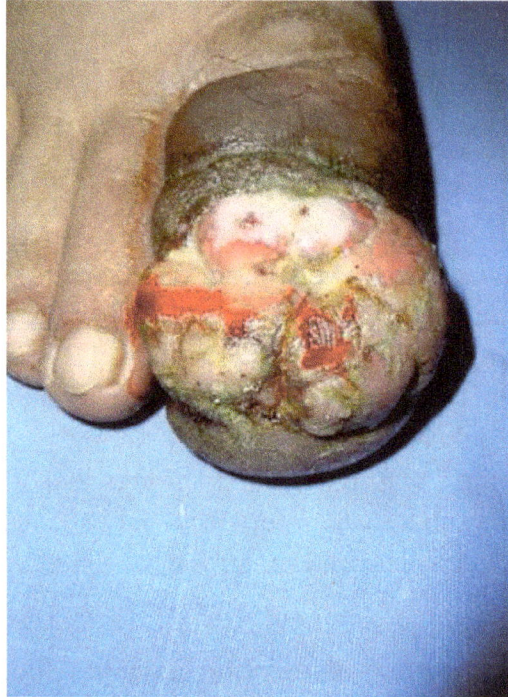

Figure 4. A subungueal tumor of a 54-year-old male patient with an advanced amelanic melanoma. ALMs are usually diagnosed in the later stages unlike SSM and LMM. It was misdiagnosed as a bleeding ulcer of progressive growth.

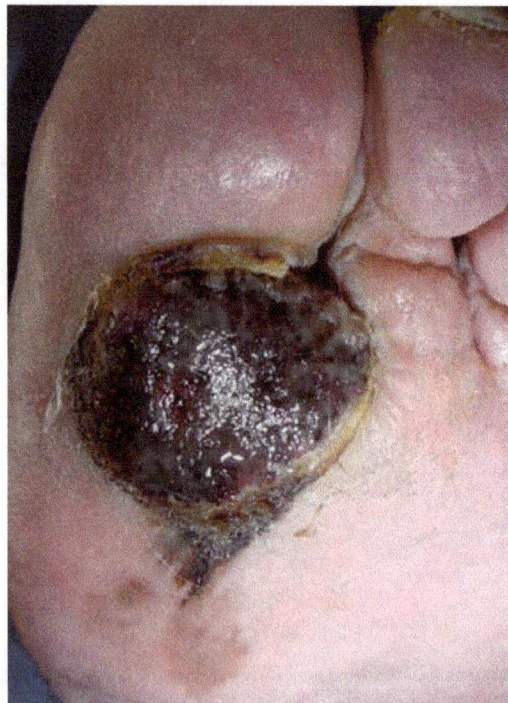

Figure 5. A plantar tumor of a 65-year-old male patient. The lower extremity is the most common anatomic location reported for mexicans. Initially this case was diagnosed as a pigmented lesion of a fast vertical phase progression.

5. Molecular alterations in melanoma

Melanoma arises through a complex process of cellular mutations and a loss of keratinocyte control over growth and differentiation. As malignant melanoma progresses, it develops through interaction between dysfunctional melanocytes and the tumor microenvironment. This in turn, allows the formation of nevocyte nests at the demal-epidermal junction and is accompanied with changes in both, keratinocytes and local adhesion molecules (29). The progression from healthy melanocyte to melanoma occurs through mutations within the tumor and through alterations of the cellular environment.

In the skin, tissue homeostasis is critical in cellular regulation and melanoma breaks this regulation through multiple processes. Defining intercellular molecular dialogues in human skin promises to provide key information about the transformation of melanocyte to melanoma. A great number of genes and proteins have been reported to play an essential role in this transformation. The most important are: B-RAF, c-KIT, PTEN, p16, p53, cyclin1, ARF, K-RAS (30).

6. Familial melanoma

It has been reported by a meta-analysis that the presence of at least one-first degree relative with melanoma increases to double or more, the risk of developing this disease.

Many genetic studies in melanoma-prone families lead to the identification of *CDKN2A* as the main familial melanoma gene. This gene is located at the chromosome 9p21 region. *CDKN2A* encodes two different proteins: INK4A (p16) and ARF (p14). In order to produce these two proteins, the use of alternative promoters and different first exons is necessary. Exon 1α is used for INK4A and 1β for ARF. The second exons of the two transcripts are translated in distinct reading frames, encoding two completely different proteins (with no amino acid homology). Nevertheless, both proteins share potent anticancer activities. *INK4A* inhibits the G1 cyclin-dependent kinases (CDKs) 4/6, which phosphorylate and inactivates the retinoblastoma protein (RB). After that, the S-phase is allowed to occur. Loss of INK4A function promotes RB inactivation resulting in cell cycle progression. *ARF* (Alternative Reading Frame) inhibits MDM2 mediated ubiquitination and degradation of p53. Loss of ARF, inactivates p53. Alterations of p16 are associated to familial melanoma in 20% and in 40% to sporadic melanoma [31].

7. Melanomas with intermitent sun exposure

As it was mentioned earlier, more than 90% of melanomas are diagnosed in white and light skinned populations. The majority of the international studies have addressed these populations, since they are at higher risk of developing melanoma. Thus, most reports are drawn from data of white and light skinned populations. The main alterations reported in SSM and NM, are B-RAF and N-RAS mutations.

7.1. BRAF

It is a tyrosine and threonine kinase that participates in the signal transduction known as Ras/Raf/MEK/ERK/MAP kinase. *BRAF* functions to regulate the MAPK/ERK pathway, which is conserved in all eukaryotes. This pathway acts as a signal transducer between the extracellular environment and the nucleus, activating downstream transcription factors to induce a range of biochemical processes including growth and differentiation, proliferation and migration associated to the ability of tissue invading [32, 33, 34]. Through direct secuentiation of PCR products, three substitutions of simple bases have been demonstrated. The most prevalent (95% of the cases) is constituted by the transversion of T1799A, occurring on exon 15 of *BRAF*, and causes the substitution of the amino acid valine for glutamic acid in position 599 (V599E). Such position has recently been modified to V600E.

Other *BRAF* mutations that cause carcinogenesis exist, such as K601E or those affecting exon 11, but they rarely occur in melanoma. A fusion of *BRAF* to *AKAP9*, by a paracentromeric inversion of the long arm of chromosome 7 has been observed in cases associated to ionized radiation exposure. This produces an oncogene, *AKAP9-BRAF*, which also results in a constitutive activation of the MAP kinase pathway [35, 36, 37].

Exon 15 BRAF mutations in melanoma were first reported in 2002. The number of reports of BRAF mutations in primary melanoma tissue increases continually. Varying prevalences in primary melanoma tissue have been detected, from 41% to 88% in SSM. These BRAF alterations alone, are not capable of demonstrating neither the immortalization of malignant cells, nor the progression of the disease further more than a nevus [37].

A pilot BRAF mutation study in ALM patients was carried out by collaboration between the Genetic Service of the General Hospital of Mexico and the Molecular Oncology Laboratory of the School of Medicine at the National Polytechnic Institute. DNA sequencing of seven ALM samples of Mexican patients (General Hospital of Mexico) showed no T1799A mutation in any of the studied samples (M. Sc. Thesis, 2012) [38].

7.2. NRAS

RAS are among the most frequently mutated oncogenes in human cancers. They show different mutation patterns and spectrums in all members: *NRAS*, *HRAS* and *KRAS*. The isoforms share a high degree of similarity, although each one displays preferential coupling to particular cancer types.

RAS play a fundamental role in the signaling pathway of MAP kinase. Extracellular signals such as hormones, cytokines, and various growth factors interact with their receptors to activate the small G-proteins of the RAS family. This pathway includes *BRAF* and it contributes to the control of cellular proliferation, particularly malignant cell proliferation. *RAS* also controls apoptosis through the PI3K-PTEN-Akt pathway.

SSM shows mutations almost exclusively in *NRAS*. A prevalence of 5% to 10% *NRAS* mutation has been reported. However for hereditary melanomas, the prevalence increases to 80%. Most cases of *NRAS* mutation are in codon 61. *NRAF* and *BRAF* mutations are mutually exclusive [39].

8. Melanoma with chronic sun exposure

There are similarities between this type of melanoma and those without sun exposure. However, there are differences with ALM since they show much lower mutational characteristics.

KIT (CD117) encodes a tyrosine kinase receptor for stem cells factor and plays a key role in melanocyte development, migration and proliferation. *KIT* is found on chromosome 4 and may be altered in a variety of different types of cancers. It is mutated in 28% of LMM, 36% in ALM, and is absent in melanomas with intermittent sun exposure. KIT over expression during the vertical growth phase of melanoma development supports the hypothesis of its participation in late stages of the disease. It is the target of several small molecules inhibitors such as imatinib, being a therapeutic target for this type of melanoma. Different roles of KIT among different types of melanoma, give additional evidence that each subtype can be considered different biologically and genetically [40].

9. Melanoma without sun exposure

ALM and mucosal melanomas have an inverse correlation among mutations of *BRAF* and *NRAS*. The increase in the copy number of Cyclin D1, CDK4, KIT and ABCB5 has also been reported.

9.1. CYCLIN D1

It is an important regulator of transition of the cell cycle for phases G1/S. It also participates in the phosphorylation of RB protein by binding kinase 4, cyclin dependent. Many studies have revealed a highly organized sequence of events indispensable for promotion of continued proliferation. The decision to continue cell cycle progression occurs when cellular RAS induces the elevation of cyclin D1. These levels are maintained through G1 phase and are necessary for the initiation of S phase, thus resulting in immediately reduced cyclin D1 levels. One requirement for DNA synthesis, is the reduction of cyclin D1 to low levels during the S phase. This forces the cell when it enters G2 phase, to induce high cyclin D1 levels once more. Thus, cyclin D1 is proposed to be a switch activator in the regulation of continued cell cycle progression [41, 42].

Cyclin D1 frequent amplification was reported in 44.4% of ALM by Sauter et al, Cyclin D1 was overexpressed in all cases with amplifications and in 20% of cases without amplification.

Cyclin D1 may be an oncogene in melanoma and that targeting its expression can be therapeutically useful in the future for ALM [42].

9.2. CDK4

It is a union protein of cyclin D1, found in chromosome 12q14. During early stages of phase G1 of the cell cycle, Cyclin D binds to kinase dependent cyclin 4 or 6 (CDK4 or CDK6) and the resulting complex "frees the brake" that limits the progression towards late G1, going into phase S. The cyclin D-CDK4/6 complex releases a potent inhibitor of the cell cycle progression: the one formed by protein pRB and inactive transcription factors. The types of melanoma having an increase in the number of copies of CyclinD1 and CDK4 have less possibilities of responding to the therapeutic target used in BRAF, such as Vemurafenib.

9.3. ABCB5

Human ATP-binding cassette transporter, also known as P-glycoprotein, is related to the subfamily of multidrug resistant genes (MDR). The ABCB subfamily includes eleven members that have different expression patterns. Whereas the functions of several transporters of the ABCB family are not known, there is some information about ABCB5 in relation to its pattern of expression or its associated function [43]. It has been described by Frank et al [44, 45] described it and it was implicated in the regulation of progenitor cell fusion (located in chromosome 7p21-15). Their study used an enriched culture of human epidermal melanocytes isolated from the foreskins of healthy donors and melanoma cell lines. They showed a higher and more intense ABCB5 expression in ALM than in SSM. Herrera-Gonzalez and her team [46], reported a 90% overexpression of ABCB5 in ALM samples of Mexican patients by using RT-PCR. A direct relationship between mRNA expression and the aggressiveness of ALM was also shown.

10. Conclusion

In regard to the progression of human cancer, it is universally thought, that it develops from a single mutated cell, followed by malignant clonal expansion secondary to additional genomic and genetic alterations. As the malignant cells continue to acquire these alterations, tumor subclones with distinct phenotypic advantages (47) for its progression may be produced: for example invasion, proliferation, ability to colonize different organs, etc. In many cancers, regulation of specific signaling molecules also goes awry, affecting a host of other proteins and cellular processes.

In recent years, the histological and phenotypic characteristics of ALM combined with its high proportion among melanomas in Afro-Americans, Asian and Latin Americans, has confirmed the thought that this histological type of melanoma may differ biological and molecularly from its most common counterparts, recognized by its sun exposure and its greater frequency among Caucasians. While ALM is characterized by a high frequency of focal amplifications (mainly involving CCND1, CDK4) and deletions, the most common cutaneous melanomas exhibit few changes in the number of genetic copies. In a similar way, while *BRAF* and *NRAS* are mutated in 50% and 20% of the cases respectively, mutation in *KIT* (which codifies the tyrosine kinase receptor) seems to be absent in the most common cutaneous melanoma. However, BRAF mutations in ALM constitute approximately 16% of the cases reported by Curtin et al. [40, 41]

A systematic sequencing was used for the human genome sequence. New technologies allow sequencing of randomly generated DNA fragments from cancer genomes and thus detect alterations and copy number variation as well as base substitutions, to identify most somatic mutations in an individual cancer genome. Pleasance et al, sequenced the complete genome of the COLO-829 cell line, an immortal and cancer derived from a metastasis of a melanoma from a 43 year-old-male. In their study they identified 33,345 somatic base substitutions [48, 49]

The study of Turajlic et al. [50] is the first to characterize the mutational spectra in ALM. They used a whole genome sequencing to characterize punctual somatic mutations and structural variation in a primary acral melanoma and its lymph node metastasis. Evidence of transcription-coupled repair was suggested by the lower mutational rate in the transcribed regions and expressed genes. Primary melanoma and metastasis, at the level of global gene copy number alterations, loss of heterozygosity and single expressed genes are very similar[50].

These results may be controversial since their sequenced results were on the genome of only one patient. They cite that despite the perception that acral skin is sun protected, the dominant mutational signature reveals sun damage. We judge that there is no solid data regarding the presence of solar exposure on sites where ALM is developed.

Studies suggest that ungual matrix does not provide a complete protection against UV radiation and it has previously been suggested that UVB can penetrate the human nail [51]. There are substantial variations in the number and pattern of mutations in individual cancers reflecting different exposures, DNA repair defects and cellular origins [52, 53]. It is also possible that characteristics of different mutations are induced by the inefficiency of pyrimidine dimers repaired by excision of nucleotide due to the presence of a mutation in ERCC5 [54, 55].

Several studies support the hypothesis that ALM is a different genetic subtype and its inherent heterogeneity represents a challenge in the era of directed therapy [56].

Author details

R. Barra-Martínez[1], N.E. Herrera-González[2], F. Fernández –Ramírez[3] and L.A. Torres[1]

1 Oncology Unit of General Hospital of Mexico, Mexico

2 Molecular Oncology Laboratory. Postgraduate Section. Superior School of Medicine, IPN, Mexico

3 Genetic Unit of General Hospital of Mexico, Mexico

References

[1] Alfeirán RA, Escobar AG Epidemiologia del melanoma de piel en México. Rev IN-CAN | (1999) 44(4): 168-174.

[2] Fernández CSB, León AG, Herrera TMC, Salazar SE, Sánchez DMR, Alcalá ORB et al. Perfil epidemiológico de los tumores malignos en México. Dir. Gral. Epidem. Secretaría de Salud México, D.F. (SINAIS / SINAVE / DGE / SALUD). (2011). p. 46 - 138.

[3] Vásquez MI, Villanueva LCG, Meraz R MA, Magaña M, Herrera GN. Biología molecular del melanoma. Actas Dermatol & Dermatopatol Méx. (2005); 5:5 - 15.

[4] Garbe C., Peris K, Hauschild A, Saiag P. Middleton M, Spatz A. Diagnosis and treatment of melanoma: European consensus-based interdisciplinary guideline Eur J of cancer (2010); 46: 270-283.

[5] Vázquez MI, Meraz RM, Magaña M, Sánchez GD, Herrera-González NE. Quimiorresistencia en el melanoma. Informe preliminar. Act Dermat y Dermapat (2006);6: 8-10

[6] Lascano AR, Kuznitzky R, Cuestas E, Mainard C et al. Factores de riesgo para melanoma cutáneo. Estudio de casos y controles en Córdoba, Argentina. Medicina (Buenos Aires). (2004); 64 (6) : 504-508

[7] Yuji Yamaguchi, Vicent J. Hearing. Melanocytes and their diseases. Cold spring harb perspect med. (2014); 4 : a017046

[8] De la Fuente GA, Ocampo CJ. Melanoma Cutáneo. Gac Méd Méx. (2010); 146: 126 – 135.

[9] Martínez SH, Vega GM, Toussaint CS, Gutiérrez VR, Orozco TR, León E, et al. El primer Consenso Nacional de Expertos en Melanoma. GAMO. (2005); 4: 11 – 13.

[10] Hayat MJ, Howlader N, Reichman ME y Edwards KB. Cancer statistics, trends, and multiple primary cancer analyses from the Surveillance, Epidemiology, and End Results (SEER) Program. The Oncologist (2007);12: 20 – 37.

[11] Geller CA y Swetter S. Screening and early detection of melanoma. CA Cancer J Clin (2011); 61:69-77.

[12] Massachusetts Institute of Technology (2014). Eumelanin's secrets: Discovery of melanin structure may lead to better sun protection. *Sciencedaily*. Retrieved January, 2015 from www.sciencedaily.com/releases/2014/05/140522115754.htm

[13] Chen, C.T., Chuang, J. Cao, V. Ball, D. Ruch, and M. J. Buehler. "Excitonic effecs from geometric order and disorder explain broadband optical absorption in eumelanin" Nature communications 5 (2014): 3859

[14] Nagore E, Botella ER, Requena C, Serra G, Martorell A, Hueso L, et al. Perfil clínico y epidemiológico de los pacientes con melanoma cutáneo según el grado de exposición solar de la localización del melanoma. Act Dermosifil (2009); 100: 205-211

[15] Rouhani P, Hu S, Kirsner RS. Melanoma in Hispanics and Black Americans. Cancer Control (2008); 15: 248-253

[16] Boriani, F O'Learly, Tohill M, Orlando A. EUR REB MED PHARMACOL SCI (2014); 08:1990-1996

[17] Schmerling R, Loria D, Cinat G, Ramos W, Cardona F, Sánchez J, Martínez-Said H, Buzaid A. Cutaneus melanoma in Latin America: the need for more data..Rev Panam Salud Publica. (2011);30(5):431-8

[18] Hernández ZS, Medina BA, López-Tello SA, Alcalá PD. Epidemiología del cáncer de piel en pacientes de la Clínica de Dermato-oncología del Centro Dermatológico Dr. Ladislao de la Pascua. Rev Mex Dermatol. (2012); 56: 30-37.

[19] Reed WB, Becker S, SR., Becker S, JR., Nickel WR. Giant Pigmented Nevi, Melanoma, and Leptomeningeal Melanocytosis: A Clinical and Histopathological Study. Arch Dermatol. (1965); 91(2):100-119.

[20] Arrington JH III, Reed RJ, Ichinose H, Krementz ET. Plantar lentiginous melanoma: a distinctive variant of human cutaneous malignant melanoma. Am J Surg Pathol. (1977); 1:131-143.

[21] Bradford PT, Goldstein AM, McMaster ML, Tucker MA. Acral Lentiginous Melanoma Incidence and Survival Patterns in the United States, 1986-2005. Arch Dermatol. (2009); 145: 427-434.

[22] C. Pereda, V. Traves, C. Requena, C. Serra-Guillén. B. Llombart, O. Sanmartín, C. Guillén, E. Nagore. Clinical presentation of acral lentiginusos melanoma: a descriptive study. Actas dermo-sifiliograficas (2012) 104: 220-226

[23] Feibleman CE, Stoll H, Maize JC. Melanomas of the palm, sole, and nailbed: a clinicopathologic study. Cancer. (1980); 46: 2492-2504.

[24] Phan A, Touzet S, Dalle S, Ronger-Salve S, Balme B, Thomas L. Acral lentiginous melanoma: a clinicoprognostic study of 126 cases. Br J Dermatol. (2006); 155: 561-569.

[25] Ghadially FN, trauma and melanoma production. Nature (1966); 211: 1199

[26] Troyanova P. The role of trauma in the melanoma formation. J Boun (2002); 7: 347-350

[27] Ranwala S, Hunt C, Modi G, Krishnan B, Orengo I. Amelanotic subungual melanoma after trauma: an unusual clinical presentation. Dermatol online j (2011); 17:8

[28] Zanhg N., Wang. L, Zhu.G., Sun. D., He. H., Luang. Q., Liu. L., Hao. F., Lee. C., Gao. P. The associatiom between trauma and melanoma in the Chinese population: a ret-

rospective study. J of the European Academy of Dermatology and Venereology. (2013).

[29] Hsu M, Meier F, Herlyn M. Melanoma development and progression: a conspiracy between tumor and host. Differentiation (2002) 70: 522-536

[30] Herrera-González Norma Estela. "Interaction between the Immune System and Melanoma", Recent Advances in the Biology Therapy and Management of Melanoma" (2013)

[31] Young, R. J., Waldeck, K., Martin, C., Foo, J. H., Cameron, D. P., Kirby, L., Do, H., Mitchell, C., Cullinane, C., Liu, W., Fox, S. B., Dutton-Regester, K., Hayward, N. K., Jene, N., Dobrovic, A., Pearson, R. B., Christensen, J. G., Randolph, S., McArthur, G. A. and Sheppard, K. E. Loss of CDKN2A expression is a frequent event in primary invasive melanoma and correlates with sensitivity to the CDK4/6 inhibitor PD0332991 in melanoma cell lines. Pigment Cell & Melanoma Research, (2014), 27: 590–600.

[32] Sullivan RJ, Flaherty KT. BRAF in Melanoma: Pathogenesis, Diagnosis, Inhibition, and Resistance. J of Skin Cancer 2011; (2011): 1 – 8.

[33] Avruch J. MAP kinase pathways: the first twenty years. Biochim Biophys Acta. (2007); 1773:1150-1160.

[34] Vidwans SJ, Flaherty KT, Fisher DE, Tenenbaum JM, Travers MD, Shrager J. A Melanoma Molecular Disease Model. PLoS One (2011); 6: 1 – 10.

[35] Ciampi R, Nikiforov YE. Alterations of BRAF gene in human tumors. Endocr Pathol. (2005);16: 163-172.

[36] Zafon C y Obiols G. Vía de señalización dependiente de la proteincinasa de activación mitogénica. De las bases moleculares a la práctica clínica. Endocrinol Nutr. (2009); 56(4):176-186

[37] Cantwell-Dorris ER, O'Leary JJ, and Sheils OM. BRAFV600E: Implications for Carcinogenesis and Molecular Therapy. Mol Cancer Ther. (2011); 10: 385 – 394.

[38] Barra-Martínez R. Estudio de la mutación de T-1799A BRAF en melanoma acral lentiginoso y nodular de pacientes del Hospital General de México 2010. Maestría en Ciencias de la Salud. Sección de Posgrado. Escuela Superior de Medicina, IPN.

[39] Jakob, J. A., Bassett, R. L., Ng, C. S., Curry, J. L., Joseph, R. W., Alvarado, G. C., Rohlfs, M. L., Richard, J., Gershenwald, J. E., Kim, K. B., Lazar, A. J., Hwu, P. and Davies, M. A. (2012), NRASmutation status is an independent prognostic factor in metastatic melanoma. Cancer, 118: 4014–4023.

[40] Curtin JA, Busam K, Pinkel D, Bastian BC. Somatic activation of KIT in distinct subtypes of melanoma. J Clin Oncol. (2006); 24:4340- 4346.

[41] Curtin JA, Fridlyand J, Kageshita T, Patel HN, Busam KJ, Kutzner H, et al. Distinct sets of genetic alterations in melanoma. N Engl J Med. (2005); 353:2135-2147

[42] Sauter. E., Yeo Un-Cheol., Streem. A., Zhu. W., Litwin. S., Tichansky. E., Pistritto. G., Nesbit. M., Pinkel. D., Herlyn. M., Bastian. B. Cyclin D1 Is a Candidate Oncogene in Cutaneus Melanoma. The American Journal of Cancer. (2002):62;3200-3206.

[43] Ambudkart. S., Dey. S., Ihrycyna. C., Ramachandra. M., Pastan. I., Gottesman. M. Biochemical cellular and pharmacological aspects of the multidrug transported. Pharmacol Toxicol. (1999); 39:361-98.

[44] Frank N, Pendse S, Lapchak P, Margaryan A., Schlain D., Doeing C, et al. Regulation of progenitor cell fusion by ABCB P-glycoprotein, a novel human ATP- binding cassette transporter. J Biol Chem. (2003); 278:47156–47165.

[45] Frank N, Margaryan A, Huang Y, Schatton T, Waaga-Gasser AM, Gasser M et al. ABCB5-mediated doxorubicin transport and chemoresistance in human malignant melanoma. Cancer Res. (2005); 65: 4320–4333.

[46] Vásquez-Moctezuma I, Meraz-Ríos MA, Villanueva-López CG, Magaña M, Martínez-Macias R, Herrera-González NE. ATP-binding cassette transporter ABCB5 gene is expressed with variability in malignant melanoma. IPN. Actas Dermosifil. (2010); 101: 341-348.

[47] Yancovitz Molly, Adam Litterman, Joane Yoo, Elise Ng, Richard L. Shapiro et al. Intra- and Inter-Tumor heterogeneity of $BRAF^{V600E}$ mutations in primary and metastic melanoma. PLoS ONE (2012); 07(1); e29336

[48] Pleasance, E.D., Cheetham, R.K., Stephens, P.J., McBride DJ, Humphray SJ, Greenman CD et al. A comprehensive catalogue of somatic mutations from a human cancer genome. Nature. (2010); 463: 191–196.

[49] Lee JT, Li L, Brafford PA,Van Den Eijnden M, Halloran MB. PLX4032, a potent inhibitor of the B-Raf V600E oncogene, selectively inhibits V600E-positive Melanomas. Pigment Cell & Melanoma Res.(2010); 23: 820–827.

[50] Turajlic S, Furney SJ, Lambros MB, Mitsopoulos C, Kozarewa I, Geyer FC, et al. Whole genome sequencing of matched primary and metastatic acral melanomas. Genome Res (2012) 22:196–207.

[51] Parker SG, Diffey BL. The transmission of optical radiation through human nails. Br. J. Dermat (1983); 108:11-16.

[52] Greenman C, Stephens P, Smith R, Dalgliesh GL, Hunter C, Bignell G, et al. Patterns of somatic mutation in human cancer genomes. Nature. (2007); 446: 153–158.

[53] Stratton MR, Campbell PJ, Futreal PA. The cancer genome. Nature. (2009); 458:719–724.

[54] Pfeifer GP, You YH, Besaratinia A. Mutations induced by ultraviolet light. Mutat. Res. (2005); 571:19–31.

[55] Gaddameedhi S, Kemp MG, Reardon JT, Shields JM, Smith-Roe SL, Kaufmann WK et al. Similar Nucleotide Excision Repair Capacity in Melanocytes and Melanoma Cell. Cancer Res. (2010); 70: 4922- 4930

[56] Furney SJ, Turajlic S, Fenwick K, Lambros MB, MacKay A, Ricken G, et al. Genomic characterisation of acral melanoma cell lines. Pigment Cell Melanoma Res. (2012); 25; 488–492.

Permissions

All chapters in this book were first published in MELANOMA, by InTech Open; hereby published with permission under the Creative Commons Attribution License or equivalent. Every chapter published in this book has been scrutinized by our experts. Their significance has been extensively debated. The topics covered herein carry significant findings which will fuel the growth of the discipline. They may even be implemented as practical applications or may be referred to as a beginning point for another development.

The contributors of this book come from diverse backgrounds, making this book a truly international effort. This book will bring forth new frontiers with its revolutionizing research information and detailed analysis of the nascent developments around the world.

We would like to thank all the contributing authors for lending their expertise to make the book truly unique. They have played a crucial role in the development of this book. Without their invaluable contributions this book wouldn't have been possible. They have made vital efforts to compile up to date information on the varied aspects of this subject to make this book a valuable addition to the collection of many professionals and students.

This book was conceptualized with the vision of imparting up-to-date information and advanced data in his field. To ensure the same, a matchless editorial board was set up. Every individual on the board went through rigorous rounds of assessment to prove their worth. After which they invested a large part of their ime researching and compiling the most relevant data for our readers.

The editorial board has been involved in producing this book since its inception. They have spent rigorous hours researching and exploring the diverse topics which have resulted in the successful publishing of this book. They have passed on their knowledge of decades through this book. To expedite this challenging task, the publisher supported the team at every step. A small team of assistant editors was also appointed to further simplify the editing procedure and attain best results for the readers.

Apart from the editorial board, the designing team has also invested a significant amount of their time in understanding the subject and creating the most relevant covers. They scrutinized every image to scout for the most suitable representation of the subject and create an appropriate cover for the book.

The publishing team has been an ardent support to the editorial, designing and production team. Their endless efforts to recruit the best for this project, has resulted in the accomplishment of this book. They are a veteran in the field of academics and their pool of knowledge is as vast as their experience in printing. Their expertise and guidance has proved useful at every step. Their uncompromising quality standards have made this book an exceptional effort. Their encouragement from time to time has been an inspiration for everyone.

The publisher and the editorial board hope that this book will prove to be a valuable piece of knowledge for researchers, students, practitioners and scholars across the globe.

List of Contributors

David N. Brindley and Matthew G. K. Benesch
Signal Transduction Research Group, Department of Biochemistry, University of Alberta, Heritage Medical Research Center, Edmonton, Alberta, Canada

Mandi M. Murph
Department of Pharmaceutical and Biomedical Sciences, The University of Georgia, College of Pharmacy, Athens, Georgia, USA

Jin Wang, Duane D. Miller and Wei Li
Department of Pharmaceutical Sciences, College of Pharmacy. The University of Tennessee Health Science Center, Memphis, TN, USA

Estelle Leclerc
North Dakota State University/Department of Pharmaceutical Sciences, USA

Jennifer Makalowski and Hinrich Abken
Center for Molecular Medicine Cologne (CMMC), University of Cologne, Germany
Dept. I Internal Medicine, University Hospital Cologne, Cologne, Germany

Luis Resende
Veterinary Faculty, Lusófona University, Lisbon, Portugal

Joana Moreira
Department of Veterinary Sciences, University of Trás-os-Montes and Alto Douro, Portugal

Justina Prada and Isabel Pires
Animal and Veterinary Research Centre (CECAV), Department of Veterinary Sciences, University of Trás-os-Montes and Alto Douro, Portugal

Felisbina Luisa Queiroga
Center for Research and Technology of Agro-Environment and Biological Sciences (CITAB), Department of Veterinary Sciences, University of Trás-os-Montes and Alto Douro, Portugal

Monica Neagu and Carolina Constantin
Immunobiology Laboratory, Victor Babes National Institute of Pathology, Bucharest, Romania

R. Barra-Martínez and L. A. Torres
Oncology Unit of General Hospital of Mexico, Mexico

N. E. Herrera-González
Molecular Oncology Laboratory. Postgraduate Section. Superior School of Medicine, IPN, Mexico

F. Fernández –Ramírez
Genetic Unit of General Hospital of Mexico, Mexico

Index